Biomedical Engineering and Instrumentation

Biomedical Engineering and Instrumentation:

BASIC CONCEPTS AND APPLICATIONS

Joseph D. Bronzino

The Vernon Roosa Professor of Applied Science Trinity College

Director of the joint Trinity College/Hartford Graduate Center
Biomedical Engineering Program
Hartford, Connecticut

Contributing authors:

Michael R. Neuman, Ph.D., M.D.
Depts. of Reproductive Biology
and Biomedical Engineering
Case Western Reserve University

Frank M. Galioto Jr., M.D.
Children's Hospital National Medical Ctr.
Washington, D.C.

Robert Howard, Director
Biomedical Engineering
Children's Hospital National Medical Ctr.
Washington, D.C.

George V. Kondraske, Ph.D.
The University of Texas at Arlington

Roy B. Davis III, Ph.D.
Assistant Professor of Engineering
Trinity College
Hartford, Connecticut

Richard P. Spencer
Dept. of Nuclear Medicine
Univ. of Connecticut
Health Center
Farmington, Connecticut

Fazle Hosain
Dept. of Nuclear Medicine
Univ. of Connecticut
Health Center
Farmington, Connecticut

Robert A. Peura, Ph.D.
Biomedical Engineering Program
Worcester Polytechnic Inst.
Worcester, Massachusetts

Kenneth D. Taylor, Ph.D.
United Technologies Corp.

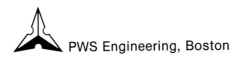

PWS Engineering, Boston

PWS PUBLISHERS

Prindle, Weber & Schmidt • 🦫 • Duxbury Press • ♠ • PWS Engineering • ⚜ • Breton Publishers • ⚙
Statler Office Building • 20 Park Plaza • Boston, Massachusetts 02116

To my parents Joseph and Antoinette Bronzino and my wife Barbara

PWS Publishers is a division of Wadsworth, Inc.

Printed in the United States of America

86 87 88 89 90—10 9 8 7 6 5 4 3 2 1

Library of Congress Cataloging-in-Publication Data

Bronzino, Joseph D.
  Biomedical engineering and instrumentation.

  Includes bibliographies and index.
  1. Biomedical engineering. 2. Medical instruments and
apparatus. I. Title. [DNLM: 1. Biomedical Engineering—
instrumentation. 2. Biomedical Engineering—
trends. 3. Computers. QT 34 B869b]
R856.B75 1986   610′.28   85-21464
ISBN 0-534-06492-2

ISBN 0-534-06492-2

Sponsoring Editor—Ray Kingman
Editorial Assistant—Jane Parker
Designer: Richard Kharibian
Composition: Carlisle Graphics
Printing and Binding: R.R. Donnelley & Sons Co.
Production: Miller/Scheier Associates
Production Coordination: Helen Walden

Preface

Purpose

In the United States today, modern medical care is extremely dependent upon technology. Since the end of World War II, the disciplines of medicine and engineering have merged continuously. This evolutionary process has given birth to the profession of biomedical engineering and has led to increased cooperation between engineers and physicians in developing new and better devices to monitor, diagnose, and treat their patients. Since this trend is likely to continue, the development of modern medical instruments will increasingly become an interdisciplinary activity. Further, throughout the next decade, the availability of the latest microcomputer-based technology is expected to dominate the field of biomedical instrumentation. Many medical tools will essentially become "smart" processors serving as the entry point for medical data into computerized systems. As a result, microcomputer technology will certainly have a significant impact upon the very nature of the acquisition and processing of almost all physiological information. These developments require that integrated interdisciplinary approaches be promoted to incorporate the latest technology into modern biomedical instrumentation systems.

Audience

Today, new technological developments virtually surround health care professionals as they tend to the well-being of their patients. The roles of the physician and nurse have been drastically altered; in addition to their responsibilities to manage and administer to the needs of their patients, they must understand the operation of a wide variety of new electronically based medical instruments. This change has increased the need for all health professionals to have some technological background. It has clearly become imperative that students interested in careers in the health care field become more knowledgeable about some of these new technologies and their application to and impact on patient care.

Similarly, engineering students interested in applying their talents in instrumentation design and information processing must, in turn, embrace increased exposure and understanding of the function of physiological systems. Further, since microprocessor-based medical instruments will probably become commonplace throughout the next decade, engineering professionals will need to understand clinical procedures as well as the flow of information within the clinical environment. With this background, more efficient and effective instrumentation systems for the collection, processing, storage, analysis, and retrieval of medically related information can be designed.

With this environment in mind, this book provides an integrated, interdisciplinary context for understanding modern techniques in the design, development, and application of biomedical instrumentation. To achieve these objectives, the introductory material is concise, yet comprehensive, treating each application in sufficient depth to let the reader understand the overall clinical and engineering problems being addressed. The result is a text that can serve as a reference to all members of the health care profession and as an instructional vehicle for undergraduate biomedical engineering students.

Joseph D. Bronzino

Contents

Part Five

Diagnostic Support Systems   277

Part Six

Medical Technology and Ethical Issues   431

Biomedical Engineering and Instrumentation

Part One

Introduction to Bioengineering and Bioinstrumentation

Biomedical Engineering: An Interdisciplinary Profession

Joseph D. Bronzino, Ph.D., P.E.

The Vernon Roosa Professor of Applied Science,
  Trinity College
Director of the Joint Trinity College/Hartford Graduate
  Center
Biomedical Engineering Program
  Hartford, Connecticut

INTRODUCTION

In a relatively short period of time, technology has affected every facet of our lives, and never has this effect been more apparent than in the area of medicine and the delivery of health care services. Although primitive humans practiced the art of medicine, the evolution of a technologically based health care system is a decidedly new phenomenon. The establishment of the modern hospital as the focal point of this highly technical system, with the "specialist physician" as its primary proponent, has come about only in this century.

Technology has particularly molded medical care, and in the process engineering professionals have become intimately involved in many medical ventures. As a result of many efforts to develop a common basis for the interaction of professionals from different scientific cultures, the discipline of biomedical engineering has emerged as a vital activity. Being an integrating medium for two dynamic professions, medicine and engineering, this discipline has the broad objective of assisting in the struggle against illness and disease by providing tools and techniques for research, diagnosis, and treatment.

As an important new discipline, biomedical engineering has its own history and set of guiding principles that must be understood if any dialogue between disciplines is to flourish. Only when this communication exists can individuals function as a "team" to solve the difficult problems confronting the health care delivery system in this country and to explore the possibilities for improved diagnosis and therapy so necessary for the maximum development of the medical arts. To facilitate this dialogue, this chapter will review the impact technology has had on health care delivery, discuss the evolution of the field of biomedical engineering, and present the roles biomedical engineers can play in the modern health care system.

THE EVOLUTION OF THE MODERN HEALTH CARE SYSTEM

The Beginnings

Primitive humans considered diseases to be "visitations," the whimsical acts of affronted gods or spirits. As a result, medical practice was the domain of the witch doctor and the medicine man and medicine woman. Yet even as magic became an integral part of the healing process, the cult and the art of these early practitioners were never entirely limited to the supernatural. These individuals, by using their natural instincts and learning from experience, developed a primitive science based upon empirical laws. For example, through acquisition and coding of certain reliable practices, the arts of herb doctoring, bonesetting, surgery, and midwifery were advanced. Just as primitive humans learned from observation that certain plants and grains were good to eat and could be cultivated, so the healer or shaman observed the nature of certain illnesses and then passed on their experience to other generations.

Evidence indicates that the primitive healer took an active, rather than simply intuitive interest in the curative arts, acting as a surgeon, a user of tools. For instance, skulls with holes made in them by trephiners have been collected in various parts of Europe, Asia, and South America. These holes were cut out of the bone with flint instruments to gain access to the brain. Although one can only speculate about the purpose of these early surgical operations, magic and religious beliefs seem to be the most likely reasons. Perhaps this procedure liberated from the skull the malicious demons who were thought to be the cause of extreme pain (as in the case of migraine) or attacks of falling to the ground (as in epilepsy). That this procedure was carried out on living patients, some of whom actually survived, is evident from the rounded edges on the bone surrounding the hole, indicating that the bone had grown again after the operation. These survivors also achieved a special status of sanctity, so that after their death pieces of their skull were used as amulets to ward off convulsive attacks. From these beginnings, the practice of medicine has become integral to all human societies and cultures.

It is interesting to note the fate of some of the most successful of these early practitioners. The Egyptians, for example, have held Imhotep, the architect of the first pyramid (3000 B.C.), in great esteem through the centuries, not as a pyramid builder, but as a doctor. Imhotep's name signified "he who cometh in peace" because he visited the sick to give them "peaceful sleep." This early physician practiced his art so well that he was deified in the Egyptian culture as the god of healing.

Egyptian mythology, like primitive religion, emphasized the interrelationships between the supernatural and health. The mystic sign *Rx,* which still adorns all prescriptions today, has a mythical origin, the legend of the Eye of Horus. It appears that as a child Horus lost his vision after being viciously attacked by Seth, the demon of evil. Then Isis, the mother of Horus, called for assistance to Thoth, the most important god of health, who promptly restored the eye and its powers. As a result of this intervention, the Eye of Horus became the Egyptian symbol of godly protection and recovery, and its descendant Rx serves as the most visible link between ancient and modern medicine (Atkinson 1956).

The concepts and practices of Imhotep and the medical cult he fostered were duly recorded on papyri and stored in ancient tombs. One scroll (dated c. 1500 B.C.), acquired by George Elbers in 1873, contains hundreds of remedies for numerous afflictions ranging from crocodile bite to constipation. A second famous papyrus (dated c. 1700 B.C.), discovered by Edwin Smith in 1862, is considered to be the most important and complete treatise on surgery of all antiquity. These writings outline proper diagnoses, prognoses, and treatment in a series of surgical cases. These two papyri are certainly among the outstanding writings in medical history.

As the influence of ancient Egypt spread, Imhotep was identified by the Greeks with their own god of healing, Aesculapius. According to legend, Aesculapius was fathered by the god Apollo, during one of his many earthly visits. Apparently Apollo was a concerned parent, and, as is the case for many modern parents, he wanted his son to be a physician. He made Chiron, the centaur, tutor Aesculapius in the ways of healing. Chiron's student became so proficient as a healer that he soon surpassed his tutor and kept people so healthy that he began to decrease the population of Hades. Pluto, the god of the underworld, complained so violently about this course of events that Zeus killed Aesculapius with a thunderbolt and in the process promoted Aesculapius to Olympus as a god.

Inevitably mythology has become entangled with historical facts, and it is not certain whether Aesculapius was in fact an earthly physician like Imhotep, the Egyptian. However, one thing is clear; by 1000 B.C., medicine was already a highly respected profession. In Greece the Aesculapia were temples of the healing cult and may be considered among the first hospitals. In modern terms, these temples were essentially sanatoriums that had strong religious overtones. In them, patients were received and psychologically prepared, through prayer and sacrifice, to appreciate the past achievements of Aesculapius and his physician priests. After the appropriate rituals, they were allowed to enjoy "temple sleep." During the night, "healers" visited their patients, administering medical advice to clients who were awake or interpreting dreams of those who were sleeping. In this way, patients became convinced that they would be cured by following the prescribed regimen (diet, drugs, or blood-letting). On the other hand, if they remained ill, it would be the result of their lack of faith. With this approach, patients, not treatments, were at fault if they did not get well. This early use of the power of suggestion was effective then and is still important in medical treatment today. The notion of "healthy mind, healthy body" is still encountered today.

One of the most celebrated of these "healing" temples was on the island of Cos, the birthplace of Hippocrates, who as a youth became acquainted with the curative arts through his father, also a physician. Hippocrates was not so much an innovative physician as a collector of all the remedies and techniques that existed up to that time. Since he viewed the physician as a scientist instead of a priest, Hippocrates also injected an essential ingredient into medicine: scientific spirit. For him diagnostic observation and clinical treatment began to replace superstition. Instead of blaming disease on the gods, Hippocrates taught that disease was a natural process, one that developed in logical steps, and that symptoms were reactions of the body to disease. The body itself, he emphasized, possessed its own means of recovery, and the function of the physician was to aid these natural forces. Hippocrates treated each patient as an original case to be studied and documented. His shrewd descriptions of diseases are models for physicians even today. Hippocrates and the school of Cos trained a number of individuals who then migrated to the corners of the Mediterranean world to practice medicine and spread the philosophies of their preceptor (Sigerest 1951). The work of Hippocrates and the school and tradition that stem from him constitute the first real break from magic and mysticism and the foundation of the rational art of medicine. However, as a practitioner, Hippocrates represented the spirit, not the science, of medicine, embodying the good physician: the friend of the patient and the humane expert.

As the Roman Empire reached its zenith and its influence expanded across half the world, it became heir to the great cultures it absorbed, including their medical advances. Although the Romans themselves did little to advance clinical medicine (the treatment of the individual patient), they did make outstanding contributions to public health. For example, they had a well-organized army medical service, which not only accompanied the legions on their various campaigns to provide "first aid" on the battlefield but even established "base hospitals" for convalescents at strategic points throughout the empire. Also the construction of sewer systems and aqueducts were truly remarkable Roman accomplishments, which provided their empire with the medical and social advantages of sanitary living. The medical men's insistence on clean drinking water and unadulterated foods effected the control and prevention of epidemics. However primitive, it made urban existence possible. Unfortunately, without adequate scientific knowledge about diseases, all the preoccupation of the Romans with public health could not avert the periodic medical disasters, particularly the plague, that mercilessly befell its citizens.

Initially, their Roman masters looked upon Greek physicians and their art with disfavor. However, as the years passed, the favorable impression these disciples of Hippocrates made upon the people became widespread. As a reward for their service to the peoples of the Empire, Caesar (46 B.C.) granted Roman citizenship to all Greek practitioners of medicine in his empire. Their new status became so secure that when Rome suffered from famine that same year, these Greek practitioners were the only foreigners not expelled from the city. On the contrary, they were even offered bonuses to stay!

Ironically, Galen, who is considered the greatest physician in the history of Rome, was himself a Greek. Honored by the emperor for curing his "imperial fever," Galen became the medical celebrity of Rome. He was arrogant and a braggart and, unlike Hippocrates, reported only successful cases. Nevertheless, he was a remarkable physician. For Galen, diagnosis became a fine art; in addition to taking care of his own patients, he responded to requests for medical advice from the far reaches of the empire. He was so industrious that he wrote more than 300 books of anatomical observations, his selective case histories, the drugs he prescribed, and his boasts. His version of human anatomy, however, was misleading because he objected to human dissection and drew his human analogies solely from the studies of animals. However, because he so dominated the medical scene and was later endorsed by the Roman Catholic Church, Galen actually inhibited medical inquiry. His medical views and writings became both the "bible" and "the law" for the pontiffs and pundits of the ensuring Dark Ages (Calder 1958).

With the collapse of the Roman Empire, the Church became the repository of knowledge, particularly of all scholarship that had drifted through the centuries into the Mediterranean. This body of information, including medical knowledge, was literally scattered through the monasteries and dispersed among the many orders of the Church.

The teachings of the early Roman Catholic Church and the belief in divine mercy made inquiry into the causes of death unnecessary and even undesirable. Members of the Church regarded curing patients by rational methods as sinful interference with the will of God. The employment of drugs signified a lack of faith by the doctor and patient, and scientific medicine fell into disrepute. As a result, for almost a thousand years, medical research stagnated. It was not until the Renaissance in the 1500s that any significant progress in the science of medicine occurred. Hippocrates had once taught that illness was not a punishment sent by the gods, but a phenomenon of nature. But now, under the Church and a new God, the older views of the supernatural origins of disease were renewed and promulgated. Since disease implied demonic possession, the sick were treated by the monks and priests through prayer, laying on of hands, exorcism, penances, and exhibition of holy relics: practices officially sanctioned by the Church.

Although deficient in medical knowledge, the Dark Ages were not entirely lacking in charity toward the sick poor, for the Christian physicians treated the rich and poor alike. The Church actually assumed responsibility for the sick. The evolution of the modern hospital began with the advent of Christianity and is considered a major contribution of monastic medicine. The rise in A.D. 335 of Constantine I, the first of the Roman emperors to embrace Christianity, all pagan temples of healing were closed, and hospitals were established in every cathedral city. The word *hospital* comes from the Latin *hospes,* meaning "host" or "guest"; the same root has provided *hotel* and *hostel.* These first hospitals were simply houses where weary travelers and the sick could find food, lodging, and nursing care. All these hospitals were run by the Church, and the art of healing was practiced by the attending monks and nuns.

As the Christian ethic of faith, humanitarianism, and charity spread throughout Europe and then to the Middle East during the Crusades, so did its "hospital system." However, trained "physicians" still practiced their trade primarily in the homes of their patients, and only the weary travelers, the destitute, and those considered hopeless cases found their way to hospitals. Conditions in these early hospitals varied widely. Although a few were well financed and well managed and treated their patients humanely, most were essentially custodial institutions to keep troublesome and infectious people away from the general public. In these establishments, crowding, filth, and high mortality among both patients and attendants were commonplace. Thus, the hospital was an institution to be feared and shunned.

The Renaissance and Reformation in the fifteenth and sixteenth centuries loosened the Church's stronghold on both the hospital and the conduct of medical practice. During the Renaissance, "true learning," the desire to pursue the true secrets of nature including medical knowledge, was again stimulated. The study of human anatomy was advanced and the seeds for further studies were planted by the artists Michelangelo, Raphael Dürer, and, of course, the genius Leonardo da Vinci. They viewed the human body as it really was, not simply as a text passage from Galen. The Renaissance painters depicted people in sickness and pain, sketched in great detail, and in the process, demonstrated amazing insight into the workings of the heart, lungs, brain, and muscle structure. They also attempted to portray the individual and to discover emotional as well as physical qualities. In this stimulating era, physicians began to approach their patients and the pursuit of medical knowledge in similar fashion. New medical schools, *similar* to the most famous of such institutions at Salerno, Bologna, Montpillier, Padua, and Oxford, emerged. These medical training centers once again embraced the Hippocratic doctrine that the patient was human, disease was a natural process, and commonsense therapies were appropriate in assisting the body to conquer its disease.

During the Renaissance, these fundamentals received closer examination, and the age of measurement began. In 1592, when Galileo visited Padua, Italy, he lectured on mathematics to a large audience of medical students. His famous theories and inventions (the thermoscope and the pendulum, in addition to the telescopic lens) were expounded upon and demonstrated. Using these devices, one of his students, Sanctorius, made comparative studies of the human temperature and pulse. A future graduate of Padua, William Harvey, later applied Galileo's laws of motion and mechanics to the problem of blood circulation. This ability to measure the amount of blood moving through the arteries helped to determine the function of the heart (Calder 1958).

Galileo encouraged the use of experimentation and exact measurement as scientific tools that could provide physicians with an effective check against reckless speculation. Quantitation meant theories would be verified before being accepted. Individuals involved in medical research incorporated these new methods into their activities. Body temperature and pulse rate became measures that could be related to other symptoms to assist the physician in diagnosing specific illnesses or disease. Concurrently, the development of the microscope amplified human vision, and an unknown world came into focus.

Unfortunately, new scientific devices had little impact upon the average physician, who continued to blood-let and to disperse noxious ointments. Only in the universities did scientific groups band together to pool their instruments and their various talents.

In England, the medical profession found in Henry VIII a forceful and sympathetic patron. He assisted the doctors in their fight against malpractice and supported the establishment of the College of Physicians, the oldest purely medical institution in Europe. When he suppressed the monastery system in the early sixteenth century, church hospitals were taken over by the cities in which they were located. Consequently, a network of private, nonprofit, voluntary hospitals came into being. Doctors and medical students replaced the nursing sisters and monk-physicians. As a result, the professional nursing class became almost nonexistent in these public institutions. Only among the religious orders did "nursing" remain intact, further compounding the poor lot of patients confined within the walls of the public hospitals. These conditions were to continue until Florence Nightingale appeared on the scene years later.

Still another dramatic event was to occur. The demands made upon England's hospitals, especially the urban hospitals, became overwhelming as the population of these urban centers continued to expand. It was impossible for the facilities to accommodate the needs of so many. As a result, during the seventeenth century two of the major urban hospitals in London, St. Bartholomew's and St. Thomas, initiated a policy of admittting and attending to only those patients who could possibly be cured. The incurables were left to meet their destiny in other institutions such as asylums, prisons, or almshouses.

Humanitarian and democratic movements occupied center stage primarily in France and the American colonies during the eighteenth century. The notion of equal rights had come of age, and as urbanization spread, American society concerned itself with the welfare of all its members. Medical men broadened the scope of their services to include the "unfortunates" of society and helped to ease their suffering by advocating the power of reason and spearheading prison reform, child care, and the hospital movement. Ironically, as the hospital began to take up an active, curative role in medical care in the eighteenth century, the death rate among its patients did not decline but continued to be excessive. In 1788, for example, the death rate among the patients at the Hotel Dru in Paris, thought to be founded in the seventh century, and the oldest hospital in existence today, was nearly 25 percent. These hospitals were lethal not only to patients, but also to the attendants working in them, whose own death rate hovered between 6 and 12 percent per year.

Essentially one could imagine that the hospital remained a place to avoid. Under these circumstances, it is not surprising that the first American colonists postponed or delayed building hospitals. For example, the first hospital in America, the Pennsylvania Hospital, was not built until 1751, and the City of Boston took over two hundred years to erect its first hospital, the Massachusetts General, which opened its doors to the public in 1821 (Crichton 1970).

Not until the nineteenth century could hospitals claim to benefit any significant number of patients. This era of progress was due primarily to the improved nursing practices fostered by Florence Nightingale on her return to England from the Crimean War. She demonstrated that hospital deaths were caused more frequently by hospital conditions than by disease. During the latter part of the nineteenth century, she was at the height of her influence, and few new hospitals were built anywhere in the world without her advice. During the first half of the nineteenth century, Nightingale forced medical attention to focus once more on the care of the patient. Enthusiastically and philosophically she expressed her views on nursing: "Nursing is putting us in the best possible condition for nature to restore and preserve health." And again: "The art is that of nursing the sick. Please mark, not nursing sickness" (Marks and Bealty 1972).

Although these efforts were significant, hospitals remained, until this century, institutions for the sick poor. In the 1870s, for example, when the plans for the projected Johns Hopkins Hospital were reviewed, it was considered quite appropriate to allocate 324 charity and 24 pay beds. Not only did the hospital population before the turn of the century represent a narrow portion of the socioeconomic spectrum, but it also represented only a limited number of the type of diseases prevalent in the overall population, In 1873, for example, roughly half of America's hospitals did not admit contagious diseases, and many others would not admit incurables. Furthermore, in this period, surgery admissions in general hospitals constituted only 5 percent, with trauma (injuries incurred by traumatic experience) making up a good proportion of these cases.

American hospitals a century ago were rather simple, in that their organization required no special provisions for research or technology and demanded only cooking and washing facilities. In addition, since the attending and consulting physicians were normally unsalaried, and the nursing costs were quite modest, the great bulk of the hospital's normal operating expenses was for food, drugs, and utilities. Not until the twentieth century did "modern medicine" in the United States come of age. And, as we shall see, technology played a significant role in its evolution.

The Modern Health Care System

Modern medical practice is a relatively new phenomenon. Before 1900, medicine had little to offer the average citizen since its resources were mainly physicians, their education, and their little black bags. At this time physicians were in short supply, but for different reasons than exist today. Costs were minimal, demand small, and many of the services provided by the physician could also be obtained from experienced amateurs residing in the community. The individual's dwelling was the major site for treatment and recuperation, and relatives and neighbors constituted an able and willing nursing staff. Babies were delivered by midwives, and those illnesses not cured by home remedies were left to run their fatal course. Only in this century did the tremendous explosion in scientific knowledge and technology lead to the development of the American "health care system" with the hospital as its focal point, and the specialist physician and nurse as its most visible operatives.

In the twentieth century the advances made in the basic sciences (chemistry, physiology, pharmacology, and so on) began to occur much more rapidly. Indeed, this is an era of intense interdisciplinary cross-fertilization. Discoveries in the physical sciences have enabled medical research to take giant strides forward. For example, in 1903, William Enthoven devised the first electrocardiograph and measured the electrical changes that occurred during the beating of the heart. In the process, Enthoven initiated a new age for both cardiovascular medicine and electrical measurement techniques.

Of all the new discoveries that now followed one another like intermediates in a chain reaction, the most significant for clinical medicine was the development of x-rays. When W. K. Roentgen described his "new kinds of rays," the human body was opened to medical inspection. Initially these x-rays were used in the diagnosis of bone fractures and dislocations. In the United States x-ray machines brought this "modern technology" to most urban hospitals. In the process, separate departments of radiology were established; the influence of their activities spread, with almost every department of medicine (surgery, gynecology, and so forth) advanced with the aid of this new tool. By the 1930s, x-ray visualization of practically all the organ systems of the body was possible by the use of barium salts and a wide variety of radiopaque materials.

The power this technological innovation gave physicians was enormous. The x-ray permitted them to diagnose a wide variety of diseases and injuries accurately. In addition, being within the hospital, it helped trigger the transformation of the hospital from a passive receptacle for the sick poor to an active curative institution for all the citizens of the American society.

When reviewing some of the most significant developments in health care practices, one is astounded to find that they have occurred fairly recently, that is, within the last 50 years. Consider, for example, that electroencephalography (EEG), the recording of the electrical activity of the brain, was not available until 1929, when it was developed by Hans Berger. The information this instrumentation technique has provided has proved to be as important in the diagnoses of cerebral disease as the electrocardiograph (ECG) has been in heart disease.

Further, not until the introduction of sulfanilamide in the mid-1930s and penicillin in the early 1940s was the main danger of hospitalization, that is, cross-infection among patients, significantly reduced. With these new drugs in their arsenals, surgeons were permitted to perform their operations without prohibitive morbidity and mortality due to infection. Also consider that, even though the different blood groups and their incompatibility were discovered in 1900 and sodium citrate was used in 1913 to prevent clotting, the full development of blood banks was not practical until the 1930s, when technology provided adequate refrigeration. Until that time, "fresh" donors were bled and the blood transfused while it was still warm (Knowles 1973).

As technology in the United States blossomed so did the prestige of American medicine. From 1900 to 1929 Nobel Prize winners in physiology or medicine came primarily from Europe, with no American among them. In the period 1930 to 1939, just prior to World War II, seven Americans were honored by this award. From 1945 to 1975, 39 American life scientists earned similar honors. Most of these efforts were made possible by the advanced technology available to these scientists.

The employment of the available technology assisted in advancing the development of complex surgical procedures. The Drinker respirator was introduced in 1927 and the first heart-lung bypass in 1939. In the 1940s, cardiac catheterization and angiography (the use of a cannula threaded through an arm vein and into the heart with the injection of radiopaque dye for the x-ray visualization of lung and heart vessels and valves) were developed. Accurate diagnoses of congenital and acquired heart disease (mainly valve disorders due to rheumatic fever) also became possible, and a new era of cardiac and vascular surgery began.

Another child of this modern technology, the electron microscope, entered the medical scene in the fifties, providing significant advances in visualizing relatively small cells. Body scanners to detect tumors arose from the same science that brought societies reluctantly into the atomic age. These "tumor detectives" utilizing radioactive material became commonplace in newly established departments of nuclear medicine in all hospitals.

The impact of these discoveries and many others was profound. The health care system that consisted primarily of the "horse and buggy" physician was gone forever, replaced by the doctor backed by and centered around the hospital, as medicine began to change to accommodate the new technology. Thus, it can be seen that the modern hospital in its contemporary, familiar form is essentially 50 years old.

Following World War II, the evolution of comprehensive care greatly accelerated. The advanced technology that had been developed in the pursuit of military objectives now became available for peaceful applications with the medical profession benefiting greatly from this rapid surge of technological "finds." For instance, the realm of electronics came into prominence. The techniques for following enemy ships and planes, as well as providing aviators with information concerning altitude, air speed, and the like, were now used extensively in medicine to follow, for example, the subtle electrical behavior of the fundamental unit of the central nervous system, the neuron, or to monitor the beating heart of a patient.

Science and technology have leap-frogged past one another throughout recorded history. Anyone seeking a causal relation between the two was just as likely to find technology the cause and science the effect with the converse also holding true; as gunnery led to ballistics and the steam engine to thermodynamics, so powered flight led to aerodynamics (Susskind 1973). However, with advent of electronics, this causal relation between technology and science changed to a systematic exploitation of scientific research, the pursuit of knowledge, sometimes undertaken with technical uses in mind.

The list becomes endless when one reflects upon the devices produced by the same technology that permitted humans to stand on the moon. What was considered science fiction in the 1930s and the 1940s has now become reality. For devices continually changed to incorporate the latest innovations, which in many cases became outmoded in a very short period of time. Telemetry devices used to monitor the activity of a patient's heart freed both the physician and the patient from the wires that previously restricted them to the four walls of the hospital room. Computers, similar to those that controlled the flight plans of the *Apollo* capsules, now inundate our society. Medical researchers have put these electronic brains to work performing complex calculations, keeping records, and even controlling the very instrumentation that sustains life. The citations, the technological discoveries, are endless and have enabled medical research to gain an insight into the functioning of the human organism that would otherwise be impossible.

"Spare parts" surgery has also become possible. With the first successful transplantation of a kidney in 1954, the concept of artificial organs gained acceptance and officially came into vogue in the medical arena. Technology to provide prosthetic devices, such as artificial heart valves and artificial blood vessels, developed. Even an artificial heart program to develop a replacement for a defective or diseased human heart began. These technological innovations radically altered surgical organization and utilization. The comparison of a hospital in which surgery was a relatively minor activity, as it was a century ago, to the contemporary

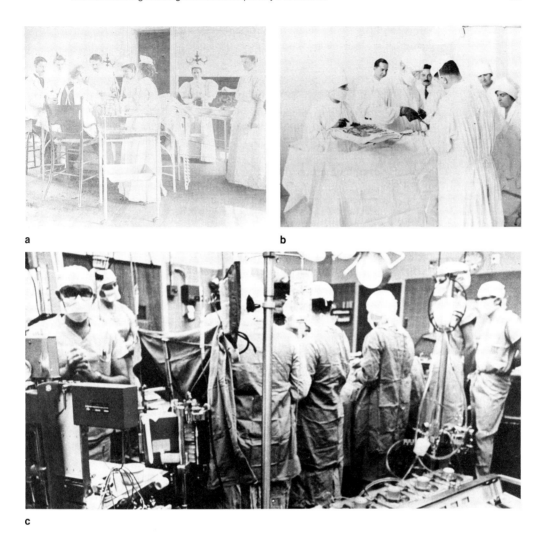

Figure 1.1 Changes in the operating room. (a) The surgical scene at the turn of the century. (b) The surgical scene in the mid-1920s and early 1930s. (c) The surgical scene today (from Bronzino, JD: *Technology for Patient Care,* St. Louis: C. V. Mosby, 1977).

hospital, in which surgery plays a prominent role, suggests dramatically the manner in which this technological effort has revolutionized the health profession and the institution of the hospital (Figure 1.1).

Through this evolutionary process, the hospital became the central institution providing medical care. Because of the complex and expensive technology that could be based only in the hospital (Figure 1.2) and the education of doctors oriented both as clinicians and investigators toward highly technological norms, both the patient and the physician were pushed even closer to this center of attraction. In addition, the effects of the increasing maldistribution and apparent shortage of physicians during the 1950s and 1960s also forced the patient and the physi-

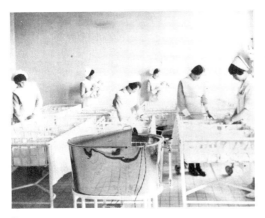
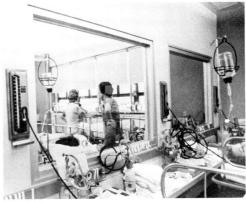

a   b

Figure 1.2 Technological innovations in the neonatal intensive care unit. (a) Continuous personal attention was necessary in the early 1920s. (b) Today computerized systems continuously monitor vital signs (courtesy of the Saint Francis Hospital and Medical Center, Hartford, Connecticut).

cian to turn increasingly to the ambulatory clinic and the emergency ward of the urban hospital in time of need.

These emergency wards today handle not only an ever-increasing number of accidents (largely related to alcohol and the automobile) and somatic crises such as heart attacks and strokes, but also problems resulting from the social environments that surround the local hospital. Respiratory complaints, cuts, bumps, and minor trauma constitute a significant number of the cases seen in a given day. Added to these individuals are those who live in the neighborhood of the hospital and simply cannot afford their own physician. Often such individuals enter the emergency ward for routine care of colds, hangovers, and even marital problems (Knowles 1973).

Demand for treatment in the emergency room increased even further as health was increasingly perceived as a birthright rather than a privilege. Although ambulatory clinics and emergency wards were expanded in response to this demand, people continued to appear in great numbers, thus straining the system. At the same time, urban hospitals were hard-pressed to meet both the increasing demands of an expanding population and the need for modern surgical facilities and intensive care units complete with electronic monitoring devices, specialized nurses, and technicians.

As a result of these developments, the hospital has evolved as the focal point of the present system of health care delivery. The hospital, as presently organized, specializes in highly technical and complex medical procedures. This evolutionary process became inevitable as "technology" produced increasingly sophisticated equipment that private practitioners or even large group practices were economically unequipped to acquire and maintain. Only the hospital could provide this type of service. The steady expansion of scientific and technological innovations

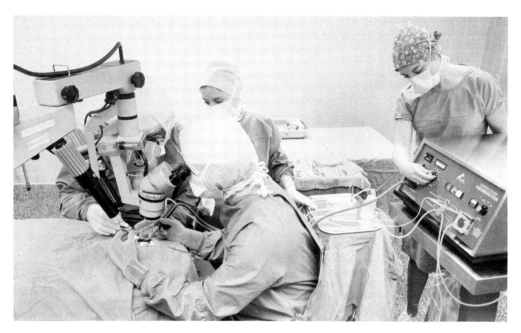

Figure 1.3 Modern American medicine depends heavily on technological innovation and its implementation (courtesy of the Hartford Hosptial, Hartford, Connecticut).

has necessitated specialization for all health professionals (physicians, nurses, and technicians) and the housing of advanced technology within the walls of the modern hospital (Figure 1.3). As Dr. John H. Knowles, former director of the Massachusetts General Hospital, pointed out:

> Through the recent expansion of emergency room facilities and ambulatory clinics, through liaison with extended care facilities, nursing homes, and through the establishment of neighborhood centers, it [the hospital] can continually extend its interest actively to the community, and in the process, keep down costs and reach more people in need. This type of development or extensions of the hospital will enable it to remain the community major institution for the coordination of health planning (Knowles 1973).

Technology will have an ever-increasing role in achieving these goals. In recent years, technology has struck medicine like a thunderbolt, providing far more advances in the last 50 years than in the previous 2,000. In a culture steeped in science, this trend will continue. However, the social and economic consequences of this vast outpouring of information and innovation must be fully understood if this technology is to be exploited effectively and efficiently.

For the future, technology offers great potential for affecting health care practices. It can provide health care for those individuals in remote rural areas by means of closed-circuit television health clinics with complete communication links to a regional health center. Development of multiphasic screening systems can provide preventive medicine to vast majority of our population and restrict admission to the hospital to those needing the diagnostic and treatment facilities housed there. Automation of patient and nursing records can inform physicians of the status of patients during their stay at the hospital and in their homes. With the creation of a central medical records system, anyone moving or becoming ill away from home can have records made available to the attending physician easily and rapidly. These are just a few of the possibilities that illustrate the potential of technology in creating the type of medical care system that will indeed be accessible, be of high quality, and be reasonably priced for all Americans.

BIOMEDICAL ENGINEERING: SOME DEFINITIONS

There is general agreement that engineering methods and technology offer significant potential for increasing the effectiveness and efficiency of health care. Many of the problems confronting health professionals today are intimately related to the skills of the engineer, because they contain the fundamental aspects of device and systems analysis, design, and practical application, all of which lie at the heart of engineering technology. These health-oriented design problems range from very complex large-scale constructs such as automated clinical laboratories, multiphasic screening, and hospital information systems to such small and "simple" devices as electrodes and transducers. They encompass the many complexities of remote monitoring and telemetry and include the requirements of emergency vehicles, operating rooms, and intensive care units. These various tasks represent a true challenge to modern technology.

Biomedical engineering is among the most recent additions to the technological professions. Since the concepts, knowledge, and approaches of virtually all engineering disciplines can be employed to meet the needs of the medical profession, from research to patient care, the opportunities for interaction between engineers and health professionals are many and varied.

Although the scope of biomedical engineering is considered by many to be quite clear, many conflicting opinions concerning the field can be traced to disagreements about its definition. It is, therefore, necessary to define and emphasize the distinctions among the following terms: *biomedical engineering, bioengineering,* and *clinical* (or *medical*) *engineering* (Goldsmith 1965; Mendelsohn 1968; Plonsey 1973; Johns 1975; Bronzino 1977a).

The most comprehensive of these three distinctive terms is *biomedical engineering,* that branch of applied science concerned with solving and understanding problems in biology and medicine using principles, methods, and approaches drawn from engineering science and technology. *Bioengineering,* on the other hand, is usually viewed as a basic research-oriented activity using the tools and concepts of the physical sciences to develop a better understanding of biological-physiological systems. It does not primarily address clinical problems. In contrast, *clinical engineering* is primarily a discipline involving the clinical aspects of health care delivery and patient care (Davis 1964; Oakes 1975; Bronzino 1977b).

Implicit in the definition of biomedical engineering is its broad scope. It ranges from theoretical, nonexperimental undertakings to state-of-the-art applications. It can encompass research, development, implementation, and operation. Accordingly, as with medical practice itself, no single person can acquire expertise that encompasses the entire field of biomedical engineering. As a result, there has been an explosion of biomedical specialists to cover this broad spectrum of activity. Yet, because of the interdisciplinary nature of this activity, the need for considerable interplay and overlapping of interest and effort remains.

Biomedical engineering emerged from the technology boom of the 1950s as a primary response to the requirements for modern instrumentation in biomedical research (Rushmer 1972; Gowen 1973). The initial activity of the early practitioners in this area consisted of specific branches of engineering reacting to the many challenging problems posed by the medical field. Because of the initial successes of these individuals in meeting the obvious needs for quantitation in biological and medical research and the envisioned potential of "space age" technology applied to the medical arena, the 1960s saw the initiation of graduate programs in biomedical engineering. These programs were designed specifically to induce "multidisciplinary professionals" to engage in medical research. The federal government stimulated this effort to train "hybrids" (individuals skilled in medicine and engineering) when branches of the National Institute of Health (NIH) established training grants in engineering for graduate students providing considerable depth in the life sciences. These individuals, it was hoped, could function as independent investigators studying specific life science problems. Thus, the highly trained "biomedical engineer" was expected to bridge the gap between the health professional and the conventionally trained engineer.

As a result of the efforts of these new professionals, a major involvement of biomedical engineering in basic research on a wide variety of medical topics characterized the mid-1960s. Medical research benefited significantly from these efforts. New materials to perfect artificial hearts and other prosthetic devices and mathematical models to provide greater insight into the mechanisms involved in many physiological systems were developed. Telemetry devices monitored patients, and computers entered the life science laboratory. These early technological innovations, however, found few mass markets, and many early medical instrumentation packages and systems were used in the health care setting before they were thoroughly tested. Many of these initial attempts failed and in the process actually retarded the entrance of technology into the field of health care. All this occurred at a time when the health care industry itself was undergoing major changes.

As a society we had come to expect the delivery of health care by the family physician, but social changes and population growth had shifted the focus of the health care system to preventive medicine and the establishment of clinics and group practices as the major approaches for better health care. During the past 25 years, technology has accelerated this process by making available new treatment techniques that function well and are economically feasible for clinical and hospital consumption. As a result, markets for the many biomedical devices have expanded, and the biomedical equipment industry has continued to grow.

CLINICAL ENGINEERING COMES OF AGE

With the advent of the 1970s, a new area of activity for biomedical engineers also began to form. In the process of benefiting patients, medical electronics also created significant problems, including incompatibility of devices manufactured by independent companies, design deficiencies, incomplete technical operating instructions, hazards to the safety of patients and employees from improper repair and maintenance of equipment, difficulty of training personnel at all levels in proper operation of equipment, and management difficulties in making appropriate decisions concerning the choice, use, and care of complex instrumentation.

To address these problems engineers entered the clinical scene to participate in the ongoing activities of clinics and hospitals as members of the health care team. As a result, a major expansion in the area of clinical engineering began. In the process, the Veterans Administration became convinced that clinical engineers were vital to the overall operation of their hospital system and divided their hospital system into "Biomedical Engineering Districts" with a chief biomedical engineer in charge of the overall clinical engineering activities within that district. Clinical engineers were hired for the centralized clinical engineering departments that were established in larger hospitals (those having more than 300 beds), to enable those facilities to utilize the technology already available within the hospitals more effectively and to incorporate new technology more efficiently.

The increased momentum of this clinical engineering movement stimulated the infusion of further technology into the patient care arena. Throughout the 1970s and early 1980s, computers and automated clinical systems were widely used in many clinical settings. Automated clinical laboratories, data collection and management systems, patient monitoring systems, and multiphasic health screening, to name just a few, are now commonplace. In the future it is anticipated that clinical engineers will become increasingly involved in developing interactive communication systems to link the various parts of the health care delivery system together into one cohesive unit. Although some doubt that technology can be successful in reducing costs, clinical engineers have become indispensible in making health care delivery possible on the vast scale presently required and expected in the future. It has therefore become necessary to have an engineer in the house.

The presence of engineering professionals within the hospital environment requires a fundamentally different kind of philosophy, one that advocates a team approach carried beyond the development of instrumentation. With an "in-house" engineer, such teamwork may start quite simply. For example, a physician or nurse may need assistance in learning how to operate a new instrument. Since they do not have time to experiment and cannot afford to make errors, they invite the engineer to participate in the first trial. The engineer teaches the physician and nurse about the subtleties of the instrument and, in turn, experiences a first lesson in clinical (or patient) variability. From such informal beginnings, true interdisciplinary processes are developed and exploited (Bronzino 1974).

In recent years, clinical engineering has become an established discipline as the role of the engineer in the hospital has gained importance (see Figure 1.4). These new in-house engineering tasks performed within the hospital include (1) supervision, proper operation, and safety of instruments; (2) design of engineering

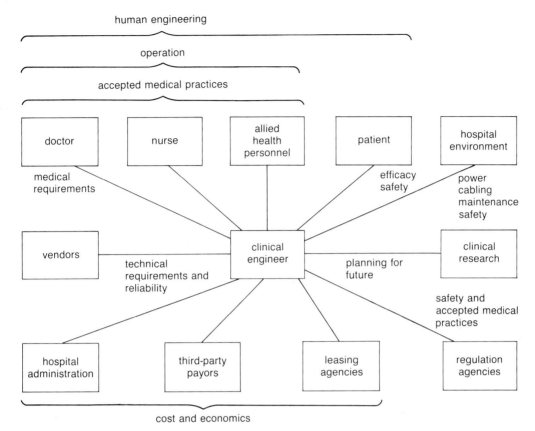

Figure 1.4   The tasks and activities of the clinical engineer
(courtesy of Oakes, JB, the Johns Hopkins Hospital,
Baltimore, Maryland).

systems and components of systems not commercially available; (3) specification
and purchase of new equipment; (4) training of staff on its proper use; and (5) introduction of industrial or management engineering techniques to optimize information handling. A clinical engineer can be described as an engineer who is able to
perform these tasks in a health care facility and who has the knowledge and experience to work as a partner with health professionals to plan and implement appropriate programs for improving health care delivery. Their acceptance in hospitals
can open the door to new types of engineering, medical interactions that will have
a significant and beneficial impact on health care delivery (Oakes 1975).

The hospitals that have established clinical engineering departments also recognize the need for these individuals to service an administrative function. Consequently, the present view is not simply to ensure that the equipment is maintained
and certified as safe, but rather to provide the hospital administration with an objective opinion of equipment function, purchase, application, overall system analysis, and preventive maintenance policies (Figures 1.5 and 1.6). With the in-house
availability of such talent and expertise the hospital is in a far better position to
manage its technical resources more effectively (Jacobs 1975). Additional benefits

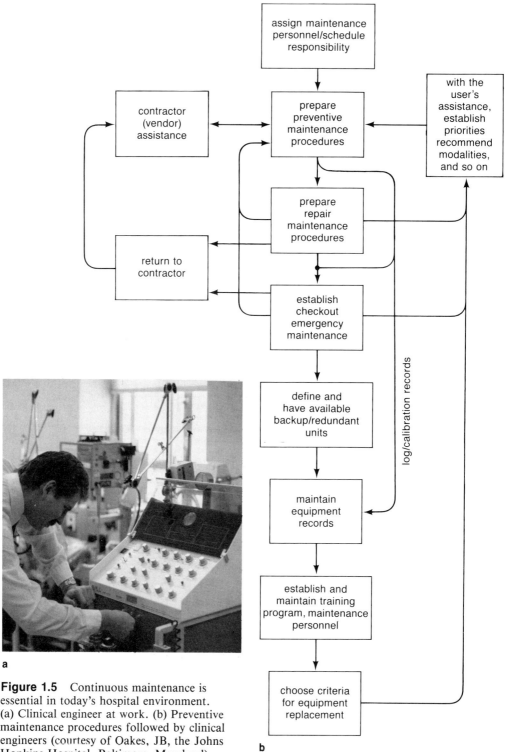

a

Figure 1.5 Continuous maintenance is essential in today's hospital environment. (a) Clinical engineer at work. (b) Preventive maintenance procedures followed by clinical engineers (courtesy of Oakes, JB, the Johns Hopkins Hospital, Baltimore, Maryland).

b

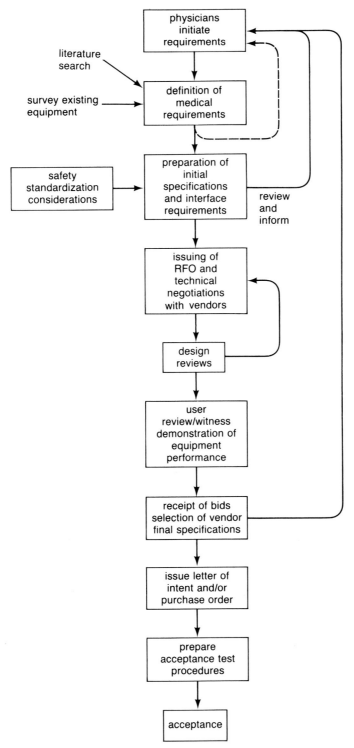

Figure 1.6 Steps in the purchase of new equipment (courtesy of Oakes, JB, the Johns Hopkins Hospital, Baltimore, Maryland).

result from involving clinical engineers in the decision-making process for buying or replacing equipment or identifying problems within the health care delivery system that can be solved with existing engineering technology. Often individuals who have neither the necessary training nor background spend too much or too little time in selecting and evaluating medical equipment and systems. The presence of a clinical engineer to assist in this area saves valuable time for patient care. These are all appropriate activities for the clinical engineer.

ROLE OF THE BIOMEDICAL ENGINEER

In its broadest sense, then, biomedical engineering involves training essentially three types of individuals: (1) the clinical engineer in health care, (2) the biomedical design engineer for industry, and (3) the research scientist (Bronzino 1971; Bronzino 1977a). Presently, one might also distinguish among three specific roles these biomedical engineers can play (Wolff 1967). Each is different enough to merit a separate description. The first type, the most common, might be called the "problem solver" (Figure 1.7). This biomedical engineer (most likely the clinical engineer or biomedical design engineer) maintains the traditional service relationship with the life scientists, who originate a problem that can be solved by applying the specific expertise of the engineer. For this problem-solving process to be efficient and successful, however, some knowledge of each other's language and a ready in-

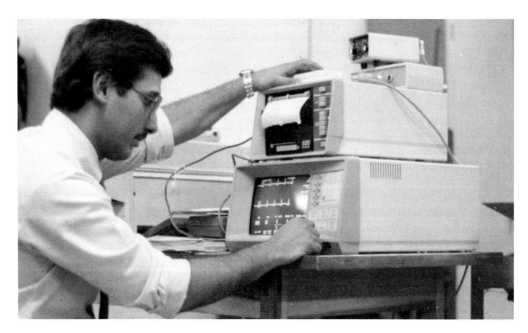

Figure 1.7   A problem solver in the clinical environment of the hospital (courtesy of the Saint Francis Hospital and Medical Center, Hartford, Connecticut).

terchange of information must exist. Biomedical engineers must understand the biological situation to apply their judgment and contribute their knowledge toward the solution of the given problem, as well as to defend their methods in terms that the life scientist can understand. If they are unable to do these, they do not merit the "biomedical" prefix.

The second type, who is much rarer, might be called the "technological entrepreneur" (most likely a biomedical design engineer in industry). This individual assumes that the gap between the technological education of the life scientist or physician and present technological capability has become so great that the life scientists cannot pose a problem that will incorporate the application of existing technology. Therefore, technological entrepreneurs examine some portion of the biological or medical front and identify areas in which advanced technology might be advantageous. Thus, they pose their own problem and then proceed to provide the solution, at first conceptually and then in the form of hardware. Finally, these individuals must convince the medical community that they can provide a useful tool because, contrary to the situation in which problem solvers find themselves, the entrepreneur's activity is speculative at best and has no ready-made customer for the results. If the venture is successful, however, whether scientifically or commercially, then an advance has been made much earlier than it would have through the conventional arrangement. Because of the nature of their work, technological entrepreneurs should have a great deal of engineering and medical knowledge as well as experience in numerous medical systems.

The third type of biomedical engineer, the "engineer-scientist" (most likely the basic researcher), is not concerned with the invention or construction of hardware at all. These individuals are primarily interested in applying engineering concepts and techniques to the investigation and exploration of biological processes. The most powerful tool at their disposal is the construction of an appropriate physical or mathematical model of the specific biological system under study. Through simulation techniques and available computing machinery, they can use this model to understand features that are too complex for either analytical computation or intuitive recognition. In addition, this process of simulation facilitates the design of appropriate experiments that can be performed on the actual biological system, whose results can, in turn, be used to amend the model. Thus, by an iterative process of this kind, increased understanding of a biological mechanism results.

This mathematical model can also predict the effect of these changes on a biological system in cases where the actual experiments may be tedious, very difficult, or dangerous. The researchers are thus rewarded with a better understanding of the biological system, and the mathematical description forms a compact, precise language easily communicated to others. The activities of the engineer-scientist inevitably impinge upon instrument development because to perform the biological side of the experimental work, the exploitation of sophisticated measurement techniques is often necessary. It is essential that engineer-scientists work in a biological environment, particularly when their work may ultimately have a clinical application. It is not enough to emphasize the niceties of mathematical analysis and lose the clinical relevance in the process. This biomedical engineer is, thus, the true partner of the biological scientist and is rapidly becoming an integral part of the "teams" being formed in many institutes to develop techniques and experiments that will unfold the mysteries of the life system (Weed 1975; Couter 1980; Wolf and Berle 1981).

Each of these roles envisioned for the biomedical engineer requires a different attitude, as well as a specific degree of knowledge about the biological environment. However, each engineer must be a skilled professional with a significant expertise in engineering technology. Therefore, in preparing new professionals to enter this field at these various levels, engineering education is being challenged to develop programs that will provide an adequate exposure to and knowledge about the environment, without sacrificing essential engineering skills. As we continue to move into a period characterized by a rapidly growing population, rising social and economic expectations, and a need for the development of more adequate techniques for the prevention, diagnosis, and treatment of disease, development and employment of biomedical engineers have become a necessity. This is true not only because they may provide an opportunity to increase our knowledge of living systems, but because they constitute promising vehicles for expediting the conversion of knowledge to effective action.

The ultimate role of the biomedical engineer, like that of the nurse and physician, is to serve society. This is not just a skilled technical service but one in the highest professional sense. To use this new breed effectively, health care practitioners and administrators should be aware of the needs for these new professionals and the roles for which they are being trained. The great potential, challenge, and promise in this endeavor promise technological and intellectual as well as humanitarian benefits for humankind.

REFERENCES

Atkinson, D. T. 1956. *Magic, myth and medicine.* New York: Fawcett. p. 18.

Bronzino, J. D. 1971. The biomedical engineer—the roles he can play. *Science* 174:1001–1003.

Bronzino, J. D. 1974. Engineers as OR team members. *AORN Journal* 20:1053–1058.

Bronzino, J. D. 1977. *Technology for patient care.* St. Louis: Mosby.

Bronzino, J. D. 1977. How to educate clinical engineers—the internship approach. *J Clin Eng* 2(1):73–78.

Calder, R. 1958 *Medicine and man.* London: Allen and Unwin.

Couter, S. S. 1980. The professional development degree for biomedical engineers. *J Clin Eng* 5:299–302.

Crichton, M. 1970. *Five patients—the hospital explained.* New York: Knopf.

Davis, J. F. 1964. Medical engineering. *Int Sci Technol* 33:18–32.

Goldsmith, A. N. 1965. Biomedical engineering. *IEEE Spectrum* 2:46–56.

Gowen, R. J. 1973. Biomedical engineering education in perspective. *Eng Educ* 64:175–176.

Jacobs, J. E. 1975. The biomedical engineering quandry. *IEEE Trans Biomed Eng* 22:100–106.

Johns, R. J. 1975. Current issues in biomedical engineering education. *IEEE Trans Biomed Eng* 22:107–110.

Knowles, J. 1973. The hospital. *Sci Am* 229:128–137.

Marks, G., and Bealty W. K. 1972. *Women in white.* New York: Scribner's.

Mendelsohn, E. I. 1968. The prehistory of biomedical engineering. *Dimensions Biomed Eng* 7:7–48.

Oakes, J. B. 1975. Clinical engineering—the problems and the promise. *Science* 190:239–242.

Plonsey, R. 1973. New directions for biomedical engineering. *Eng Educ* 64:117–179.

Rushmer, R. 1972. *Medical engineering projections for health care delivery.* New York: Academic.

Sigerest, H. E. 1951. *A history of medicine.* New York: Oxford University Press.

Susskind, C. 1973. *Understanding technology.* Baltimore: The Johns Hopkins University Press.

Weed, H. R. 1975. Biomedical engineering—practice or research. *IEEE Trans Biomed Eng* 22:110–114.

Wolf, S., and Berle B. B. 1981. *The technological imperative in medicine.* New York: Plenum.

Wolff, H. S. 1967. Bioengineering, *Biomed Eng* 2:547–549.

Part Two

Basic Physiology and Biomedical Instrumentation Devices

CHAPTER 2

Biosensors: Transducers, Electrodes, and Physiological Systems

Michael R. Neuman, Ph.D., M.D.

Departments of Reproductive Biology and Biomedical
    Engineering
Case Western Reserve University
Cleveland, Ohio

INTRODUCTION

One of the major contributions of biomedical engineering to the life sciences and clinical medicine has been in biomedical instrumentation. Advances in this field have resulted in the development of new types of biomedical instruments and the development of numerous clinical approaches, such as electronic patient monitoring, an important aspect of critical care medicine, as well as a variety of devices to assist individuals with disabilities. Biomedical instrumentation involves three basic functions, as illustrated in Figure 2.1. Since the sensor or transducer portion of the instrument effects the interface with the physiological system being measured, biosensors represent an essential component of any biomedical instrumentation system. As the primary vehicle for converting a specific biological, chemical, or physical event into an electrical signal, the biosensor must accomplish this transduction process without altering, that is, perturbing, the very event it is measuring. Consequently, they are extremely important, for without them we would be unaware of the changing dynamics of the physical, chemical, and biological worlds. Since biosensors deal with a variety of specific quantities, physiological considerations are as important as those of engineering design when dealing with biosensors for medical instruments.

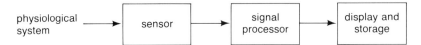

Figure 2.1   Block diagram of a general instrumentation system.

Medical electronic instrumentation has benefited from the information explosion in electronic technology. Self-contained medical electronic instruments today can carry out complex signal processing that only recently required a separate computer. The highly sophisticated processing capabilities of today's instruments, however, still require high-quality signals at the instrument input. Such signals must come from sensors that act as the interface between the biological organism and the rest of the instrument. Thus the field of sensors for biomedical electronic instruments represents an important area of research, development, and manufacturing in biomedical engineering. This chapter will highlight some of the progress in this area in recent years and look at sensing techniques that may be important in the future.

Once the biosensor converts the physiological information being measured into an electronic signal it is handled by the second major block of the instrumentation system, the signal processor. The *signal-processing section* of the instrument takes the electronic signal from the sensor and amplifies, filters, and operates upon it to produce an electrical signal capable of operating the output devices or providing a display. This signal processing can be as elementary as simply amplifying the signal, or it can be much more complex, involving the design and utilization of extensive hardware and software packages to provide appropriate, reliable outputs for the measurement being made.

The *output* section of the basic medical instrument is similar to the sensor section in that it provides an interface between electrical signals and a biological system. In this case, the biological system is the health care provider. The function of the output section of a medical instrument is to convert the processed electrical signals into a form that people using the instrument can observe and, in some cases, to store the information for future observation and analysis. Typical output devices used in a medical instrumentation system are the cathode-ray tube (CRT) for visual observation of signals in graphic or alpha-numeric form, the graphic chart recorder for observation and permanent records of signals, and the magnetic tape recorder for analog or digital records of signals that are observed and analyzed at a later time.

It is to be emphasized from this brief, general description of a biomedical instrumentation system that an intimate understanding of the quantities being measured is important in designing each of the three major blocks of the system. To make physiological measurements properly, then, one must clearly understand the interaction between the sensor and the biological system. Only then can one minimize the measurement errors that in turn may affect clinical decisions. One purpose of this chapter is therefore to provide a review of the basic physiological events, along with the basic concepts involved in the development of biosensors (transducers) and electrodes for physiological measurement.

PHYSIOLOGICAL SYSTEMS: GENERAL CLASSIFICATIONS

A *physiological system* consists of a group of interconnected or interdependent organs that work together to perform a specific function or group of functions in the body. The functions of a physiological system are represented in general by the block diagram of Figure 2.2. Here, a set of input variables controls another set of output variables generated by the system. In a way, this process is similar to our generalized medical instrument since the physiological system must have sensors to detect and measure the input variables. The physiological system also processes information and produces outputs in response to these inputs. Unlike medical instruments, however, humans do not always understand the operation of a physiological system. We are only beginning to learn how certain parts of the body are able to sense physiologic variables and convert them into signals within the nervous system. Although we do not really know exactly how the nervous system processes these signals, we do have a reasonably good idea of the physiological outputs from many of the systems in the body.

Mammals have many physiological systems. Often, a particular organ belongs to more than one system since individual organs may be involved in many different functions. To appreciate this point, let us briefly review some of the major physiological systems encountered in mammals and define their functions.

Nervous System

The nervous system is the major communicator of the body, allowing various organs to interact with one another and permitting the body to react to its environment and to make adjustments based upon internal and external factors. The nervous system, as such, can be a part of other systems of the body, although this is not necessary. It is divided into the *central nervous system*, the brain and spinal cord; and the *peripheral nervous system*, those nerves and ganglia not in the brain or spinal cord. Peripheral nerves play an important role in sensation and motor control. The *autonomic nervous system* is that portion of the central and peripheral nervous systems regulating the activity of smooth muscle, cardiac muscle, and glands. It comprises the sympathetic and parasympathetic divisions. The *sympa-*

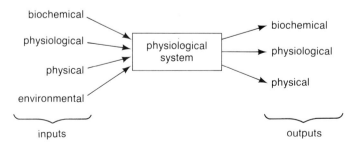

Figure 2.2 A general physiologic system from the standpoint of input and output variables.

thetic division tends to act in a broad manner to prepare the body for conditions resulting from emergencies and requiring a vigorous and immediate response. The *parasympathetic* division, on the other hand, acts more discretely upon individual organs or regions of the body and is more involved in vegetative functions such as digestion and rest. (For further details on the nervous system, see Chapter 5.)

Cardiovascular System

The cardiovascular portion of the body, consisting of the heart and blood vessels, is concerned with the circulation of the blood and is also referred to as the *circulatory system*. Its primary role is to supply nutrients to peripheral tissue and to remove waste products. It also serves in communication in that it transports hormones from the glands of the endocrine system to the organs that resond to them. (More details on the cardiovascular system can be found in Chapter 3.)

Respiratory System

The organs of the respiratory system enable the cardiovascular system to exchange gases with the air. This system includes the airway (nose, pharynx, larynx, and trachea), the bronchial tree, and the lungs. Muscles associated with breathing such as the diaphragm and intercostal muscles can also be considered a part of this system. (For more details, see Chapter 4.)

Endocrine System

The endocrine system is similar to the autonomic nervous system in that it is involved in regulation and control of visceral function, but it is generally slower in response than the nervous system. It acts by secreting hormones that are transported by the cardiovascular system. Endocrine glands control such general body functions as growth, metabolism, and reproduction.

Gastrointestinal System

Sometimes referred to as the *digestive system*, the gastrointestinal system is concerned with the ingestion and digestion of food, as well as the elimination of the residues of digestion. In addition to those organs having direct contact with ingested food, it includes the liver, gallbladder, and pancreas. These organs function in the production of substances to aid in digestion.

Urogenital System

The urogenital system comprises the organs acting in the production, storage, and elimination of urine, as well as those involved in the process of reproduction.

Thus, in reality, it consists of two separate systems. The urinary and the reproductive systems are considered together because several organs are common to both.

Musculoskeletal System

The musculoskeletal system also comprises two distinct systems, the muscular and the skeletal. The former consists of all of the voluntarily controlled muscles of the body; the latter involves the bone and cartilage.

Hematopoietic System

The hematopoietic system consists of organs involved in the production of the blood. It includes the bone marrow, spleen, and lymphatic tissue.

Integumental System

The skin and its appendages such as hair and nails make up the integumental system. Among other processes it is involved in the protection of the body from its environment.

The preceding summary of systems is by no means complete. Not only do other systems of the body perform specific functions, but often these systems can be divided into subsystems as well. Overlap between different physiological systems is extensive, with organs being common to more than one system. One example is the kidney, an important organ in the urinary system, which also plays an important role in the regulation of blood pressure; thus, it is a part of the cardiovascular system as well.

BASIC PHYSIOLOGICAL MEASUREMENTS AND TECHNIQUES

An important aspect of the study of physiology and of diagnostic medicine is the measurement of the function of physiological systems and subunits of the systems, such as individual organs or even cells. These measurements enable health professionals to understand the functions of the systems and to determine when the systems fail to function properly through disease or other causes. Physiological systems are measured in several ways. One can begin by making a physical measurement of system components. For example, one way that a physician diagnoses an upper respiratory infection (cold) is to palpate (feel) the lymph nodes of the neck to determine whether they have become enlarged, indicating increased activity in fighting infection. This is an example of measuring the physical size and shape of an organ as a means of learning more about it. One can also measure some of the output variables from a physiological system. For example, a measure of the blood pressure can help to illustrate the effectiveness of the heart in pumping blood and the peripheral resistance of the circulation.

One can also look at inputs to physiological systems to determine whether the systems are dealing with the input information properly. For example, following a meal, the pancreas should increase the amount of insulin secreted into the blood in response to the increase in blood glucose (sugar) resulting from digestion of the food. This insulin causes the blood glucose level to fall as glucose is transported into the cells of the body. If the pancreas is unable to respond to this input after a meal, the blood glucose will initially increase but will then decrease less rapidly; thus, by measuring the time course of blood glucose following the ingestion of a known amount of sugar (glucose tolerance test), one can determine whether the pancreas is functioning properly or whether the disease diabetes may be present.

The preceding example also represents another common form of measurement of the behavior of a physiological system: the response of the system to a standard input. In this case, ingestion of a known amount of glucose is the standard input. Other standard inputs frequently used in diagnostic medicine are the familiar eye chart, auditory stimuli, and tap with a reflex hammer. Measurements can be made with an input to the physiological system that represents a stress to the body. These types of measurements are referred to as *stress tests*, and one of the most familiar is the evaluation of the heart in which a subject undergoes a known stress by exercising on a treadmill. Stress testing is useful not only in determining normal operation of a physiological system or component of that system, but in establishing the limits of the range of this normal operation.

Measurements on physiological systems can also involve determining the physical and chemical properties of the environment of the body and determining whether the physiological response is appropriate for that environment. Physiologists are interested in the body's response to heat and cold stress, and the behavior of the body in the presence of other physical stresses such as zero gravity are currently of great interest in aviation and space medicine.

Of the many specific ways to make the measurements described in the previous section, this section will concentrate on some frequently applied examples of important measurement systems. References on medical instrumentation will provide more detailed descriptions and more diversified measurements (Webster 1978; Bellville and Weaver 1969; Hill and Dolan 1976).

Medical instrumentation systems fall into two general categories: those that measure physical quantities and those that measure chemical quantities. The section of the instrumentation system that is primarily concerned with these differences is the sensor, or transducer. Physical sensors usually convert a physical variable into an electrical signal that, as previously discussed, the remainder of the instrumentation system processes. Chemical variables, on the other hand, can either be converted directly into an electrical signal or into a physical quantity that in turn is transduced to an electrical signal by another physical transducer.

Physical Transducers

Physical quantities of physiological interest range from geometric variables such as displacement through energy-related variables such as temperature to more complex physical variables such as pressure and flow. Transducers for each of these general areas are important in medical instrumentation, with many different types of sensors employed for these variables. A sample of some of these sensors is indicated in Table 2.1, which includes some of the different classifications for physical sensors and lists examples of sensors for particular measurements. As the table indicates, some physical variables can be converted to other physical variables that are sensed by transducers for the new variable. Thus some sensors measure apparently unrelated physical variables. For example, strain gauges, which are displacement sensors, can measure force, acceleration, or pressure when they are incorporated into sensor systems that convert these physical variables into a displacement. Such a system for measuring weight will be illustrated later in this chapter. Other examples of these sensors and their applications will be presented in the following sections.

Sensors of geometric variables

Geometric variables of general physiological interest include displacement, area, and volume. Table 2.1 includes some of the sensors in this category. Because of the many applications of these types of measurements, this chapter will consider only two.

Table 2.1 Sensors of physical biomedical variables

I. Geometric variables

   A. Linear and angular displacement
      1. Variable resistance devices such as variable resistance controls and linear slide wires
      2. Strain gauges such as metal foil, semiconductor, and mercury in a compliant tube
      3. Mutual inductance coils
      4. Linear variable differential transformer (LVDT)
      5. Variable capacitance devices
      6. Piezoelectric materials
      7. Optical analog and digital encoders
      8. Ultrasonic transit time measurement
      9. Magnetic field strength measurement
     10. Radiation intensity from point or other well-defined sources using radiation such as light, x-ray, radioactive particle, ultrasound, or other electromagnetic waves

   B. Area
      1. Magnetic induction coil in which induced voltage is proportional to area of the coil
      2. Light intensity where the intensity of scattered light is proportional to the cross-sectional area of the scattering particles or the intensity of transmitted light decreases as scattering particle area increases
      3. Signals from two or more displacement sensors processed to a given area
      4. Medical imaging techniques such as x-ray or computer axial tomography giving cross-sectional areas

   C. Volume
      1. Imaging in two or more planes
      2. Electrical conductivity
      3. Flow differences from two or more sensors
      4. Spirometry for gas volumes
      5. Pressure changes in closed chambers as in plethysmography
      6. Mass determinations as from displaced fluids
      7. Signals from three or more displacement sensors processed to a given volume

Table 2.1   (continued)

II. Kinematic Variables

    A. Velocity
1. Ultrasonic and laser Doppler velocimetry
2. Magnetic induction with a fixed magnetic field and a movable coil or vice versa
3. Taking the time derivative of any displacement signal to give the velocity component in the direction of the displacement

    B. Acceleration
1. Piezoelectric accelerator
2. Displacement of a mass on a spring
3. Taking the second time derivative of any displacement signal to give the acceleration component in the direction of the displacement

III. Radiation and sound intensity

    A. Light
1. Photoelectric-effect phototube
2. Photomultiplier tube
3. Semiconductor photodiodes
4. Phototransistors
5. Photoconductive cells
6. Photovoltaic cells

    B. Nuclear radiation
1. Geiger-Müller tube
2. Ionization chamber
3. Scintillation counter
4. Semiconductor radiation detectors
5. Photographic film

    C. Infrared radiation
1. Bolometers
2. Semiconductor infrared detection diodes
3. Thermopiles
4. Infrared image converters

    D. Sound and ultrasound
1. Piezoelectric crystals and other materials
2. Electromechanical microphones
3. Optical phonocardiographic sensors
4. Hot wire anemometer

IV. Force and tactile sense

    A. Force
1. Load cells
2. Displacement of materials with known elastic properties
3. Piezoelectric materials

    B. Tactile sense
1. Strain gauge arrays
2. Piezoresistive materials
3. Optical sensor arrays
4. Capacitive sensor arrays

Table 2.1 (continued)

V. Temperature

    A. Direct contact
        1. Thermal volume expansion thermometers (common mercury in glass thermometer)
        2. Metallic electrical resistance thermometers
        3. Thermistors (semiconductor electrical resistance thermometers)
        4. Thermocouples
        5. Semiconductor *pn* junction diodes
        6. Liquid crystals

    B. Thermal radiation (see III.C, infrared radiation)

VI. Hemodynamic variables

    A. Pressure
        1. Fluid column manometer
        2. Unbonded strain gauge sensor
        3. Capacitive membrane displacement sensor
        4. Semiconductor piezoresistive sensor
        5. Bourdon tube connected to a displacement sensor
        6. Fiber-optic reflectance photometer and reflecting diaphragm

    B. Flow
        1. Indicator techniques such as Fick and indicator dilution methods
        2. Thermal conductivity and convective cooling, as in hot wire anemometer
        3. Electromagnetic flow meter
        4. Ultrasonic pulse propagation time and Doppler frequency shift
        5. Pressure drop across a known resistance
        6. Plethysmography
        7. Nuclear magnetic resonance and magnetic resonance imaging.

VII. Mass

    A. Direct sensor
        1. Resonant frequency of a structure on which materials can be absorbed
        2. Mass spectrometer at the atomic level

    B. Indirect sensors
        (indirect measurements through sensors of other variables such as the force of an object in a gravitational field)

VIII. Electromagnetic variables

    A. Potential and current
        1. Biopotential electrodes
        2. Magnetometers

    B. Impedance
        1. Current-voltage relationships of a set of biopotential electrodes, some of which are driven with a known excitation current
        2. Reflectance of radio frequency electromagnetic radiation

    C. Magnetic fields
        1. Induction coils
        2. Hall effect devices
        3. SQUID magnetometers

Ultrasonic displacement sensors.   During childbirth, the obstetrician is interested in knowing the dilation (opening) of the uterine cervix to assess the progress of the birth process. The standard clinical method of measuring the extent of cervical dilatation before birth is examining the cervix by the obstetrician's fingers. Experienced clinicians can accurately estimate the opening of the cervix by what they feel, but this practice does not really represent an objective measurement. Researchers in reproductive medicine have developed various transducers to allow them to measure cervical dilatation objectively. One example is the ultrasonic displacement gauge (Zador et al. 1976). The velocity of ultrasound in soft tissue varies only a small amount from one type of tissue to another. It has been found experimentally to be 1.48 millimeter (mm) per microsecond (μs) at body temperature. Since the uterine cervix and the fetal head are primarily soft tissue, and the cervix is approximately circular as it is dilating around the fetal head, one can place small ultrasonic transducers at diametrically opposite sides of the cervix as illustrated in Figure 2.3. Here, the obstetrician has placed a small ultrasound piezoelectric transducer at the 3 o'clock and 9 o'clock positions on the cervix. Piezoelectric transducers are *reversible transducers*, in that when they are excited by an electrical signal, they can produce ultrasound; when excited by ultrasound, they produce an electrical signal.

In measuring cervical dilatation, one of the piezoelectric transducers is excited by a very short, moderate-voltage electrical pulse that causes the transducer to generate a burst of ultrasound. This burst propagates through the cervix and the fetal head and excites the transducer on the other side of the cervix, which generates a small electrical signal. The time duration between the generation of the ultrasonic burst and its reception at the second transducer is proportional to the separation of the transducers. This separation can then be determined from

$$d = ct \qquad (2.1)$$

where d = separation of the two transducers

  t = time for the ultrasound signal to propagate from one sensor
     to another

  c = velocity of propagation of ultrasound in soft tissue

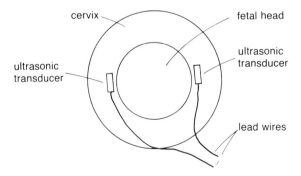

Figure 2.3   Diagram of the dilating uterine cervix, showing the placement of miniature ultrasonic transducers for measuring cervical dilatation.

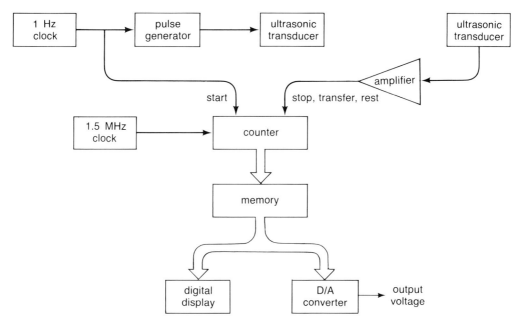

Figure 2.4 Block diagram of the ultrasonic cervimeter.

The electronic signal processor of this ultrasonic cervimeter essentially applies equation (2.1) to provide an output voltage proportional to the displacement which can be recorded on a chart recorder or displayed on an analog or digital meter.

Figure 2.4 illustrates this signal processor. A clock controls the entire process. Timing pulses are generated at a rate of one per second, and each pulse triggers the excitation pulse that generates the burst of ultrasound. The clock pulse also starts a counter consisting of a register connected to a second clock that generates a pulse every $0.68~\mu s$. The interval between pulses thus corresponds to the time the ultrasonic burst requires to propagate 1 mm through the tissue. Thus the number in the counter register corresponds to the distance that the ultrasonic burst has propagated from the transmitting transducer. When this burst reaches the receiving ultrasonic transducer, this sensor generates a small voltage that is amplified and stops the counter. The number in the counter register represents the distance that the ultrasonic burst has traveled from the transmitting transducer to the receiver. This number is transferred to a storage register and displayed on the analog and digital readouts of the instrument while the counter is reset to zero to await the transmission of the next ultrasonic burst.

Figure 2.5 is a typical record from an ultrasonic cervimeter monitoring a patient in labor. The advantage of such an instrument over the manual method is that once the transducers are applied to the patient, feeling the cervix is not necessary, so the patient experiences less inconvenience and discomfort. The risk of infection decreases as a result of decreasing internal examinations. The instrument also provides highly objective, nearly continuous data, compared to the subjective spot samples obtained by the manual method.

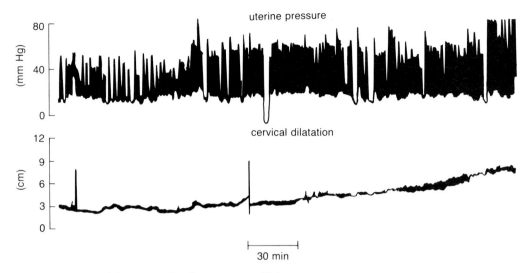

Figure 2.5   Example of a progress-of-labor curve as measured by the ultrasonic cervimeter.

Plethysmography

It is desirable to have patients move following surgery to prevent pooling of blood in the veins of the legs which can lead to clot formation. Such clots can break away and cause blockage of the pulmonary vessels. Such pulmonary emboli can be so severe as to cause sudden death; therefore, detecting their presence is important. A noninvasive procedure used for this purpose is plethysmography, measuring the change in volume of a limb when the venous outflow from that limb is occluded, and then the occlusion is removed. If venous clots are present, the blood requires more time to leave the limb than when all venous channels are open.

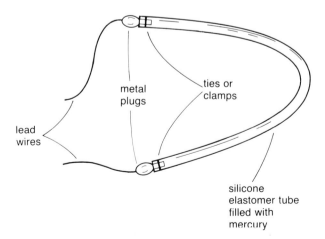

Figure 2.6   A Whitney elastic strain gauge.

One of the simplest ways to measure changes in the volume of a limb is through the use of mercury in silicone rubber strain gauge (Brakkee and Vendrik, 1966). The basic structure of this gauge as illustrated in Figure 2.6 consists of a thin wall, small diameter silicone rubber tube that has been filled with mercury. Metal plugs connected to lead wires are inserted into each end of the tube, so that they directly contact the mercury. The electrical resistance of the mercury column between the two metal plugs will be

$$R = \rho \frac{l}{A} \tag{2.2}$$

where ρ is the resistivity of mercury

l is the length of the column of mercury

A is the cross sectional area of the column of mercury.

The volume V of the mercury column is the product of A and l; thus, the resistance can be written as

$$R = \rho \frac{l^2}{V} \tag{2.3}$$

When the strain gauge is stretched to a new length l_1 the resistance R_1 becomes

$$R_1 = \frac{\rho l_1^2}{V} \tag{2.4}$$

where

$$l_1 = l + \Delta l$$

Thus, one can relate the increase in resistance of the strain gauge to its elongation Δl by

$$R_1 = \rho \frac{[(l^2 + 2l \Delta l + (\Delta l^2)]}{V} \tag{2.5}$$

$$\Delta R = R_1 - R = \rho \frac{2l \Delta l + (\Delta l)^2}{V} \tag{2.6}$$

Although this shows that change in resistance is nonlinearly related to the increase in length, it can be approximated as being linear for $\Delta l << 1$. Thus, by measuring the resistance one can determine the extent that the strain gauge has been stretched.

In venous occlusion plethysmography using mercury strain gauges the change in circumference rather than the actual volume change is measured. One or more strain gauges are wrapped around the leg as illustrated in Figure 2.7. A sphygmomanometer cuff is placed around the leg proximal (closer to the body center) to the strain gauge(s) as shown. The strain gauge is attached to an unbalanced Wheatstone bridge curcuit, with the output voltage from the bridge connected to a

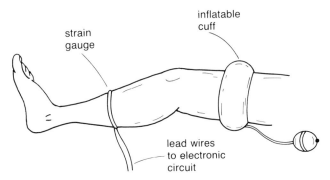

Figure 2.7   Application of a Whitney strain gauge and a sphygmomanometer cuff to the leg for venous occlusion plethysmography.

chart recorder, so that the resistance of the strain gauge and hence the circumference of the limb can be recorded as function of time. An initial base line voltage (resistance or circumference) is established on the recording, and then the cuff is pumped to a pressure of approximately 50 mmHg to occlude the venous return from the limb without seriously interfering with arterial blood flow. The limb thus can receive blood but cannot allow it to drain back off, so its volume and hence its circumference increase, as illustrated by the recording of Figure 2.8. Eventually, the venous pressure reaches 50 mmHg and venous blood can one again flow through the cuff. The leg volume saturates, and the output voltage becomes approximately constant over time. At this point, the cuff is released, and the blood stored in the leg flows out through the veins, causing the volume and hence the circumference to return to its initial value. The rate at which this occurs is determined by the rate at which the blood can flow out through the veins. If clots are present,

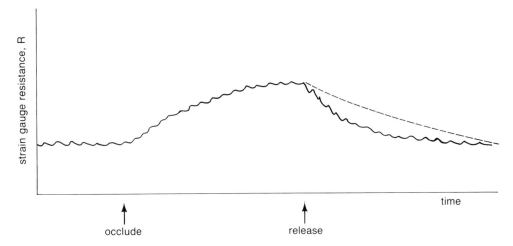

Figure 2.8   A venous occulsion plethysmogram from the arrangement illustrated in Figure 2.7. The solid curve indicates normal circulation. The dashed curve shows the response when venous clots are present.

this rate will be significantly lower than it would be in the absence of clots. Thus, by measuring the rate of return to the initial volume, a physician can determine whether venous clots are present in a patient.

As seen in Table 2.1, there are other types of sensors of geometric factors such as those described previously. The most familiar of these in medical instrumentation are the linear or rotary slide wire (variable resistance), wire strain gauge, foil strain gauge, mutual inductance coils, linear variable differential transformer, and variable capacitors. All of these transducers convert a geometric displacement into an electrical signal that can be related to the displacement as it was in the two preceeding examples.

Force sensor

Sensors of force are useful in several types of physiological measurements. These include electronic laboratory methods for measuring body weight, grasping force, isometric muscle contractions, and analyzing gait (Chapter 6). The usual method of measuring force is to convert the force to a small displacement and measure that displacement. The following paragraphs consider an electronic scale as an example of this type of measurement.

An electronic scale is basically a platform placed upon a load cell, as illustrated in Figure 2.9. The essential part of the load cell is an element that changes shape with the application of force. This change in shape, measured by a displacement transducer, relates to the applied force in a reproducible, preferably linear way. As an example, let us consider a simple cantilever as the load cell. Figure 2.10 shows such a structure, with the cantilever attached to the base of the scale at one end and the platform at the other; as a force is applied by placing a weight on the platform, the cantilever bends. Thus, the top surface of the cantilever becomes slightly longer, while its bottom surface is somewhat compressed. A semiconductor strain gauge (Dean 1962) can detect this small change in length of either the top or bottom or both surfaces. In this example, it is attached to the bottom surface.

The principle of operation of semiconductor strain gauge is somewhat similar to that of the mercury strain gauge described previously, except that the mercury gauge can undergo much greater displacements than can the semiconductor gauge. On the other hand, semiconductor strain gauges have much higher sensitivity; that is, their resistance changes approximately 40 times more than do mercury strain gauges for the same small change in length. The semiconductor strain

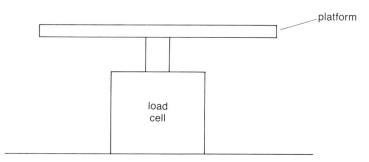

Figure 2.9   The basic structure of an electronic scale.

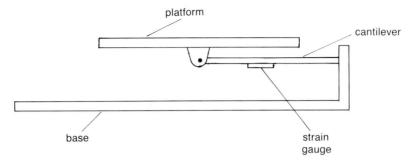

Figure 2.10   Structure of an electronic scale that uses a cantilever beam and strain gauge as the load cell.

gauges are also considerably smaller than mercury strain gauges and can be mass-produced by using integrated circuit technology.

The change in resistance for a semiconductor strain gauge is proportional to the *strain*, the change in length per unit length, that it undergoes, which in turn is proportional to the deflection of the cantilever beam. A lightweight, uniform cantilever beam with an applied force at one end will deflect according to the following equation (Trathen 1964):

$$\delta = \frac{L^3}{3\zeta} F \qquad (2.7)$$

where δ = deflection of free end of beam

$\quad L$ = beam length

$\quad \zeta$ = flexural rigidity of beam (a constant),

$\quad F$ = applied force at free end of beam or in other words the weight of the object on the platform.

The strain on the surface of the beam is proportional to this deflection. Thus, the electrical signal coming from the strain gauge can be made directly proportional to the weight on the platform. This signal can then be processed electronically and used, for example, to provide a digital readout of the weight. Electronic scales of this type can range from a consumer item for home use that has a resolution of 1 lb to a sensitive laboratory balance with a resolution of a fraction of a milligram.

Sensors of hemodynamic variables

Two of the most important and also most difficult variables to measure are blood pressure and flow. These quantities represent important variables of the cardiovascular system. Although today there are several direct, invasive methods of measuring them, effective and practical ways to measure them noninvasively have yet to be developed. The following examples illustrate two of the most popular sensors of these variables.

Blood pressure.   The direct measurement of blood pressure is an important method of continuously monitoring this variable in intensive care medicine. The method involves hydrostatically coupling an external pressure transducer to a major artery by passing one end of a *catheter*, a small open flexible tube, filled with physiological saline solution through the skin and into the lumen of an artery. The other end of the catheter is connected to a pressure sensor. The fluid in the catheter then transmits the pressure from the artery to the pressure transducer, where it is measured.

Figure 2.11 shows a typical pressure transducer. The top part, known as the *dome*, is a closed chamber that is directly connected to the catheter. One wall of the chamber consists of a thin diaphragm that can be deflected by the force resulting from the pressure difference between the fluid in the chamber and atmospheric pressure on the outside. For a circular diaphragm fixed along its circumference, the maximum deflection of the center can be approximated for small deflections (Cobbold 1974):

$$d = \frac{3(1 - \mu^2)R^4(\Delta P)}{16Et^3} \tag{2.8}$$

where d = displacement of diaphragm center
μ = Poisson's ratio
R = diaphragm radius
t = diaphragm thickness
E = Young's modulus for the diaphragm
ΔP = pressure difference across diaphragm

Strain gauge displacement sensors measure this diaphragm deflection. The center of the diaphragm is connected to four unbonded wire strain gauges located in the body of the transducer that measure the displacement of the diaphragm. The strain gauges are attached such that two are lengthened when pressure increases, and the other two have their tension and thus length reduced. When these four

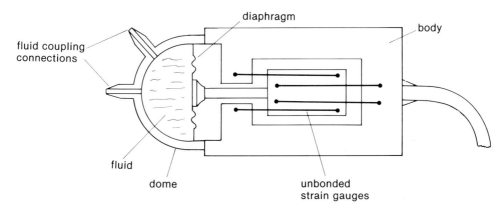

Figure 2.11   Structure of a pressure transducer using four unbonded strain gauges in a bridge configuration.

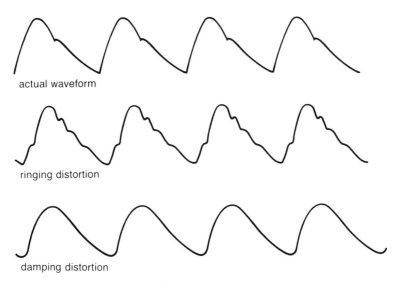

actual waveform

ringing distortion

damping distortion

Figure 2.12   Resonances in the pressure transducer–catheter system can cause ringing distortion in an arterial pressure waveform. Trapped air bubbles in the catheter or a partial obstruction can cause dumping.

strain gauges are connected as a Wheatstone bridge, the output voltage is proportional to the displacement of the diaphragm, and hence the pressure in the chamber. Because the chamber is coupled through the catheter to the artery, the Wheatstone bridge output voltage is indeed proportional to arterial pressure (Geddes 1970).

We have described this device in terms of hydrostatic pressures. The arterial blood pressure, however, is a time-varying pressure that follows a complex pattern between systolic and diastolic pressure over the course of time between two heartbeats. Accurate reproduction of this waveform at the pressure transducer entails several considerations. The fluid in the catheter and in the pressure transducer dome has a mass associated with it. The catheter, if it is flexible, and the dome and diaphragm have an associated compliance. Thus the fluid column and pressure transducer behave very much as a mass on a spring. The system has a resonant frequency, which is often sufficiently low to cause some distortion of the arterial blood pressure waveform. The system can also generate artifact in responding to sharp changes in pressure. For example, a step function in pressure often produces ringing at the resonant frequency of the system, further distorting the waveform. It is, therefore, important when using such a system to consider not only static behavior of the transducer, but also the dynamic behavior of the transducer-catheter system. Figure 2.12 illustrates the difference in waveform that can occur just as a result of a difference in the fluid coupling system used for the measurement.

A pressure sensor that does not require the fluid coupling components eliminates problems associated with the catheter and pressure transducer dome by miniaturizing the pressure sensor so that it can be located in the artery at the site of the pressure measurement. Such a sensor, needless to say, must be much smaller than the one illustrated in Figure 2.11. This requires that the diaphragm also is much

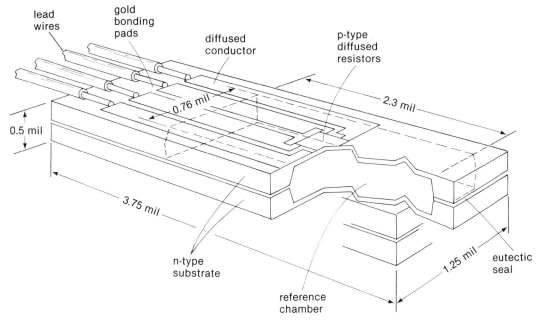

Figure 2.13   A miniature pressure transducer developed by
W. H. Ko and colleagues that was fabricated by using
integrated circuit technology (reproduced from Ko [1979] with
permission).

smaller; therefore, if unbonded wire strain gauges are used to measure the diaphragm deflection, the sensitivity is considerably lower than it would be for the external type of pressure sensor. Equation (2.8) illustrates this point, since the displacement is directly proportional to the fourth power of the diaphragm radius.
Thus, a miniature pressure transducer for inter-arterial application must employ
displacement sensors with the highest possible sensitivity. Such a sensor, as pointed
out earlier, is the semiconductor strain gauge. Figure 2.13 illustrates a minature intravascular pressure sensor developed by Ko and colleagues (1979) that uses a silicon diaphragm with silicon strain gauges formed in it using microelectronic techniques. The overall sensor is 1.25 by 0.5 by 3.75 mm and thus occupies a very small
volume. Since the diaphragm is only a fraction of this size, its deflection will be
very small, and this sensor can be considered to be noncompliant. It will therefore
have a very high resonant frequency that should be well outside the frequency
range of normal physiolocial signals. Thus sensors such as this will provide effica-
cious signals from various biological sources. (Neuman 1982; 1984) has demonstrated applications of this sensor in the uterus and lower uninary tract.

Blood Flow.   The measurement of blood flow has had great interest for
biomedical engineers. A sensor cannot have direct contact with the blood since this
could lead to the formation of clots and emboli. Although some sensors have been
placed on catheters in the bloodstream, most flow transducers such as are used for
measuring a fluid flowing through a pipe are not appropriate here.

   One of the most common methods of measuring blood flow is the electromagnetic flow meter, illustrated in its simplest form in Figure 2.14. A cuff around

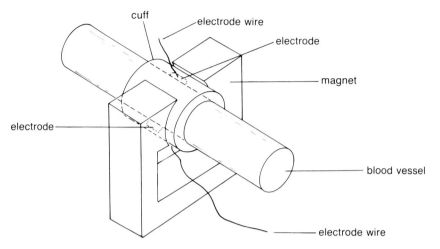

Figure 2.14   Schematic illustration of an electromagnetic
flow probe.

the blood vessel being measured has an associated magnetic field that passes
through the blood vessel normal to its axis. This magnetic field can be produced by
a permanent magnet or an electromagnet, this latter method being more desirable
because it can generate time-varying fields. The blood has many components,
some of which are charged particles such as inorganic ions and proteins. These
charged particles flowing through the magnetic field are deflected by the force generated in a direction normal to both the magnetic field and the blood flow directions. This force is given by the vector equation:

$$\bar{F} = q\bar{V} \times \bar{B} \tag{2.9}$$

where $\bar{F}$ = vector force
  q = electrical charge on particle
  $\bar{V}$ = vector velocity of particle
  $\bar{B}$ = vector magnetic field through vessel

Because positive charges are deflected toward one side of the vessel and negative
charges toward the other, an electric field is set up across the vessel in the direction
of the deflecting force. This field results in a potential difference across the vessel;
when the magnetic field is constant, this potential difference is proportional to the
velocity of the blood flowing through the transducer. Placing two small electrodes
on the surface of the blood vessel as illustrated in Figure 2.14 allows one to measure this potential difference and to determine the velocity of the blood.

The transducer must be designed to fit snugly around the blood vessel, with
the electrodes in good contact with it. This arrangement also has the effect of con-
straining the blood vessel to have a fixed diameter, and hence, a fixed cross-
sectional area, since it cannot expand with increasing blood pressure as it would if
the cuff were not present. Thus, the placement of the flow transducer establishes
the cross section of the vessel, and the volume flow is proportional to the blood ve-

locity. Thus the voltage induced at the electromagnetic flow probe electrodes will be proportional to flow.

This method of measuring blood flow is primarily used in the research laboratory. A frequent application of it is in measuring stroke volume and cardiac output. A flow transducer around the aorta at the point where it exits from the heart allows all blood flowing out of the heart, except that entering the coronary arteries, to pass through the transducer and be measured. The flow signal can be electronically integrated over a single heartbeat to measure the stroke volume, or over a longer period to measure cardiac output.

Like pressure transducers, electromagnetic flow measurements have technical difficulties. In addition to artifact produced by the placement of the flow transducer around the blood vessel, its presence, which to some extent constricts the vessel, may alter the flow. When the flow through relatively small arteries is measured, the transducer is often much larger and more massive than the segment of vessel it is measuring. Thus, it can easily shift in position and begin to crimp the vessel, thereby reducing its cross section and the blood flow.

The description of the basic principle of the electromagnetic blood flow transducer applies to a transducer with a constant magnetic field. Thus, a steady voltage appears between the electrodes when the blood velocity is constant. In addition to this flow-induced voltage, often an artifact voltage is associated with the electrodes themselves, and it may be sizable with respect to the flow-induced voltage. It is also a dc voltage; thus significant errors can occur when dc magnetic fields are used. For that reason, many electromagnetic flow meters today utilize alternating current (ac) magnetic fields. In this way, the flow-induced voltage is an ac voltage at the same frequency as the applied magnetic field, and the electrode artifact is a dc voltage that is easily removed in processing the signal.

The other types of blood flow sensors in use today are listed in Table 2.1. These include ultrasonic transit time and Doppler shift flow meters and thermal flow probes. Noncontinuous measurements of blood flow can be performed by various indicator dilution methods, and these are frequently employed clinically. Recent ultrasonic and nuclear magnetic resonance techniques have demonstrated that obtaining flow information noninvasively is possible, but much more research and development are needed in this area (Webster 1978).

Thermal Measurements

A great variety of measurements related to the thermal energy of a biological system are possible. These include temperature, heat flux, thermal conductivity, and thermal radiation. Of these, temperature is the most commonly measured. It is a clinically important physiological variable and one of the four basic vital signs used in the clinical assessment of patients.

The sensor is the most important component of a temperature measurement system. In actuality a temperature measurement instrument indicates the temperature of the sensor. Thus the problem in biomedical measurements of temperature is maintaining the temperature sensor at the physiological temperature to be measured. The easiest way to do this is to keep the temperature sensor in direct contact with the structure whose temperature is being measured. This in itself is not sufficient, however, since the temperature sensor may alter the temperature of the tissue in contact with it. For example, if the sensor is initially at a lower temperature than the tissue being measured, when it is brought into contact with that tissue, heat flows from the tissue to the temperature sensor. If this heat cannot be replaced by thermal energy conducted into the tissue or metabolically generated thermal energy in the tissue, the act of placing the temperature sensor into contact with the tissue cools it and thus gives an incorrect temperature reading. For this reason the effective thermal mass of the temperature sensor should always be much lower than that of the tissue it is measuring. Furthermore, it is important that the thermal resistance between the actual temperature sensor and the tissue being measured be as low as possible.

Common sensors of temperature used in biomedical instrumentation include: (1) the thermistor, (2) metallic wire resistance temperature sensors, (3) thermocouples, (4) semiconductor *pn* junctions, and (5) temperature-sensitive materials, such as liquid crystals, that change their physical properties. Of these, the thermistor is the most common temperature sensor in biomedical instrumentation. It consists of semiconducting metal oxides sintered into a variety of physical sizes and shapes. These range from very small bead thermistors that are spherical and have diameters as small as 0.1 mm to large flat disks having diameters of several centimeters. Electrodes and lead wires provide electrical contact to the thermistor material, and the electrical resistance of the thermistor is measured through these contacts. Semiconductor materials have electrical resistances that decrease as their temperature increases. The thermistor materials were developed to maximize the change in resistance with temperature over the temperature range of interest while maintaining a high degree of electrical stability to avoid resistance changes from

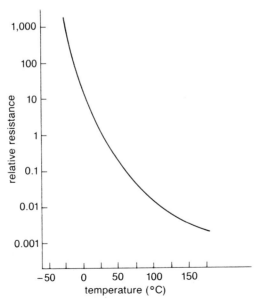

Figure 2.15   Typical resistance versus temperature curve for a thermistor.

other sources or simply aging of the material itself. Achieving such characteristics is not simple, and hence the actual formulations of the various thermistor materials used by different manufacturers as well as the process used to stabilize their electrical characteristics are closely held secrets.

A typical curve based on resistance as a function of temperature for a thermistor is shown in Figure 2.15. Note the negative temperature coefficient of resistance and the nonlinear relationship between resistance and temperature. This relationship can be approximated by

$$R = R_0 e^{\beta \left(\frac{1}{T} - \frac{1}{T_0} \right)} \tag{2.10}$$

where R = resistance at temperature T

β = a constant

R_0 = resistance measured for the thermistor at the reference temperature T_0.

Typical thermistors have negative temperature coefficients of resistance of approximately 5 percent per degree Celsius (°C) at room temperature.

A clinical electronic thermometer is a typical thermistor-based temperature measurement instrument. Figure 2.16 shows the basic block diagram of such an instrument. The sensor in this instrument consists of a probe that contains a thermistor. The design of this probe is an important factor in the overall instrument performance. The mass of the probe and thermistor must be small to give a rapid response time, yet the probe must be sturdy to withstand repeated uses. Thus an engineering compromise is necessary since these two requirements usually oppose one another. Furthermore, if the instrument is used on a number of different subjects, cleaning and sterilizing the probe between each use is not practical. Thus a disposable, sterile protective film covers the probe and is changed from one patient to the next. This cover also must have a low thermal mass as well as a high thermal conductivity to prevent severely reducing the response time of the instrument. It also must be sturdy so that it can be placed on the probe without rupturing, which would destroy its protective function.

The purpose of the signal-processing electronics in this instrument is to convert the electrical resistance of the thermistor to a voltage related to its temperature

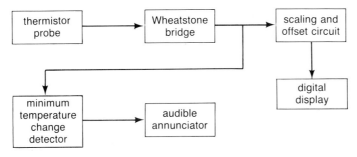

Figure 2.16 Block diagram of an electronic thermometer.

and to provide this voltage to a readout device, usually a digital display that indicates temperature. An unbalanced Wheatstone bridge circuit in which the thermistor constitutes one arm of the bridge achieves this purpose. If the bridge is designed appropriately, the nonlinearity in the Wheatstone bridge voltage output as a function of resistance can compensate for the nonlinearity of the thermistor over a temperature range of up to 40 °C so that the output voltage of the bridge has a linear relation to temperature. The remainder of the electronic circuit has to scale this signal so that the output device will show the correct number that corresponds to the measured temperature.

Another function, contained in some electronic thermometers, is a circuit to determine when the temperature sensor reaches equilibrium so that the indicated temperature can be read. Such a circuit can look at the temperature every second and compare the latest reading with several previous ones. If the differences are less than 0.1 °C, the temperature is considered to be stable. The operator is advised that the temperature can be read, usually by a short tone.

Other temperature instrumentation described at the beginning of this section is based upon this type of instrument in that measurements of thermal conductivity, heat flux, and radiation all involve making temperature measurements. This signal is processed to give the quantity to be measured based upon the sensor design.

Electromagnetic Measurements: Biopotential Electrodes

Many different electrical variables have been measured from biological organisms. These include electrical potentials, electrical current, electrical resistance and impedance, and magnetic fields. Of these the measurement of biopotentials and biological impedances is most common. Clinical medicine routinely uses devices based upon these measurements. The electrocardiogram is an example of a biopotential that is frequently measured. It results from electrical fields and currents in the body generated by the depolarization and contraction of cardiac muscle cells. By looking at an electrocardiogram, a physician can determine much information about the status and rhythm of the heart.

The cardioscope.   An example of an instrument for displaying the electrocardiogram is the cardioscope, illustrated in the block diagram of Figure 2.17. In this case electrodes perform the sensor function. These electrodes make electrical contact with the body. In the body, electric current is carried by means of ions, whereas in metal electrodes and electronic circuitry electrons carry the current.

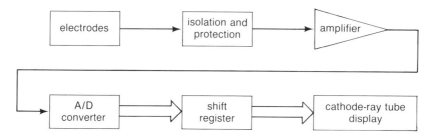

Figure 2.17   Block diagram of a cardioscope.

Thus the electrode must convert an ionic current to an electronic current. To do this an oxidation-reduction reaction must occur at the electrode-body interface. In this reaction charge is transferred between the electrode and the body, either by the oxidation of atoms of the electrode material

$$M \rightleftharpoons M^{n+} + n(e^-) \tag{2.11}$$

where M = a metal atom
n = an integer
(e^-) = an electron

or by oxidation or reduction of ions in the body that contact the electrode surface:

$$A^{n-} \rightleftharpoons A + n(e^-) \tag{2.12}$$

where A^{n-} = an ion in the electrolytic solution

When such reactions occur, the concentration of reactants and products will be different at the electrode-body interface than they are deeper in the body. This will result in charge build-up at the interface as schematically illustrated in Figure 2.18. This layer of charged species plays a strong role in the electrode's electrical characteristics. Its electrical behavior can be modeled as a parallel resistance-capacitance circuit that can contribute a significant series impedance at low frequencies. This layer is also responsible for much of the electrical noise- and motion-induced artifact seen from the electrode. This latter is a result of electrode movement with respect to the charge layer that produces voltage in much the same way as would moving the plates of a charged capacitor. This motion artifact presents many problems when one desires to measure biopotentials from active subjects, for example, during exercise tolerance testing.

Many different types of biopotential electrodes are available today. Figure 2.19 shows the structure of a disposable biopotential electrode designed for use

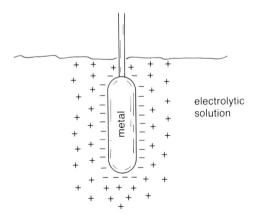

Figure 2.18   Illustration of a metal electrode immersed in an electrolytic solution showing the build-up of charge at the electrode-electrolyte interface.

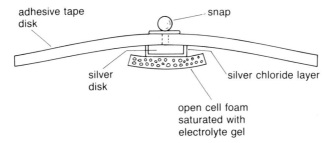

Figure 2.19   Cross-sectional view of the structure of a
disposable bipotential electrode used for cardiac monitoring.

with a cardiac monitor or a cardioscope. The electrode itself is a silver disk. Frequently this is a silver-plated garment snap rather than a solid piece of silver for
economic considerations. An open-celled sponge covering the disk is saturated
with a water-based gel containing inorganic ions to establish contact between the
electrode and the skin. This sponge separates the metallic electrode from the skin
and keeps the relative motion between the electrolyte gel and the electrode small to
minimize motion artifact. Finally, the electrode includes a ring of an adhesive tape
material to hold it in place on the skin. A lead wire with a female garment snap
connector at its end connects the electrode to the electronic signal processor and
display portions of the instrument. This type of electrode is inexpensive and can be
discarded after a single use.

The remainder of the cardioscope is illustrated in the block diagram of Figure 2.17. The amplitude of the electrocardiogram at the electrodes is approximately 1 to 2 millivolts (mV) and depends upon the position of the electrodes between which it is measured. This signal is amplified by the cardioscope. Since
higher voltages may be generated in the patient from defibrillation or occasionally
even static electricity, an isolation and protection circuit precedes the amplifier to
block these transient voltages from causing amplifier damage. In addition electrical leakage currents from the cardioscope electronics must be prevented from
passing through the patient to avoid the hazards of microshock. The isolation and
protection circuit carries out this function, as well.

Although the output from the amplifier could directly drive a cathode-ray
tube (CRT) oscilloscope to display the electrocardiogram waveform, most modern
cardioscopes digitize the output and use it to fill a first in–first out shift register.
This register in turn is scanned at a more rapid rate to provide a continuous display
on the CRT screen. This has the advantage over the conventional oscilloscope of
providing a display that does not fade and moves across the screen in the same way
it would if it were recorded on the strip chart recorder of an ordinary electrocardiograph. With this type of cardioscope it is also possible to stop the electrocardiogram at any point by stopping input to the shift register. This capability allows a
more detailed analysis of the pattern on the screen.

Other types of biopotential instruments used in clinical medicine include the
electromyograph, which measures electrical activity associated with muscle contraction; the *electroencephalograph,* which measures the electrical activity of the

brain from surface electrodes placed on the head; and the *electronystagmograph,* which electrically measures nystagmus, an involuntary rapid movement of the eye (Geddes 1972).

Electrical Impedance Measurements.   As a second example of the uses of biopotential electrodes, let us consider impedance measurements in biological tissue. Electrical impedance measurements have become important for research and clinical measurement in animal and human subjects. In these measurements the electrical impedance is measured between two or four electrodes placed on a particular part of the body. This impedance can be related to geometric changes such as result from physical movement of the electrodes or from changes in the electrical properties of the tissue between the electrodes. This latter effect is of most interest in clinical applications.

One of the most common applications of electrical impedance instrumentation in medicine is in infant apnea monitors. These devices are used to monitor continuously the respiratory efforts of infants by detecting changes in the electrical impedance across their chest. The instrument also determines when apnea, the cessation of breathing, occurs. If apnea lasts for more than a predetermined amount of time, the instrument sounds an alarm. Biopotential electrodes are the sensor elements in electrical impedance instrumentation systems. The electrical impedance between a pair of electrodes placed on opposite lateral sides of the chest is determined by the skin, the muscles of the chest wall, the lungs, the heart, and the blood in all of these tissues. Changes in electrical impedance seen between the chest electrodes are determined by changes in conductivity and admittance of the various structures, since geometrical variations between the electrodes are relatively small. The most significant changes are in the lungs and heart, with a smaller change also occurring in the vascular compartments of all the tissues.

Let us consider the lungs first. From the standpoint of electrical impedance, the lungs can be considered to have two components: tissue and air. At maximum expiration the ratio of tissue to air is highest; since tissue has a much lower impedance than air (which is a good insulator), one would expect that the impedance across the lungs would be lowest at maximum expiration. At maximum inspiration the tissue to air ratio in the lungs has its lowest value, and hence the lungs should have their highest electrical impedance. Thus by measuring the electrical impedance variation of the lungs, one can determine whether pulmonary ventilation is taking place and apnea is absent. If it were possible to put electrodes directly onto lungs that were electrically isolated from adjacent tissues, one would see a relatively large change in electrical impedance with ventilation. Because we are constrained to place the electrodes onto the surface of the chest, the change in impedance actually observed is considerably less as a result of the electrical shunting effects of the other tissues. In actual practice the impedance variations seen with breathing are no greater than 0.5 percent of the baseline impedance value. Unfortunately impedance variations due to movement in the tissues that provide the shunt pathways can be greater than this, thereby causing artifact that can greatly impair the meaurement of respiration and apnea. Furthermore, impedance variations at the interface between the electrodes and the body can also be larger than the impedance variations with respiration during motion, and this too can severely compromise the usefulness of impedance instrumentation.

The other physiological sources of electrical impedance variation in the chest are the heart and blood. Variations in blood volume in the heart during the cardiac cycle and to a lesser extent blood volume in the chest vasculature cause changes in the electrical impedance. In this case the blood has a lower impedance than the other tissues of the chest, and so the impedance across the chest decreases during diastole and increases during systole. This change in impedance is usually less than that associated with respiration, and although these changes can be quantitatively measured to estimate cardiac output noninvasively (Nyboer 1970), the effects of motion and other sources of artifact strongly influence the results.

Figure 2.20 is a block diagram of an electrical impedance type of apnea monitor. The electronic circuit supplies a constant-current amplitude 20- to 100-

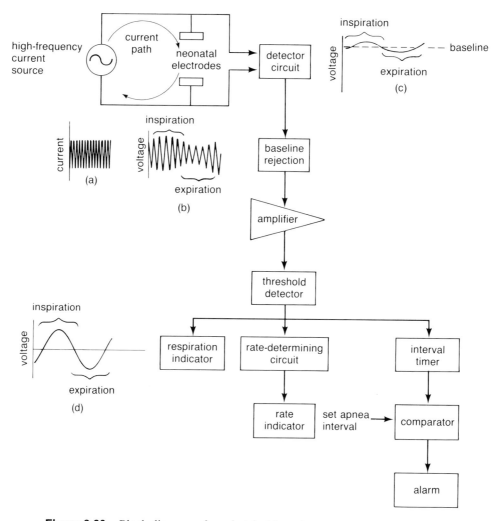

Figure 2.20   Block diagram of an electrical impedance type of infant apnea monitor (from M. R. Neuman, R. Huch, and A. Huch. 1984. The neonatal oxycardiogram, *CRC Crit. Rev. in Biomed Eng* 11:77).

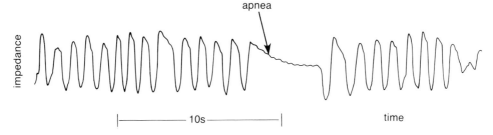

Figure 2.21 Typical respirogram signal from an electrical impedence apnea monitor as illustrated in Figure 2.20.

Kilohertz (kHz) sinusoidal signal to the electrodes so that a voltage proportional to the transthoracic impedance appears across them. Exciting the electrodes at a frequency of greater than 20 kHz minimizes the impedance associated with the interface between the electrodes and the body. This can then minimize some of the motion artifact associated with this interfacial impedance, but it will not eliminate it. Because the impedance variations associated with respiration are so small, it is especially important that the constant-current alternating current (ac) source be very stable. Variations in its amplitude of 0.1 to 0.5 percent may appear similar to variations in transthoracic impedance due to respiration and may therefore lead to measurement errors.

The remainder of the signal processing circuitry detects the amplitude variations in the voltage between the electrodes and converts it to a voltage proportional to the magnitude of the transthoracic impedance signal. This is amplified and passed through a circuit to recognize respiration patterns (Neuman 1984). When there are no breaths, a timer is started; once this timer reaches a preset interval corresponding to the duration of apnea to be detected, an alarm sounds. There may also be a respiration rate meter circuit that displays the breathing rate of the subject. Some apnea monitors also display the breathing waveform on a CRT screen. They may include a cardiac monitor as well, using the same electrodes as sensors for both signals.

A typical infant respiration pattern as measured by electrical impedance is shown in Figure 2.21, which indicates a short apnea. Note that during the apnea the weaker impedance variations due to cardiovascular sources are visible. This example illustrates that infant respiration patterns can be quite complex and that signal processing to determine respiration rate and apnea accurately is not a simple problem. For this reason presently available infant apnea monitors leave much to be desired in terms of sensitivity and specificity in detecting and alarming on true apnea episodes.

Chemical Sensors

Because living cells are essentially chemical systems, the chemistry of complete organisms is important not only in understanding their operation but also as a means of monitoring when things go wrong. Two general types of chemical sensors interest biomedical engineers: devices that determine the activity or concentration of substances in aqueous solutions and those that determine the concentration of gaseous elements and compounds. These transducers convert the chemical signal into an electrical one that can be processed by a biomedical instrumentation system. Table 2.2 outlines many chemical sensors of physiologically significant variables. The following sections present some examples of chemical sensors that are of interest to biomedical engineers and illustrate their applications.

Amperometric sensors

The amperometric chemical sensing system employs an electrochemical cell in which the substance to be determined undergoes a chemical oxidation-reduction reaction that either consumes or liberates electrons. The reaction takes place at one of the electrodes of the cell, and so the number of electrons involved determines the electrical current at that electrode. This current is in turn porportional to the availability of the chemical substances being sensed, and so the current can be used as a method of measuring the concentration of that substance.

As an example, let us consider the polarographic determination of the partial pressure of oxygen. Figure 2.22 illustrates the basic electrochemical cell, which consists of a noble metal cathode such as gold and a silver anode. These are placed in an aqueous electrolytic solution containing the chloride ion such as physiological saline (0.9 percent sodium chloride in water, a concentration equivalent to the extracellular fluid in the body). Oxygen is also dissolved in this electrolyte. Biasing this electrochemical cell with the voltage source shown produces reactions at the cathode and anode when the voltage is sufficiently high to provide enough energy to drive them. Oxygen can be reduced at the cathode according to the following chemcial reaction:

$$O_2 + 2H_2O + 4(e^-) \rightleftharpoons 4OH^- \tag{2.13}$$

In this reaction, which is a simplification of an actual several-step reaction, oxygen is reduced to hydroxyl ions, and electrons are taken from the cathode. This reaction requires approximately 0.4 volts (V) of bias voltage and consumes oxygen, water, and electrons. Since the latter two components are in good supply, oxygen is the rate-limiting species in the reaction, and the reaction rate should be proportional to oxygen availability.

At the anode, silver from the electrode is oxidized to the silver ion, and electrons are liberated to the anode. The silver ions immediately combine with chloride ions in solution to form the low-solubility compound silver chloride, which precipitates on the electrode surface. This reaction requires approximately 0.22 V of bias voltage:

$$Ag \rightleftharpoons Ag^+ + (e^-)$$
$$\qquad \quad \llcorner\!\!\longrightarrow + Cl^- \rightarrow AgCl\!\downarrow \tag{2.14}$$

Thus the total cell requires a minimum of 0.62 V of bias voltage; once this minimum valve is exceeded, electrons from reaction (2.12) are supplied to the an-

Table 2.2   Sensors of chemical biomedical variables

I. Amperometric sensors
   A. Oxygen cathode
   B. Clark oxygen electrode
   C. Polarograph
   D. Potentiostat

II. Potentiometric sensors
   A. Membrane electrodes
   B. Glass pH electrode
   C. Metal–metal oxide pH electrodes
   D. Ion-sensitive field-effect transistors
   E. Other Nernstian electrodes such as coated-wire electrodes
   F. Fuel cell sensors

III. Conductimetric sensors
   A. Direct contact conductance cell, two- or four-electrode system
   B. High-frequency noncontacting (inductive or capacitive) cell

IV. Biochemical and biological sensors
   A. Catalysis electrodes that catalyze reactions involving reactants or products that can be measured by other methods listed in this outline
   B. Enzyme electrodes that behave as the catalysis electrodes but are more specific with regard to a reactant (substrate)
   C. Electrodes with living tissue or organisms (for example, bacteria) that convert the substance to be measured to a form that can be measured by other methods listed in this outline

V. Colorimetric and other optical sensors
   A. Transmission and reflection oximetry
   B. Fiber-optic sensors with indicator dye at one end and a photometer at the other
   C. Fluorescence sensors
   D. Transmission and reflectance spectroscopy
   E. Emission spectroscopy
   F. Infrared absorption photometry and spectroscopy

VI. Other sensors and laboratory instruments
   A. Mass spectrometry
   B. Gas chromatography
   C. Nuclear magnetic resonance
   D. Immunologic assays with various indicator tags

ode and passed through the circuit to the cathode, where they are utilized in reaction (2.11). The ammeter in the circuit detects this electron current, which is proportional to the amount of oxygen being reduced at the cathode. This, in turn, is proportional to the partial pressure of oxygen in the solution. Thus the relative current through the cell can be used as a measure of oxygen tension.

Figure 2.22 shows the electrical characteristics of the cell. Note that as the voltage is increased, the current increases nonlinearly until the minimum bias voltage for the chemical reactions of 0.62 V is reached, and then we have a current plateau even though the voltage is increasing. This continues until voltages of approximately 1.1 V are reached, when additional chemical reactions involved in the breakdown of water can occur, causing a substantial increase in current. The current in the plateau region of this characteristic is proportional to the availability of oxygen and, hence, the partial pressure of oxygen. The plateau current increases as the oxygen partial pressure increases, as seen in Figure 2.23.

This type of oxygen sensor is known as a *polarographic oxygen sensor,* and the current-voltage curve shown in Figure 2.23 is known as a *polarogram*. This electrochemical cell is the basis of the Clark (1956) oxygen sensor illustrated in Figure 2.24. The Clark sensor is a miniature polarographic cell with an oxygen-permeable membrane bounding one surface. Oxygen diffuses through the membrane into the electrolyte, where it can be sensed. The membrane serves as a filter allowing oxygen and similar gases to pass through it while blocking large molecules, such as proteins, that could contaminate the electrodes. Thus this kind of cell can determine the oxygen partial pressure of whatever is located outside the membrane, gaseous or liquid. The Clark electrode is used for oxygen partial pressure measurement in instrumentation in the clinical chemistry laboratory and as instrumentation for intensive care patient monitoring. In the former application, it is part of an instrument known as a *blood gas analyzer* that determines the partial pressure of oxygen and carbon dioxide and the acid-base balance of a blood sample, usually an arterial blood sample since this blood has just returned from the lungs and indicates how well the lungs oxygenate the blood. The blood gas analyzer determines the partial pressure of oxygen in the blood by using a Clark electrode with a small chamber to hold the blood sample on the outside of the oxygen-permeable mem-

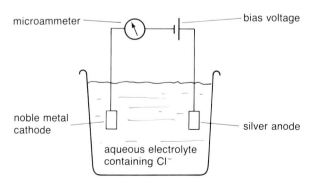

Figure 2.22   Schematic illustration of a polarographic electrochemical cell.

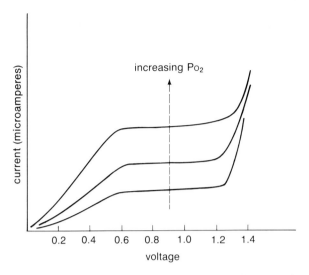

Figure 2.23 Typical polarogram from a cell such as is illustrated in Figure 2.22 for different oxygen partial pressures (Po_2) in the electrolytic solution.

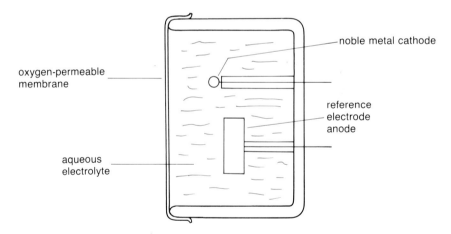

Figure 2.24 Schematic illustration of a Clark oxygen sensor.

brane (see Figure 2.25). Initially when the blood sample enters the chamber, the oxygen partial pressure in the Clark electrode and that in the blood are different. As a result, oxygen diffuses through the membrane from the high-tension side to the low-tension side. This process continues until both sides of the membrane are at the same oxygen partial pressure.

In a practical Clark electrode for use in the blood gas analyzer, the amount of electrolyte in the electrochemical cell is kept very small by having just a thin layer of it between the membrane and the anode and cathode. The solubility of oxygen

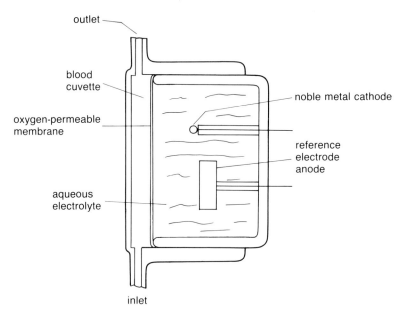

Figure 2.25   Illustration of a Clark oxygen sensor for measuring the oxygen partial pressure in a blood sample.

in the electrolyte is very small, so that only a very little oxygen need cross the membrane to change the partial pressure of oxygen in the electrolyte significantly. In contrast, the blood volume in this sensor, although small, is much greater than the electrolyte volume. Furthermore, the effective solubility of oxygen in the blood is much greater than that in the electrolyte by virtue of the hemoglobin present. Thus, bringing the oxygen tension on both sides of the membrane into equilibrium is not likely to change the partial pressure of oxygen in the blood by any significant amount even though the partial pressure of oxygen in the electrolyte can change by several tens of millimeters of mercury.

Laboratory blood gas analyzers also contain sensors for pH and the partial pressure of carbon dioxide in contact with the same blood sample. In addition, they have the capability of automatically placing a calibration standard in the sensing chamber, so that all of the sensors are periodically calibrated. The entire instrument is under microprocessor control, which not only carries out the automatic calibrations and sample measurements, but also calculates derived quantities such as base excess or deficit and hemoglobin oxygen saturation from the blood gas analysis. Some analyzers are even directly connected to a centralized computing system to return the results of the analysis to the patient's physician quickly and to store it on the patient's medical chart.

The use of the blood gas analyzer has contributed much to patient management during critical care situations, but this instrument also has limitations. Because the measurements are made on a sample of blood, they are indicative of the condition of the patient at the time the blood was drawn only, and to see changes additional samples are necessary. There is also a delay from the time the blood sample is drawn to the time the results of the measurement are returned to the physician. The blood sample must be transported from the patient and introduced into the machine, and this procedure can also lead to delays.

These limitations have been eliminated by continuous blood gas measurement techniques. These involve either utilizing an oxygen sensor that is sufficiently small to be placed within a vessel or using a technique of measuring the oxygen tension in the blood transcutaneously. This latter technique involves the use of a Clark electrode that is placed against the skin rather than in contact with a blood sample; such a system is illustrated in Figure 2.26. The Clark electrode consists of a very small cathode that is usually a disk of platinum 15 micrometers (μm) in diameter. This is surrounded by a cylindrical silver anode, 8 mm is diameter, that is separated from the cathode by a glass insulator. Both electrodes are coplanar and covered with a thin layer of a chloride ion containing electrolytic solution that may be as thin as 25 μm. This electrolytic solution is maintained in place by an oxygen-permeable membrane that is stretched over the sensor as illustrated in Figure 2.26.

The sensor is placed into direct contact with the skin so that the oxygen-permeable membrane and the skin have no air gap between them. Capillary loops that are approximately one mm beneath the surface perfuse the skin under the sensor. We can think of the blood in these capillaries as being similar to the blood in the sample chamber of the sensor in Figure 2.25. Then if we consider the skin, which is permeable to oxygen, as a part of the oxygen-permeable membrane on the Clark electrode, it should be possible to determine the oxygen tension in the capil-

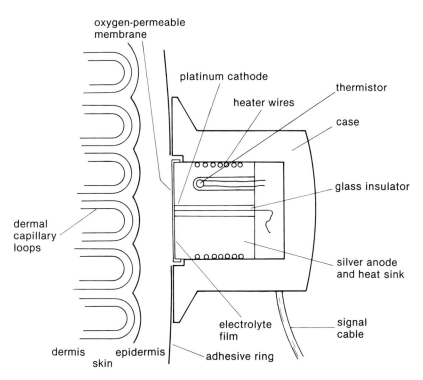

Figure 2.26 Cross-sectional view of a transcutaneous oxygen tension sensor.

lary blood once the capillary blood and the electrolyte in the Clark electrode reach equilibrium.

The measurement, however, is somewhat more complicated than the preceding description suggests. Even though it is possible to consider the skin as an oxygen-permeable membrane, its histology varies from one point to another, and so we only roughly know the geometry of this membrane. A second problem is that a portion of this layer of skin between the capillary loops and the oxygen sensor contains living, metabolizing cells that consume oxygen and give off carbon dioxide. Thus, this is not a simple oxygen-permeable membrane since it consumes oxygen as well. Perhaps the most difficult problem, however, is that this sensor, when everything is working correctly, senses the partial pressure of oxygen in the capillary blood, but we desire to know the partial pressure of oxygen in the arterial blood. Thus it is necessary to make the capillary blood look more like arterial blood than it normally does.

Fortunately this can be done to some extent through heat. Physiologists know that the human body has an intricate temperature regulation mechanism. Part of this involves using the skin to dissipate excessive heat. When an individual is in a warm environment, losing heat by conduction through the body is not easy so the circulatory system aids in providing heat loss through convection. Thus when the temperature of the environment around the body increases, cutaneous blood flow must also increase to help dissipate body heat. It turns out that heating a small portion of the skin with the transcutaneous oxygen sensor "fools" that local portion of skin into believing that the body is in a warm environment and that cutaneous blood flow must be increased to maintain temperature regulation. To do this we can heat the transcutaneous oxygen sensor itself by placing an electric heating coil around the outside of the silver anode. Thus the silver serves not only as an anode but also as a heat sink. A thermistor within the silver anode senses its temperature and controls the power supplied to the heating element so that a fixed temperature in the range of 43 to 45°C can be maintained. Thus, once the transcutaneous oxygen sensor has been in place on the skin for 15 to 20 minutes (min) and is at its elevated temperature, the capillary blood flow in the skin beneath the sensor increases greatly. At this increased flow rate the cells surrounding the capillaries have much more oxygen available to them than they would in a similar piece of nonheated skin since the perfusion is so much greater. The oxygen requirements of these cells, however, are not appreciably increased (although there is some increase due to the increased temperature), and so the oxygen partial pressure of the blood in these capillary loops more closely approximates that of the arterial blood than it would if the capillary perfusion were much lower. Thus the oxygen measured by the transcutaneous oxygen sensor more closely approximates that of the arterial blood, and this sensor can be used for continuous monitoring of blood oxygen tension in critically ill patients (Huch, Huch, and Luebbers 1981).

Several commercial transcutaneous oxygen tension instruments are in clinical use today. Figure 2.27 illustrates an instrument that measures both transcutaneous oxygen tension and transcutaneous carbon dioxide tension by utilizing a similar technique. The figure also shows an actual transcutaneous oxygen electrode. Such instrumentation is primarily used on newborn infants because the best correlations between transcutaneous and intra-arterial oxygen tensions occur in these

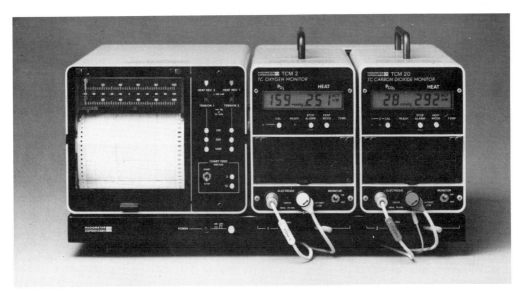

Figure 2.27 Typical transcutaneous blood gas instrument
(courtesy of Radiometer, Copenhagen).

patients. Monitors such as those illustrated in Figure 2.27 have played an important role in the technology of neonatal intensive care and are especially useful in monitoring infants in respiratory distress. Although the instruments are also used for adult patients, the high correlation between transcutaneous and intra-arterial measurements seen in the infant does not occur in this group, and the usefulness of the instrumentation is not universally accepted.

Potentiometric measurements

A second type of electrochemical cell used for biomedical measurements consists of a reference electrode in an electrolytic solution to be measured. A membrane that is permeable only to an ionic species to be measured separates this solution from a reference solution containing a known activity of that ion. The cell is completed by a reference electrode in this known reference solution. Reference electrodes are special electrochemical electrodes that maintain a very stable voltage with respect to the electrolytic solution they contact. The silver–silver chloride electrode used as the anode in the polarograph described in the previous section is an example of a reference electrode. Because the membrane separating the two solutions is permeable only to the ion we desire to measure, if the concentration of that ion is different in the solution being measured from that in the reference solution, some of that ion diffuses through the membrane in the direction of the concentration gradient. Thus, since only the ion in question can diffuse through the membrane, charge balance cannot be maintained because oppositely charged ions cannot penetrate the membrane so well. This, then, establishes an electric field across the membrane that eventually will stop the net diffusion of ions through the membrane. This also means that the electrical potential of one solution will now be different from that of the others; thus if we connect the two reference electrodes to a very high input impedance voltmeter, we can measure this potential difference as a voltage. We use a high impedance voltmeter because drawing current through this cell may cause reactions that will change the chemical composition. Since the cell and membrane can have a very high electrical resistance, drawing current can cause voltage drops that give erroneous potential differences.

The potential difference across the ion-permeable membrane is related to the logarithm of the concentration (or more correctly, the activity) of the permeable ion in the unknown solution. This relationship is described by the Nernst equation:

$$E = E_0 + \frac{RT}{nF} \ln(A^{n+}) \tag{2.15}$$

where E = potential difference
$\quad E_0$ = constant potential
$\quad R$ = universal gas constant
$\quad T$ = absolute temperature
$\quad F$ = Faraday constant

This type of sensor can have many different forms; Figure 2.28 illustrates one of the most familiar, the laboratory pH electrode. In this case the ion-permeable membrane is made of glass and frequently is a thin bubble of a very special glass. Although the actual mechanism of the hydrogen ion sensitivity of this glass is very complicated (Eisenman et al. 1966), we can approximate it by considering that the glass is permeable only to hydrogen ions. Thus if the solution inside the glass bulb

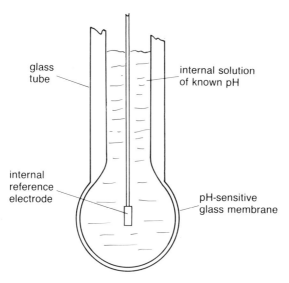

Figure 2.28   Glass membrane pH electrode used in the analytical laboratory.

has a known hydrogen ion concentration, the potential measured between this inner solution and an external solution of unknown pH is proportional to the negative logarithm of the hydrogen ion concentration (activity) in the external solution, in other words, its pH.

Hydrogen ion activity is an important variable in critical care medicine. By knowing the amount of acid (or base) in the blood, physicians can determine whether the lungs can remove carbon dioxide satisfactorily from the blood or whether the kidneys have problems in regulating acid-base balance. Frequently taking a small sample of arterial blood from patients in the intensive care unit to measure its pH is necessary. This sample is measured in the blood gas analyzer (described in the previous section) in the pH sensor of the instrument. In such a sensor as illustrated in Figure 2.29, the electrode appears to be inside-out compared to the conventional electrode shown in Figure 2.28. By making the pH glass into the form of a tube of diameter of 1 to 2 mm, it is possible to suck a small blood sample into this tube. This blood sample is also in contact with a reference electrode. The outside of the pH-sensitive glass tube contains a chamber in which the reference solution and a second reference electrode are placed. The volume of this reference solution is actually much larger than the volume of the blood sample. With this inverted design, it is possible to make pH measurements with very small blood samples. This is important, especially in the intensive care of very small premature infants since they do not have a great amount of blood volume available, and frequent sampling with larger samples could represent a serious blood loss for them.

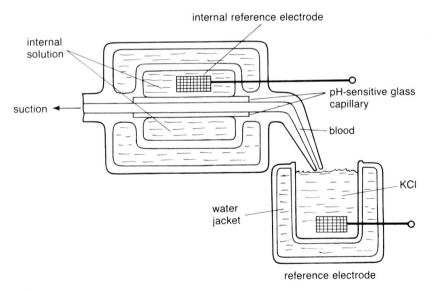

Figure 2.29 A glass pH electrode for use in a blood gas analyzer from Neuman, The Biophysical and Bioengineering Bases of Perinatal Monitoring, Part VI: Neonatal Temperature, Blood-Pressure and Blood-Gas Instrumentation, *Perinatology/Neonatology,* 3 (3): 25, (May-June, 1979) with permission.

In this blood pH instrument, the two reference electrodes are connected to a very high-impedance electronic voltmeter known as an *electrometer*. This is necessary since the glass membrane has a very high resistance, giving the overall cell a very high source resistance. The output from this signal processing circuit is then displayed on a digital readout or other output device as described previously.

Unlike oxygen and carbon dioxide, the pH of the blood cannot be transcutaneously measured because of a fundamental difference between hydrogen ions and oxygen or carbon dioxide molecules. In the case of the gas molecules, uncharged particles can diffuse through the skin and some membranes. The hydrogen ion, on the other hand, is positively charged, and even though the skin is permeable to it, every ion that diffuses through the skin moves a positive charge with it and, as in the case of the glass electrode, establishes an electric field that opposes further diffusion of additional hydrogen ions. Thus this electric field rather than the partial pressure can limit the diffusion since there is no way to balance the transported charge. This makes it impossible to have equal concentrations or activities of hydrogen ions in blood and in some sensor on the skin surface. Thus at the present time, we are limited to blood samples for clinical determinations of blood pH.

Even though it is not possible to measure blood pH transcutaneously, a miniature pH sensor that can be placed in tissue to sense the pH of the extracellular fluid continuously has been developed. In this case, other cations in the extracellular fluid, such as sodium or potassium, can diffuse across the capillary wall into the blood when hydrogen ions diffuse through the capillary wall in the opposite direction. This allows charge neutrality to be maintained, and the extracellular fluid can be at or near equilibrium with the blood with regard to pH. Thus by continuously measuring the pH of the extracellular fluid, one can get some indication of the blood acidity.

Potentiometric electrochemical measurements are not limited to pH but can be used for various other inorganic and organic ions. One can also have potentiometric measurements that do not involve a permeable membrane but rather are related to oxidation-reduction reactions as described for the amperometric technique.

Colorimetric measurements

Perhaps one of the most familiar chemical measurements is the litmus paper test for determining whether a solution is acidic or basic. In this case the color of a special dye embedded in the litmus paper indicates whether a substance is an acid or a base. An optical instrument that measures the amount of reflected light from the dye at one or more different wavelengths can also determine the color of this dye. Such an instrument provides much more quantitative data than the eye can, since it measures small changes in reflected light intensity. Any chemical reaction that can be coupled to a dye that changes color as the reaction proceeds can then be measured in this way. The numerous applications of this principle in medical instruments range from automatic blood chemistry analyzers in the clinical laboratory to relatively inexpensive devices used in the home by diabetes patients. This latter instrument furnishes a useful example of the technique.

Several manufacturers produce chemical indicator paper that contains a mixture of indicator dyes that are sensitive to glucose. When a drop of fresh blood is placed on a strip of this paper, the glucose in the blood reacts with materials in the paper and alters the color of the indicator dyes. Since the blood is opaque these color changes are not visible until it is washed away. The reactions are also time-dependent, so the color varies with the amount of time that the blood is in contact with the paper, as well.

The colorimetric glucose instrument contains a timer that is set when the operator places the blood droplet on the indicator paper. After the internally set time elapses, an alarm indicates that the blood should be washed from the paper and the paper inserted into the sensing cuvette of the instrument. Figure 2.30 is a simplified diagram of this instrument. A source of light of a specific band of wavelengths is focused onto the indicator paper. A photodetector such as a photodiode or photo-transistor receives some of the reflected light and determines its intensity. The relative intensity of reflected light quantitatively determines the color of the indicator. This in turn is related to the concentration of glucose in the blood specimen. The instrument processes the reflected light intensity and calculates the glucose concentration from it and then displays it on a digital readout.

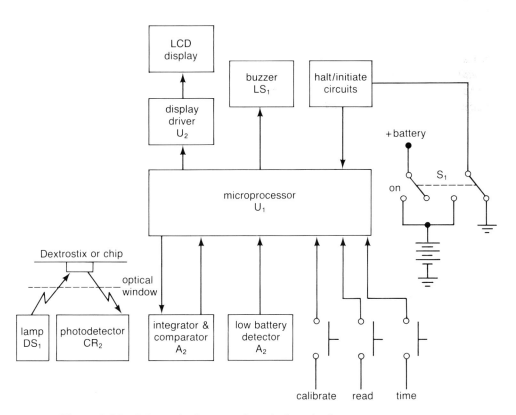

Figure 2.30 Schematic diagram of a colorimetric glucose analyzer (courtesy of Ames, Inc).

Home glucose colorimeters such as those described have been important in the control of diabetes (Sonksen et al. 1978). Patients purchase these relatively inexpensive instruments and periodically collect a droplet of blood by pricking a finger with a small, disposable lancet. By looking at the glucose level at certain times of the day patients can determine their own insulin requirements or provide the data to their physician so that their blood sugar can be more closely regulated and the risk of complications from diabetes reduced.

The preceding examples indicate some of the applications of medical instrumentation systems in the care of patients. Such systems can range from relatively simple home devices to complex intensive care monitoring systems for tertiary medical centers. From the examples described, it is apparent that the sensor plays an important role in the instrumentation system. Although the sensors described in this chapter exemplify the different types of sensors used in medical instrumentation, they do not represent a complete set. Not only are there many other types of sensors being applied in medical instrumentation, but sensors also represent a very active field of biomedical engineering research and development. Numerous academic, independent, industrial, and government laboratories are developing physical and chemical sensors for biomedical as well as other applications. Many of these utilize the basic principles described in this chapter but in new and sophisticated ways. The next section looks at some of these new techniques and indicates some of their applications to biosensors.

NEW TECHNOLOGIES FOR BIOSENSORS

The many advances in signal processing hardware and software based on large-scale integrated circuits and the microprocessor have facilitated the development of sophisticated instrumentation systems. As stated in the previous sections, it is possible to calibrate instrumentation automatically when the system is under microprocessor control, and this can be very important in overall measurement reliability. The laboratory instrumentation divides the specimens to be measured into individual portions for individual testing. Some manufacturers are even marketing robots to perform specimen manipulation and tests in the clinical laboratory. The one aspect of such instrumentation systems that still needs improvement is the sensor. Easily replaced or perhaps disposable sensors with characteristics requiring a minimum of calibration would make these instruments more efficient. Smaller sensors would allow smaller specimens to be used, a particular advantage when only small specimens are available, for example, in working with premature infants. The sensor is often one of the most costly and delicate portions of an instrument system. If it could be simplified and mass-produced, it might be possible to make small, inexpensive instruments that could be used at the patient's bedside. This would provide more rapid feedback to physicians and prevent errors related to specimen transport. Such a class of instrumentation would also be available for physicians' offices, thereby allowing them to perform tests while examining patients. This feature would eliminate the need to send the patient or specimen to another laboratory and would provide more rapid information for diagnosis and treatment.

Sensors that can meet some of these needs are currently not only under development for medical applications but for industrial applications as well, with new technologies such as photolithography, integrated circuit processing, and micromachining being applied to this type of sensor development. In the following pages, we look at some examples of what this technology makes possible.

Photolithography

The technique of photographically defining a planar geometry and then chemically etching a surface to conform to this geometry is well known in the graphic arts. Fine artists have used the technique in making prints and etchings, and publishers employ the technology in reproducing halftone black and white or color photographs on the printed page. By improving the resolution of the process, the microelectronics industry has used it to carefully define regions on semiconductors to receive doping agents to form large scale and very large scale integrated circuits. These basic photolithographic techniques are also used in inexpensive fabrication of large numbers of biosensors.

Thick-film photomasking techniques are useful in forming the electrodes of a polarographic oxygen sensor. Figure 2.31 illustrates the structure of such a sensor, in which the cathode consists of a series of twenty-four 125-μm squares formed by depositing a fork-shaped gold film. An insulating film that has slots oriented at right angles to the tines of the fork and intersects them to form the square cathodes covers the cathode. It is possible to take advantage of the low stirring artifact associated with small area cathodes but get a relatively high cathode current due to the parallel connection of 24 of them. The anode consists of a rectangular silver film.

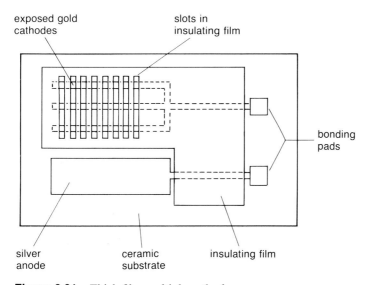

Figure 2.31   Thick-film multiple cathode oxygen sensor.

The entire structure is formed on a ceramic substrate, with leads from the cathode and anode brought to bonding pads at one end of the substrate. In insulating film also coats these leads for protection.

Sensors of this type determine the dissolved oxygen in seawater, and since seawater contains fewer proteins and other heavy molecules that can contaminate the electrode surface than does blood, it is unnecessary to make this sensor into a Clark electrode with a oxygen-permeable membrane.

Through thick-film and thin-film technologies for forming the electrode structures, large numbers of sensors can be manufactured inexpensively, with uncalibrated characteristics that are surprisingly similar. (Liu, 1980) Even with this relatively crude process, Liu found variations from sensor to sensor to be within 5 percent. These features imply that even though the initial design and tooling costs are great for this type of sensor, such costs can be amortised over a large number of manufactured sensors so that individual items are low in cost when large numbers are produced. The similarity of operating characteristics greatly simplifies the calibration procedure for individual sensors. Thus, it is possible to use a sensor such as this for a single measurement, then dispose it. In Liu's biological application of determining the dissolved oxygen in seawater, sensors used for a single measurement were discarded afterward. A similar approach is appropriate for medical measurements. For example, such a sensor could be incorporated into a cell filled with a single sample of blood placed in an instrument to read the oxygen tension and then discarded. Because the photolithographic process makes fabrication of very small sensors possible, such a disposable sample chamber and sensor combination could function on a very low volume of blood.

Integrated circuit fabrication technology

Although the fabrication of silicon integrated circuits uses some of the photomasking techniques described in the previous section, the techniques of impurity diffusion and ion implantation are also employed to construct three-dimensional impurity structures in the bulk of a silicon integrated circuit chip. The discussion of miniature pressure transducers that are used for intravascular blood pressure measurements indicated how this technology may be used for fabricating a biosensor. The sensor designed by Ko and colleagues (1979) and illustrated in Figure 2.13 involved forming four strain gauges in the diaphragm of the sensor. Unlike the photolithographic film techniques that would form the strain gauges on the surface of the diaphragm, this sensor incorporates the strain gauges within the diaphragm itself. In this case, this was done by forming a mask on the surface of the diaphragm by using photolithographic techniques and then diffusing impurities through the mask so that they enter the diaphragm having the same pattern as the opening in the mask. The impurities cause formation of *pn* junctions in the silicon, electrically isolating a small region from the bulk of the diaphragm. This region then serves as the strain gauge. The pattern used for forming the strain gauges in the diaphragm of the Ko sensor is shown in Figure 2.32. Two of the strain gauges are oriented to be sensitive to the deflection of the diaphragm, and the other two are oriented not to have this sensitivity. All four are located close together so that

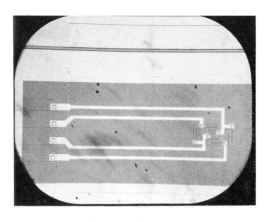

Figure 2.32   A pattern of strain gauge placement on the diaphragm of the miniature silicon pressure transducer in Figure 2.13 (Ko, 1979).

the local temperature affects them all equally. Thus because of the bridge connection the effect of temperature on the output signal from the sensor is small.

Low-resistivity channels diffused into the bulk of the silicon pressure transducer structure serve as electrical leads connecting the strain gauge elements to lead wire bonding pads on the surface of one end of the sensor. Growing a film of silicon dioxide on all surfaces except where the bonding pads for the lead wires are located passavates (protects) the surface of the sensor.

The technology of forming integrated circuits has applications in more complex structures as well. Sensors that are redundant in that they have more than one transducer element for a particular measurement are more reliable than single-element sensors. These can also provide information on the spatial distribution of the variable being measured. The same technology used to form the sensor can also form signal preprocessing electronics on the sensor itself. For example, an intravascular pressure transducer incorporating a preamplifier on the chip could allow the transmission of a stronger signal along the lead wires, to give a higher overall signal-to-noise ratio. When multiple, redundant transducers are used on a sensor, multiplexing electronics can be integrated into the sensor to allow each transducer element to be addressed without requiring a large number of lead wires to the sensor. Such a multiplexing system can even be programmed to recognize sensors in the array that have failed and to bypass their signal to prevent transmission of the erroneous data to the remainder of the signal processing electronics.

Many types of sensors can be developed through solid-state integrated circuit technology. These cover almost the entire range of sensor types mentioned in this chapter.

Micromachining

The field of micromachining has developed as a further extension of the application of microelectronic fabrication techniques to the development of biosensors. This involves, in addition to the standard integrated circuit fabrication technologies, methods to etch silicon and other semiconductor crystals isotrophically to form three-dimensional structures. One can also diffuse impurities into the semiconductor to serve as an etch stop, allowing only the semiconductor material to be etched away until the impurity is encountered. Combining these techniques with the photolithographic and diffusion technologies produces complex structures over very small dimensions, including holes, electrical conduits through a chip, thin membranes, cantilevers, and structural bridges. This technology will allow sensor designers to create unique miniature three-dimensional structures for mass production. Angell (1983) has reviewed the techniques of micromachining and its applications to biosensors. One such application is the miniature accelerometer in Figure 2.33. This sensor, which is formed from a silicon chip, consists of a cantilever beam made of silicon and contains a silicon strain gauge along its length. One end of the beam is attached to the silicon chip, and the other is free-floating with a known mass of gold deposited upon it. The beam is carved from the original silicon chip by etching around and under it using photomasks and etch stops to define both the extent of the etched-away silicon and of the cantilever beam. When this structure is accelerated in a direction normal to the surface of the chip, the beam deflects because of the inertia of the mass. The strain gauge senses this deflection, and an electrical signal proportional to the deflection and hence the acceleration results.

These new technologies for sensor development are still in the laboratory stage at the time of this writing. They, nevertheless, offer great potential for the development of mass-produced biosensors and other types of sensors at much lower costs than those that are currently used. Furthermore, such sensors can have characteristics that are reasonably reproducible. The techniques are applicable to both physical and chemical sensors and should allow these sensors to interface more readily with modern signal processing electronics. The great need for improved sensors as well as the availability of new technologies to produce them will lead to many significant developments in this important field.

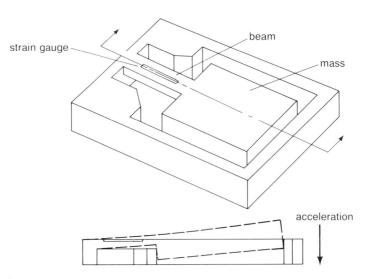

Figure 2.33 Miniature micromachined silicon accelerometer (after Angell et al. 1983. Silicon micromechanical devices. *Sci Am* 248:44).

REFERENCES

Angell, J. B., Terry, S. C., and Barth, P. W. 1983. Silicon micromechanical devices. *Sci Am* 248:44.

Bellville, J. W., and Weaver, C. S. 1969. *Techniques in clinical physiology*. New York: MacMillian.

Brakkee, A. J. M., and Vendrik, A. J. H. 1966. Strain-gauge plethysmography: Theoretical and practical notes on a new design. *J Appl Physiol* 21:701.

Clark, L. C. 1956. Monitor and control of blood tissue oxygen tensions. *Trans Am Soc Artif Intern Organs*, 2:41.

Cobbold, R. S. C. 1974. *Transducers for biomedical measurements*. New York: Wiley.

Dean, M. (ed.) 1962. *Semiconductor and conventional strain gauges*. New York: Academic.

Eisenman, G., Mattock, G., Bates, R., and Friedman, S. M. 1966. *The glass electrode*. New York: Wiley.

Geddes, L. A. 1970. *The direct and indirect measurement of blood pressures*. Chicago: Year Book.

Geddes, L. A. 1972. *Electrodes and the measurement of bioelectric events*. New York: Wiley. (1972).

Guyton, A. C. 1981. *Textbook of medical physiology*, (6th ed.), Philadelphia: Saunders.

Hill, D. W., and Dolan, A. M. 1976. *Intensive care instrumentation*. New York: Grune & Stratton.

Huch, R., Huch, A., and Luebbers, D. W. 1981. *Transcutaneous PO₂*. New York: Thieme-Stratton.

Ko, W. H. 1984. Physical Transducers. *Proc. IEEE/NSF Symposium on Biosensors,* pp 1–3.

Ko, W. H., Hynecek, J., and Boettcher, S. F. 1979. Development of a miniature pressure transducer for biomedical applications. *IEEE Trans Electron Devices* 26:1896.

Liu, C. C., Neuman, M. R., Montana K. L., and Oberdoerster M. C. 1980. Miniature Multiple Cathode Dissolved Oxygen Sensor for Marine Science Application, *Proc. 16th Conference on Marine Technology.* pp 468–72.

Montcastle, V. B. 1982. *Medical physiology*, (13th ed.). St. Louis, Mosby.

Neuman, M. R. 1982. Physical and chemical sensors for medical instrumentation. *Med Prog Technol* 9:95.

Neuman, M. R. 1984. Optimal detection of respiration and apnea by infant monitors. In *Medical Technology for the Neonate*, monograph. Arlington, Va.:AAMI. pp. 49–54.

Nyboer, J. 1970. *Electrical impedance plethysmography*. Springfield, Ill: Thomas.

Ruch, T. C., and Patton, H. D. 1965. *Physiology and biophysics*. (19th ed.). Philadelphia: Saunders.

Sonksen, P. H., Judd, S. L., and Lowy, C. 1978. Home monitoring of blood glucose—method for improving diabetic control. *Lancet*, 1:732.

Stamm, O., Latscha, U., Janacek P., and Campana, A. 1976. Development of a special electrode for continuous subcutaneous pH measurement in the infant's scalp. *Amer. J. Obstet. Gynec.*, 124: 193

Trathen, R. H. 1964. *Statics and strength of materials*. New York: Wiley. chap. 4.

Webster, J. 1978. *Medical instrumentation: Application and design*. Boston: Houghton-Mifflin.

Zador, I., Neuman, M. R., and Wolfson, R. N. 1976. Continuous monitoring of cervical dilatation during labor by ultrasonic transit time measurement. *Med Biol Eng* 14:299.

Part Three

Instrumentation Systems

CHAPTER **3**

Cardiovascular Assist and Monitoring Devices

Frank M. Galioto, Jr., M.D.

Children's Hospital National Medical Center
Washington, D.C.

INTRODUCTION

Despite significant improvements in cardiac diagnosis and treatment in recent years, heart disease remains the leading cause of death and significant disability in the United States. In 1980, over 1 million Americans died of diseases of the heart and blood vessels. The majority of these patients died of acute problems such as a heart attack or a stroke with 566,900 deaths in 1980 caused by heart attacks alone. Over 4 million living Americans either have had a heart attack or have chest pain (angina) due to heart disease (American Heart Association 1984).

The economic cost of this health problem is staggering. In 1983, the American Heart Association estimated that over $56 billion was spent on or lost due to cardiovascular disease, with the majority, over $32 billion, spent on hospital or nursing home care (American Heart Association 1984). In 1984, a slight decline in cardiac-related deaths occurred, due in part to preventative measures taken in the form of diet and exercise by an educated populace and in part to improved treatment of existing disease. Americans are now aware that hypertension, cigarette smoking, and high-cholesterol diets all predispose to heart disease and that exercise and fitness reduce one's risk.

In terms of treatment of existing heart disease, quite clearly, the cooperative efforts of the disciplines of medicine and biomedical engineering have resulted in improved survival rates. The cardiologist and cardiovascular surgeon must work together with the biomedical engineer to conduct even the most fundamental research; the combination of their skills has led to the tools of better diagnosis and more effective therapy. Consequently, this chapter focuses its attention upon the basic mechanical and electrical characteristics of heart action and evaluates the biomedical and technological innovations utilized in the monitoring and assist devices.

FUNDAMENTAL PRINCIPLES OF HEART ACTION

To explore the development, current status, and future of many of the tools of cardiology, a knowledge of the basic anatomy and physiology or function of the heart and blood vessels is necessary. The heart comprises muscular tissue organized into four chambers with four one-way valves at various levels to separate the chambers and their outflow blood vessels (Figure 3.1). The valves permit the development of different pressures within the heart to allow for low levels on the inflow site and higher levels for output.

The two upper cardiac chambers, called *atria,* receive blood from either the body or lungs and serve as booster pumps to maximize filling of the two lower chambers (*ventricles*), which in turn eject the blood out of the heart. It is useful to consider the heart and cardiovascular system as a group of pumps and valves connected in series with only one-way flow. The right atrium receives blood from the upper and lower portions of the body via the two major veins: the *inferior* and the *superior vena cava.* This blood has had oxygen removed from it by the body and needs to have that essential element of life replenished by the lungs. The right atrium pumps the blood through the tricuspid valve into the right ventricle, which in turn

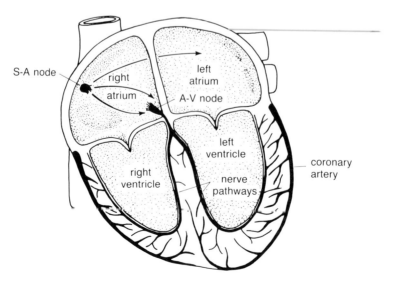

Figure 3.1   The normal heart.

develops a higher pressure and pumps the blood through the pulmonary valve into the lungs. In the lungs, the blood comes into contact with a thin interface with the air sacs, or *alveoli,* where gas exchange takes place. The blood, now rich with oxygen, returns to the left atrium, which boosts it into the left ventricle through the mitral valve. The left ventricle, the major pump for the body, now ejects the blood into the major artery, the aorta, through the aortic valve. The left ventricle is the most essential part of the heart and is the site of much of the disease affecting it. The first branches of the aorta are the *coronary arteries,* which bring oxygen-rich blood and nutrients to the heart muscle, or *myocardium.* Disease of these blood vessels causes many heart problems. After passing the coronary artery origins, the blood is distributed throughout the body, where oxygen is extracted. The entire cycle starts again with the return of blood to the right side of the heart.

The pressures produced by the various heart chambers are governed by the simple physical law that states that pressure equals flow times resistance ($P = Q \cdot R$). Each cardiac chamber and great vessel normally produces its own characteristic pressure and wave form. For the atria, these are determined by the flows into the chambers from either the body (the right atrium) or the lungs (the left atria) and by the resistance offered by the respective ventricles that receive their output. A ventricle whose myocardium has been damaged either may not relax well during diastole or may not have emptied adequately, potentially causing the atria to work harder. The ventricles, which must generate enough flow to meet the needs of the body for cardiac output, develop pressure levels proportional to the resistance offered by either the lungs or the body. The lungs usually offer very low resistance so that the right ventricular pressure is normally below 30 mmHg at peak systole. Because the left ventricle must overcome the resistance of the entire body, it typically generates a peak systolic pressure of between 110 and 140 mmHg in most adults. The pressure during cardiac relaxation and filling determines the diastolic pressure. *Systole* is thus the period of the cardiac cycle when the heart is emptying, and *diastole* the period when it is filling.

The measurement of these pressures is quite important in the assessment of health and disease. The only pressure that can be measured even indirectly without inserting an instrument or needle into the patient is the arterial blood pressure in the body. This is most simply done by the use of a sphygnomanometer (Kirkendall et al. 1980), which consists of a compression bladder, an inflating bulb or pump with a control valve to allow for slow deflation, and a manometer for reading the pressure of the bladder. A stethoscope is used to listen for the sounds of blood flow. One inflates the bladder to a pressure sufficient to stop all flow in the limb and gradually deflates it. When the sounds of flow are first heard, the manometer pressure is noted as the systolic pressure. The cuff is further deflated until the sounds of disturbed flow are not longer audible, and this is recorded as the diastolic pressure. This system is quite simple but not sufficiently accurate in critical situations.

For patients who are critically ill and require continuous measurement of blood pressure, a direct assessment is necessary. This is accomplished by an arterial line consisting of a needle or plastic cannula inserted directly into a major artery, typically the radial at the wrist. A skilled physician can usually insert this cannula directly through the skin and into the vessel without making a large incision in the skin. These puncture sites must be watched carefully for infection, bleeding, or compromise of the hand or other part of the body that depends on the artery for flow. The cannula is typically connected to a fluid-filled tube joined to a transducer for continuous measurement of blood pressure. The arterial line is also useful for the withdrawal of blood samples to assess blood pH, oxygen, and carbon dioxide content. The clinical setting for this type of monitoring is further addressed in the section on intensive care units.

To function efficiently, the cardiac pumping action must proceed in a coordinated fashion. Specialized groups of cardiac cells that generate and conduct electrical pulses effect this coordination. Electrical activity in the normal heart begins with a voltage generated by a group of excitable cells located in the right atrium and called the *sinoatrial* (S-A) *node.* This group of cells is the usual pacemaker for the entire heart. The electrical impulse spreads across both atria, causing them to contract and thus pump blood into the two ventricles. The impulse spreads next to another group of specialized cells, the *atrioventricular* (A-V) *node,* which causes a slight delay in the electrical signal so that the mechanical event of atrial contraction, which is much slower than the electrical conduction, can precede the electrical stimulation of the ventricles. This delay is essential to allow the atria to serve as booster pumps for the ventricles. After the atria have pumped, the electrical impulse spreads into the ventricles through a special pathway called the *bundle of His* and causes them to contract vigorously and pump blood out of the heart. It is essential to note that although all of the specialized cells in the heart can generate electrical stimuli, in the normal heart, the S-A node controls the overall pattern of heart activity. It is the frequency at which the S-A node generates an electrical impulse that the cardiologist detects as the heart rate. The S-A node reponds to external stimuli from the brain and other parts of the nervous system and to hormonal influences such as epinephrine to increase or decrease the heart rate. However, all impulse formation takes place in the heart itself.

Because the electrical control of cardiac activity is essential to its function, the clinician evaluating a patient for heart disease requires a means of analyzing this vital function. This analysis is based on the recording of an *electrocardiogram* (ECG) (Figure 3.2). A series of electrodes placed on the body detects the electrical signal and displays it on an oscilloscope or records it on paper. The *electrocardiograph,* the instrument used for detecting and recording the ECG, was the first biomedical device to have widespread use and was introduced into hospitals around 1910. To make these vital tracings universally useful, standards have been established so that a cardiologists in New York can interpret a tracing obtained in California without knowing the manufacturer of the machine used to make the tracing.

Each portion of the ECG tracing represents electrical activity in various parts of the heart. It is known that electrical depolarization of the atria is represented by the P wave in the ECG trace. The QRS complex comes from the depolarization of the ventricles, and repolarization of the ventricles is represented by the T wave segment. The pacemaker cells of the S-A node initiate all electrical activity, but this voltage is so small that it cannot be detected in itself by a standard ECG machine.

Standards for the size and duration of these ECG components have been established for adults and children. A larger amplitude of the QRS, for instance, reflects an increased muscle mass of a ventricle, which is called *hypertrophy.* If the electrodes are varied in their position to analyze different areas of the heart, then

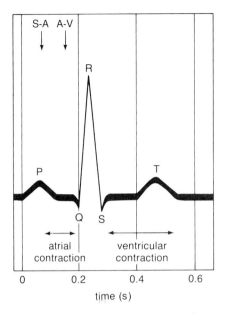

Figure 3.2   An electrocardiographic recording (ECG) from a normal heart.

specific chambers can be separately studied. In this way, a cardiologist who notes a reduction in the voltage from the left ventricle and alterations in depolarization and repolarization can make the ECG diagnosis of an *infarction,* or death of a portion of the ventricular muscle from a heart attack.

The heart rate is documented by the ECG, and the normal sequence of P–QRS–T can be analyzed. Slower heart rates than normal are called *bradycardia* and faster rates *tachycardia.* The extremes of these variations are *asystole,* or cessation of all cardiac electrical activity due to a lack of impulse formation, and *ventricular fibrillation,* which is very rapid, chaotic electrical activity conducted through the ventricles in a random and uncoordinated fashion. Since no effective mechanical cardiac action occurs in either of these states, death would result if neither were treated. Fortunately, medicine and biomedical engineering have developed specialized devices to treat these situations; e.g., the artificial pacemaker for bradycardia and the defibrillator for ventricular fibrillation. Prompt recognition of these conditions leads to appropriate therapy, and lives are regularly saved through these devices.

To detect the electrical event of the heart in the form of the electrocardiogram, electrodes convert the ionic potential in the body into electron current. The most common electrode in clinical use is a nonpolarizable silver–silver chloride device recessed in a plastic foam disk with adhesive that sticks to the skin. These recessed Ag–AgCl electrodes are mass-produced and disposable. Typically, they are placed on the chest and replaced as the adhesive dries out over the course of 24 h.

The heart generates its ECG potential as an electric field with a given magnitude and direction. This field is characterized by measuring it between a series of electrodes placed over various parts of the body. The standard 12-lead electrocardiogram represents the heart's voltage as measured between known electrode positions. For instance, standard lead I is always considered to be the voltage measured between electrodes placed on the right and left arms with the right arm always the negative pole.

Similarly, for lead AVL, the left arm electrode is considered to be positive, with the negative pole the average between the right arm and left leg. To assess the ECG voltage more accurately, a series of six standard points on the chest wall is considered to be positive electrodes, and the negative the sum of the left arm, right arm, and left leg potentials. By analyzing all 12 leads, the cardiologist reconstructs the ECG potential as an electrical signal with a mean spacial vector and magnitude.

CARDIAC MONITORING AND ASSIST INSTRUMENTATION

Cardiac Pacemakers

The use of artificial cardiac pacemakers is well established in medical practice (Judson et al. 1967). More than 500,000 pacemakers have been implanted into patients in the United States alone, making this the most common of all cardiovascular therapeutic procedures (American Heart Association 1984). The most common indication for a pacemaker is a very slow heart rate or bradycardia due to a failure of the natural pacemaker or a component of the conduction system. Patients who have bradycardia are at risk for loss of consciousness as their hearts cannot speed up in response to stress and their brains do not receive adequate blood flow.

The first animal experiments with electrical stimulation of the heart took place over 100 years ago, but the first human use of a pacemaker did not occur until 1932 (Hays 1964; Hyman 1932). At that time, a needle was passed through the chest wall into the heart of a dying patient and an electrical stimulus applied. This crude effort soon failed but led to further scientific study. In 1952, Dr. Paul M. Zoll, a cardiologist working with the engineers of the Electrodyne Company, developed an external pacemaker that pulsed energy to the heart through large electrodes placed on the chest wall (Falk et al. 1983). This system was not practical as it required such high voltages to stimulate the heart that other muscle groups also contracted, and skin burns developed. In 1957, Dr. C. Walton Lillehei paced the heart directly during heart surgery by sewing wire electrodes into the heart muscle and using an external pulse generator (Thevenet et al. 1958; Weirich et al. 1957). This effort was again successful for only a brief period. What was needed was a self-contained, battery-powered unit to be implanted in the body and connected by reliable electrodes directly to the heart.

The development of better power sources and reliable solid-state electronics led to the development of the first implantable cardiac pacemaker by Dr. William Chardack, a physician, and Wilson Greatbatch, an electrical engineer, in 1960 (Chardack et al. 1960). Their device was placed into the body and delivered at a predetermined rate an electrical impulse that was conveyed to the heart's ventricles by a wire electrode. This device could not sense the heart's own electrical activity, and some patients with this unit developed a competition between their own slow rhythm and that of the pacemaker. This effect led to the development of ventricu-lar fibrillation and death in some cases.

The next generation of pacemakers was developed to sense the heart's own rhythm and would suppress the artifical pacemaker's output to avoid this danger-ous situation. This "demand" pacemaker had electronic circuits to detect the heart's own native rhythm through the electrodes. If the heart were beating above a certain rate, typically 60 beats per minute, the pacemaker would not stimulate the heart. When the natural heart rate fell below the preset rate, the pacemaker would be instructed to send an electrical impulse to cause the heart to beat. Thus, this more intelligent unit could "sense" or detect the heart's activity and "pace" as needed. These early units did not address the need for coordinated atrial booster function because only the ventricles were being sensed and paced.

The current generation of cardiac pacemakers represents the combined ef-forts of medicine and biomedical engineering (Furman 1983; Ludmer and Gold-schlager 1984). Three problems, the electrodes, the power source, and the pulse generator with its control mechanism, will be discussed in turn. The electrodes used today all have direct contact with the heart. Two types of electrode systems are used: (1) *bipolar,* with two leads, a positive (+) and a negative (−) electrode and (2) *unipolar,* with the negative (−) electrode positioned in or on the heart and the positive electrode as one surface of the pulse generator placed under the skin of either the chest or abdomen. The electrodes are either sewn directly into the heart muscle or placed via a vein into the atrial or ventricle and into close contact with the inner lining of these chambers, the *endocardium.* Myocardial electrodes can be placed on any surface of the heart, but endocardial leads can reach only the right-sided cardiac chambers. Myocardial sew-in electrodes are shaped like corkscrews or barbs to permit firm attachment, whereas endocardial leads have tines to snare any rough surface in the right-sided chambers to achieve a firm anchor.

At present, most patients have their pacemakers implanted via a large vein and utilize an endocardial electrode system. In this technique, a chest incision into the thoracic cavity is not needed, and the postimplantation hospital stay can be quite brief. The cardiologist makes a small incision in the skin over the subclavian vein, isolates that blood vessel, and places a catheter with the tined electrode at its tip into the vessel (Figure 3.3). The cardiologist then uses a fluoroscope, an x-ray

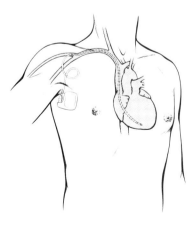

Figure 3.3   Electronic pacemaker. The catheter containing the electrodes is inserted into the heart through the right cephalic vein (from Bronzino, JD: *Technology for Patient Care,* St. Louis: C. V. Mosby, 1977).

viewing device, to pass the catheter into the heart and the precise location where pacing or sensing would be most useful. The pulse generator is then connected to the catheter leads, tested, and then placed under the skin, and the incision is closed. Many patients leave the hospital on the day following such a procedure. The electrodes and connecting wires themselves must be very strong to avoid breakage but flexible enough to permit catheter passage into the heart. The most commonly used metals today are a stainless steel alloy, Elgiloy, for the wires, with the electrodes at the tip coated with iridium or platinum.

The power sources for pacemakers have followed a similar course of improvement over the first external units, which required ac power sources. Battery life on the first implantable units was only 1 yr, after which reoperation to replace the generator was needed. Three separate avenues of biomedical research attempted to solve this problem. First, rechargable units that were implanted and charged weekly through the skin by radiofrequency stimulation were developed (Holcomb et al. 1969). These units worked quite well but were inconvenient and are no longer in widespread use as the useful life of the rechargable batteries was only 10 yr. Second, a nuclear-powered pulse generator, using the heat generated by the decay of radioactive plutonium to produce electrical energy was introduced. These units were quite heavy because of the shielding needed and had a life expectancy of 15 yr. The third and most successful approach was the development of better conventional power sources. Most units now implanted utilize a lithium-iodine battery which has a life expectancy of 15 years. These units have proved to be very reliable and can be monitored externally for signs of power source depletion (Ludmer and Goldschlager 1984).

The modern pacemaker is a far cry from the early impulse generators. The latest units available can sense the heart's own electrical activity and pace appropriately. For patients with S-A node dysfunction, the pacemaker can pace the atrium directly through an atrial electrode, allowing the heart's own conduction system to

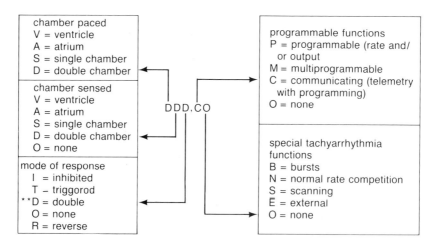

Figure 3.4   Inter-Society Commission for Heart Disease Resources (ICHD) code.

function normally. For patients with a blockage of impulse conduction between the atria and ventricles, a condition called *heart block,* the pacemaker can sense the heart's own atrial activity, and a stimulus is sent directly to the ventricle. This type of physiological pacing allows the patient's own S-A node to set the rate. Many patients have widespread conduction system disease. At various points in their conduction system, problems may occur and flexibility is needed to control the situation. These patients may initially exhibit only S-A node dysfunction and subsequently develop heart block. In response to this changing problem, the cardiologist has requested and the engineers have developed a dual-chamber programmable pacing system. Even after implantation, this unit can have its functions controlled and reprogrammed by an external device using radiofrequency commands. The functions that can be controlled are selections of the chambers to be paced, the chambers to be sensed, and the mode of response. All of these functions, including battery status, are monitored by telemetry (Sutton et al. 1980). The complexity involved necessitated the special code developed so that the cardiologist could refer to a uniform description of the modes used by modern pacemaker, the Inter-Society Commission for Heart Disease Resources (ICHD) code table (Figure 3.4) (ICHD 1983).

Typically, patients with pacemakers have the unit installed and programmed by a cardiologist. They are monitored by telemetry, even by telephone on a monthly basis, with periodic reprogramming of the pacemaker as needed. As time passes, improved electrodes, batteries, and pulse generators are expected to provide even more flexibility.

The normal heart contracts rhythmically and in a set sequence as discussed previously. In the diseased heart, especially in coronary artery disease, when the heart muscle does not receive adequate blood flow through the blocked coronary arteries, rhythm disturbances occur. These are usually limited to occasional extra beats called *ventricular extrasystoles* but can progress to the potentially lethal rhythm called *ventricular fibrillation.* This state has no orderly beat, with the ventricle overstimulated electrically to the point where mechanical activity ceases, and there is no effective cardiac pumping. Death occurs in a few minutes if this condition persists (Figure 3.5).

Defibrillators

Ventricular fibrillation is the primary cause of death from heart disease in the United States. It is usually related to coronary artery insufficiency and is commonly called a *heart attack*. This condition can respond to treatment if promptly detected before the heart muscle or other vital organs are further damaged by the lack of cardiac pumping (De Silva et al. 1980).

William B. Kouwenhoven, an electrical engineer, produced the first instrument to treat this condition in the 1930s (Geddes and Hamlin 1983). This defibrillator was designed to pass alternating current through the chest of a person with ventricular fibrillation. Significant refinements have been made since that time, but the basic principle of causing all cells of the heart to depolarize at the same time remains. All cardiac cells are made to enter their electrically silent, or refractory,

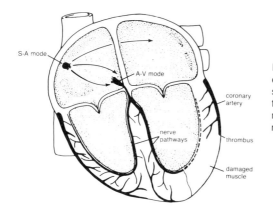

Electrical activity of damaged heart is erratic because nerve impulses can no longer flow smoothly from the atrioventricular node through the pathways that feed impulses to the ventricular muscles. Most heart-attack patients develop one or more of the arrhythmias shown.

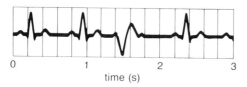

First sign of arrhythmia in the heartbeat, following a coronary heart attack, usually takes the form of a premature ventricular beat (arrow).

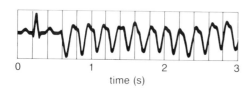

More serious arrhythmia is tachycardia, or fast heartbeat, in which ventricular impulses occur at two or three times the normal rate. If not halted, they can cause death.

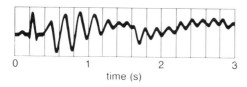

Fatal arrhythmia known as *fibrillation* can develop from tachycardia or when premature beats fall within a critical part of the T wave.

Figure 3.5 Electrical activity in the damaged heart (after Lown, B.: *Sci Am* 219:19–27, July 1984. Copyright © 1968 by *Scientific American,* Inc. All rights reserved).

period at the same time. The heart cells that recover first are presumably the normal pacemakers cells of the S-A node, restoring normal heart rhythm (Kerber et al. 1983; Tacker et al. 1974).

In 1962, Dr. Bernard Lown of Harvard University, a cardiologist, developed a direct current defibrillator that is still used today. His method (Figure 3.6) entails charging a capacitor to the desired dc voltage and then discharging it through large metal paddles passed on the patient's chest. During ventricular fibrillation, this voltage may be discharged at any time because no existing organized rhythm has to be coordinated.

The defibrillator can also correct other serious rhythm disturbances of the heart. A patient who develops a rapid but still electrically organized rhythm may have such a fast electrical stimulus that the ventricles do not have time to fill before

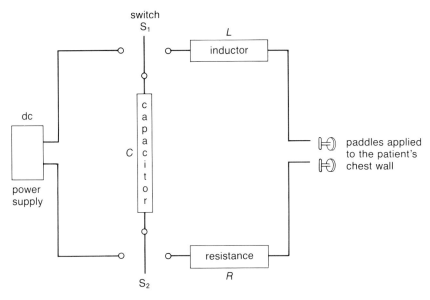

Figure 3.6   RLC defibrillator (from Bronzino, JD:
Technology for Patient Care, St. Louis: C. V. Mosby, 1977).

they are required to beat again. Two common conditions, *atrial* and *ventricular ta-chycardia,* can cause this clinical problem. A random electrical shock in this situation is not desirable because it can overstimulate the heart and cause ventricular fibrillation. To avoid this problem, the defibrillator is programmed to sense the heart's own rhythm and allow delivery of an electrical charge only at the right instant of the ECG cycle. The charge is never allowed to occur during the critical T-wave phase of the cycle, to prevent ventricular fibrillation.

In practice, the defibrillator is now part of the ambulance equipment in most areas. The paramedical team, which arrives at the home of a patient who is thought to be suffering from a heart attack, promptly attaches ECG leads to the patient, observes the rhythm, and sends a copy of the signal by radio to the physician at the hospital base. If ventricular fibrillation is apparent, cardiopulmonary resuscitation begins, and by remote direction of the physician, the defibrillator paddles are placed on the patient's chest. Ventricular fibrillation is again confirmed by analysis of the ECG signal sensed by the paddles. Good skin contact is essential to overcome the approximately 2,000-ohm (Ω) resistance of the skin, usually by an electrode gel or paste. One paddle is placed over the upper chest and the other over the lower chest, taking care to prevent the electrode gel from forming a bridge between the two paddles. The discharge switches are located in the handles of the paddles, and both must be pressed at the same time to allow the defibrillator to discharge. Assuring that no one is touching the patient prevents unwanted and dangerous shocks to the medical team. The patient is defibrillated, and within seconds, the ECG trace presumably indicates a return to a normal rhythm. Transporting the patient to the hospital for further care is then safe. This system of portable monitoring, telemetry, and defibrillation is a major reason that patients who have heart attacks now survive in greater numbers.

A recent development in the area of defibrillation has been the automatic, implantable device (Mirowski et al. 1980). This type of device can allow patients with very unstable rhythm that is only partially controlled by medication to leave the hospital and resume a more normal lifestyle. This new electronic device is designed to have two electrodes placed on the heart and is programmed to monitor cardiac electrical activity and to recognize ventricular fibrillation. If ventricular fibrillation is sensed, an internal discharge of the device can be triggered. Less energy is required for these pulses because the electrodes are in direct contact with the myocardium. Early experience with this type of device in selected patients has been encouraging, and further work is underway. Accurate sensing of the cardiac rhythm and energy storage to allow repeated discharges if needed is receiving particular emphasis.

Cardiac Monitors

The reduction in mortality of patients with cardiac diseases is related directly to the availability of a modern intensive care unit (Thibault et al. 1980). These units were initially for patients with heart disease, but now many specialized units exist for the special needs of critically ill patients with a variety of problems (Callahan and Bahn 1974). Emphasis here is on cardiac problems, but many other illnesses have been addressed in a similar fashion (Goldenheim and Kazemi 1984).

Continuous monitoring of heart rate and rhythm is essential for all patients in such a setting. Disposable electrodes with adhesive on a foam backing are usually used and are intended to be left in place for days without causing skin irritation. These electrodes are interfaced with a cardiac monitoring system. In its simplest form, this is an oscilloscope that displays the wave form of the ECG. Monitors also include alarm channels that signal when the heart rate falls below or rises above predetermined levels.

The modern monitor in the intensive care unit allows the physician and intensive care unit (ICU) nurse to monitor a series of selectable parameters, including ECG, blood pressure from an arterial line, respiration from transthoracic impedance changes, and temperature from a probe inserted into the nose or placed on the skin. The partial pressure of carbon dioxide at the airway is a parameter measured to assess ventilation. Cardiac output is usually measured by determining the pulmonary blood flow. To avoid inserting an instrument into the body, the disappearance of an inert gas from a rebreathing bag is determined. The rebreathing measure is accurate but requires some patient cooperation if the patient is not on a ventilator; otherwise, it entails an interruption of the ventilator cycle.

In most cases, cardiac output determination employs an indwelling pulmonary artery catheter and the use of thermodilution. In 1970 Swan and Ganz introduced bedside use of balloon-tipped catheters (Figure 3.7). These plastic catheters are usually introduced into a major vein directly, without an incision. They are swept along by the blood into the right atrium, through the tricuspid valve into the right ventricle, and out the pulmonary valve into the pulmonary artery (Figures 3.7b–d). The catheters are very flexible so that the manipulation required is minimal, and x-ray visualization by fluoroscopy is unnecessary. The catheter usually

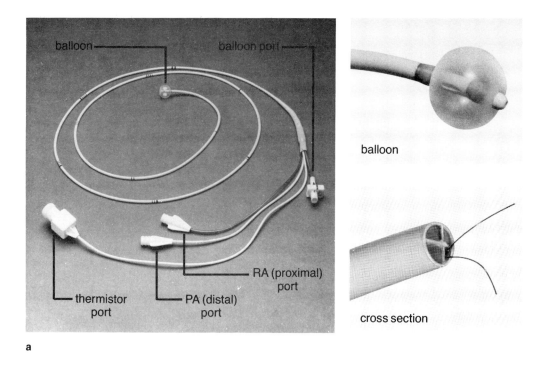

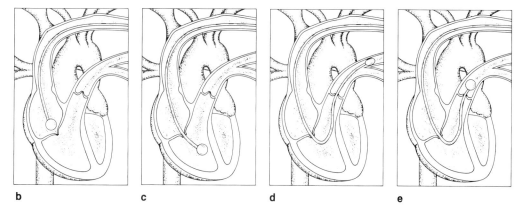

Figure 3.7   Determination of cardiac output. (a) The Swan-Ganz. (b) Right atrial pressure. (c) Right ventricular pressure. (d) Pulmonary artery pressure. (e) Pulmonary capillary wedge pressure. (b-e redrawn from *RN Magazine,* September, 1983).

floats out to a "wedge" position. As the lumen of the catheter is open at its end, and the balloon occludes the vessel farther back, the left atrium pressure is sensed in this position, as reflected in the pulmonary veins. Display of this pressure on the monitor allows analysis for signs of left heart failure. When the balloon is deflated, the pressure wave becomes that of the pulmonary artery, providing valuable information about the status of the right heart.

To measure cardiac output by thermodilution, the Swan-Ganz catheter is adapted by placing a thermistor near its distal end so that it is located in the pulmonary artery in the patient. A second lumen is created with its opening back 20 centimeters (cm) from the tip so that it is in the right atrium. The patient has a small amount of room-temperature or iced saline or dextrose solution injected through the right atrial opening. As the cold fluid passes the thermistor, the temperature drops abruptly and then progressively rises as each heart beat carries it away. This time-temperature curve is recorded, and the area under the curve translated into flow of blood per minute, the standard way of stating cardiac output. In practice, a microprocessor-controlled device connected to the thermistor computes and displays the cardiac output almost immediately after completion of the injection.

A recent addition to the intensive care unit is the central computer for continuous surveillance of all parameters, interpretation of the data produced, and appropriate warning of potentially dangerous situations (Feldman et al. 1972). The continuous survey for arrhythmias, for example, ventricular fibrillation or premature ventricular contractions, has great interest today. A decade ago, automated systems for detecting and classifying arrhythmias were still on the drawing board. However, the central computer's capacity to detect, record, store, and indicate the presence of true arrhythmias presently has extensive applications (Green et al. 1983). A typical application is admitting a patient to the ICU, attaching appropriate sensors, and programming the monitoring computer to watch for problems. For example, a patient may be suspected of having a cardiac rhythm disturbance. In an older system, the monitor would trigger an alarm only if the heart rate fell below or rose above the preset levels. If the computer is instructed to analyze the patient's ECG and premature ventricular beats begin, the physician can be alerted to the frequency and site of origin within the heart. Similarly, the blood pressures from the arterial lines and the Swan-Ganz catheter can be plotted and any abnormal trends promptly detected. Now being introduced are computer programs to assess all monitored functions and all laboratory data, including blood pH, gases, chemistry. Given information about medication, they are able to show the effect of all therapy without delay, identifying an abnormal situation promptly and facilitating appropriate action.

The modern intensive care unit depends on microprocessor-controlled monitors and central observation stations. In the early days of cardiac monitoring, patients were connected to the monitor by a series of electrodes, and only the electrocardiogram was displayed on an oscilloscope. As technology progressed, the monitor was connected to a remote station so that the ECG signal was also accessible to a central station, where a single nurse or physician could observe the ECG signals of several patients at the same time. This simple system required the constant presence of a specially trained medical specialist to interpret all of the ECG signals. Obviously when the specialist was at the bedside of one patient in the intensive care unit, the other patients' ECG signals were no longer being observed. This problem led to the develoment of the next type of monitor, which could recognize changes in heart rate.

This second generation of cardiac monitors were basically set to detect the larger voltage of the QRS complex and to count them over a period of seconds. The monitor could be set to alarm with either a flashing light or buzzer if the heart rate as detected by QRS voltage fell below or rose above a predetermined range. Now, the specialist could leave the bedside and the monitor would "watch" the patient. It soon became apparent that this system could lead to many errors. For instance, a patient's QRS voltage on the monitor might fall below the threshold of the monitor for detection because of electrode failure, so that a low heart rate signal would be triggered even if the patient were well. These units were also not flexible enough for complex rhythm disturbances, especially if multiple forms of extra beats, the precursor of ventricular fibrillation, were present.

Currently, the most modern monitoring units are microprocessor-based and modular in concept. They monitor multiple parameters at the same time and detect any alteration from the physician-designated norms for the patient. For instance, as the patient progresses, the physician may wish to observe for a change in QRS morphology and not in heart rate alone; the monitor allows this flexibility.

In the modern monitor, the input voltage is digitized as soon as the signal arrives in the monitor. This digitized signal is now free from signal alternation and allows software control of all information processing. The chip-based microprocessor carries out all functional control-based on user-determined sequences. The data input is organized for analysis and display as a digital signal, and its content is stored for future display or displayed on a priority basis. The data can be reproduced as an analog signal on the oscilloscope or specific information displayed as an alphanumeric message for the specialist.

The modular concept allows study of a series of physiological parameters on the same monitor mainframe. For instance, if all patients in an ICU needed electrocardiographic monitoring but some also needed to be monitored for respiration, blood pressure by arterial line connection, temperature by thermistor probe, and cardiac output by thermodilution, the submodule for the physiological signal input and processing would be plugged into the monitor mainframe and its output integrated into the patient's analysis profile.

The mainframe oscilloscope usually can display up to four dynamic waveforms, so that typically at any one time the ECG, arterial blood pressure, venous blood pressure, and respiration signals may be displayed. Alarm limits can be selected for each parameter and displayed as alphanumeric information. In the microprocessor or controlled monitor, alarms are of two types, medical and technical. A *medical alarm* could detect a fall in systolic blood pressure below a preset level, causing an appropriate alert signal to be sounded and displayed. A *technical alarm* would sound if an ECG electrode were disconnected or if the input voltage of the respirator signal were lost. Its program enables the entire unit to self-test all functions.

The most sophisticated feature of the state-of-the-art monitor is the arrhythmia analyzer. The microprocessor program "recognizes" the basic P–QRS–T morphology of the patient's ECG and "learns" the patient's ECG complex and then applies an algorithm for template correlation. A validation program reduces the problem of artifacts in the signal. The monitor not only recognizes a morphology abnormality but also stores it for future analysis. For example, if a patient has frequent premature ventricular beats, the monitor recognizes each one and assigns it to a template. The total number of each type of abnormal beat is recorded for recall at a later time. The abnormal beats can be recalled one at a time or as a group.

Obviously, a potentially lethal arrhythmia is immediately recognized and an alarm sounded so that prompt therapy can begin. The monitor can not only recall the abnormal rhythm but also display the 10 seconds (s) before that rhythm started so that any predisposing event can be identified and treated as well.

In most modern systems, interfaces with larger computers are integral to the system. The physician or engineer can take the processed digital sound and feed it into a central computer for integration with the other aspects of the patient's care such as laboratory tests and physical findings.

The basic monitoring system calls for hard wire connection of the patient to the monitor. This is acceptable during the acute phase of illness, but as patients recover, their need for monitoring may not lessen. Although patients are encouraged to walk about the hospital, monitoring of their status during this activity is necessary and is accomplished by telemetry.

The modern telemetry unit transmits by frequency modulation (FM) signal two channels of ECG signals simultaneously, enhancing artifact rejection. The central station receives the signal and integrates it into the same analysis program used when the patient is hard-wired. Alarms can be programmed for ECG events recognized as warnings of more major problems, allowing the staff to recall the patient from a walk and avert a potential crisis. As the entire modern monitoring package is microprocessor-based, as with advances in algorithm design, it can be retrofitted as microchips into the existing monitors, providing technology at the patient's bedside in a timely fashion and with minimal delay.

Despite their differences, manufacturers of arrthymia detection systems share a single design goal: accuracy (Nose and Levin 1970; Sadove et al. 1974). An accurate algorithm for monitoring arrhythmia is a must. Various algorithms currently provide a step-by-step computer procedure that divides the arrhythmia detection and classification processes into a number of simpler tasks. These algorithms measure QRS complexes, compare beat intervals, classify individual beats, and determine whether arrhythmias are present. Chapter 7 provides a detailed description of these computerized systems.

One of the most difficult tasks for the computer is the classification of arrhythmia patterns in the presence of artifact. Since errors usually are caused by the misclassification of noise and artifact as arrhythmias, manufacturers are keenly aware of the need to refine algorithms and reduce incidence of error. Consequently the quality of arrhythmia monitoring is judged on the basis of low false alarm rate, high ventricular beat sensitivity, flexible lead configuration requirements, uninterrupted surveillance, second-by-second heart rate update, and advanced information management capabilities that enable the medical staff to calculate drug dosages and hemodynamics.

The fairly recent modular concept is a definite asset for monitoring. Initially when a patient needed more monitoring, the medical staff wheeled in and hooked up additional equipment. A great deal of cumbersome activity arose. But now, with the availability of specifically designed modules, monitoring can be expanded easily. Since these separate plug-in units snap into the main monitor easily, requiring no additional assistance or special tools, they offer many combinations of monitoring capabilities (Figures 3.8, 3.9, and 3.10).

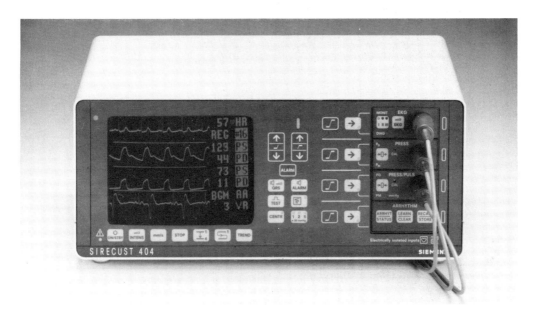

Figure 3.8 Siemens Sirecust 404 monitor with plug-in modules (courtesy of Siemens Medical Systems, Inc., Iselin, N.J.).

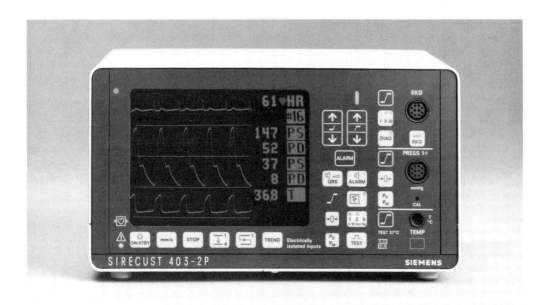

Figure 3.9 Siemens Sirecust 403-2P monitor (courtesy of Siemens Medical Systems, Inc., Iselin, N.J.).

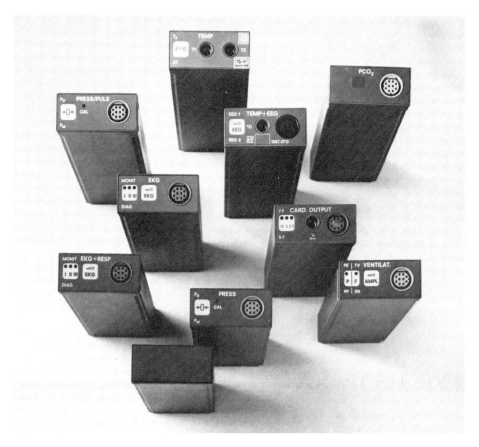

Figure 3.10   Modules that can be plugged into monitor
mainframe (courtesy of Siemens Medical Systems, Inc., Iselin,
N.J.).

Numerous companies provide state-of-the art models of cardiac monitors,
including Hewlett-Packard, Siemens, Litton, Vitatek, Marquette, Physio-control,
and Kontron.

All units display some differences in performance and safety characteristics.
Disadvantages of some monitors offset their advantages. The choice of a hospital's cardiac monitor, therefore, depends on its particular needs and requirements.
The decision to purchase a unit should take into account the features and capabilities needed to optimize patient care.

The Artificial Hearts and Assist Devices

Over 20 yr ago, it became clear to many researchers that some patients with heart
disease could not be aided by medication or surgical repair of their damaged
hearts. The heart valves could be replaced with artificial devices, but the heart
muscle (myocardium) was often so damaged that if it were not replaced, the patient would die. Two separate avenues of research to the problem were initiated.

First, the era of cardiac transplantation began. Kidney and cornea transplants from other humans had proved so successful that cardiac transplantation was studied. Dr. Norman Shumway of Stanford University performed much of the pioneering work. Dr. Christiaan Barnard undertook the first human heart transplant in South Africa on 3 December 1967. Soon, many other centers began their own programs. The most successful center remains Dr. Shumway's at Stanford. Many problems with rejection, donor organ procurement, and infection remain, but considerable progress has been made, and this approach is now an accepted part of cardiac therapy. In 1983, 172 heart transplants were performed in the United States alone, with a 1-yr survival rate of 80 percent (American Heart Association 1984).

The second area of research in the area of cardiac replacement was the development of the artificial heart. This effort was subdivided into two areas: the left ventricular assist device and total cardiac replacement. These two parallel approaches both require close cooperation between the biomedical engineer and the physician and surgeon. The success to date of these efforts are testiment to the great efforts expended by these disciplines (Akutsu 1975; Akutsu and Kloff 1958; *Jama* 1974; Bryson 1974; Gott and Klopp 1974; Harmison 1972).

The first temporary use of a mechanical device to sustain life while the heart was unable to function was the pioneering effort of J. H. Gibbon, Jr., and C. W. Lillehei at the University of Minnesota (Allen and Lillehei 1957). Their group in 1953 initiated cardiopulmonary bypass, leading to the development of open heart surgery. Their device consisted of a pump to maintain blood flow and an oxygenator to permit gas exchange when the heart and lungs were removed from the path of circulation.

The modern heart-lung machine typically consists of a double-roller pump, which propels the blood forward by a squeezing action, and either a bubble or membrane oxygenator. The roller pump is quite effective as a generator of flow, but prolonged use causes mechanical damage to the red blood cells (hemolysis). This damage is acceptable for the short periods of several hours as is typical in open heart surgery but is not suitable for prolonged periods as the damaged red cells release hemoglobin into the bloodstream, causing kidney failure. For longer periods of time, compression of the blood between the walls of flexible chambers as in the natural state is more desirable. With appropriate pressures and materials, these new types of pumps are finding use in the mechanical heart programs. It is important to remember that the materials in these new devices are sensed as foreign to the body. Although they are not rejected as biological tissue, as in the case of the heart transplant, the body does attempt to form clots on their surface (Hershgold et al. 1972). This must be avoided since it can cause the mechanism to fail. Patients with these devices must receive anticoagulants to prevent clotting as long as the mechanical device is in the circulation. Excessive amounts of these medications can promote spontaneous bleeding, producing hemorrhage in such vital organs as the brain and gastrointestinal tract. These anticoagulation precautions are also taken for patients who have received artificial heart valves; these mechanical devices are usually made of stainless steel and pyrolized carbon and would cause clots if the patient were not receiving anticoagulants. In other situations, the materials selected are used to promote clots and a reaction by the body to coat the material completely with the body's own tissue. These materials are used for vascular grafts and for patches within the heart to close a hole caused by a birth defect. In these cases, a knitted Dacron material promotes ingrowth by the body's own tissues. Within 6 wk, the body completely encases the Dacron fibers and uses the patch as the framework for the body's own "patch" (McGoon 1982).

Both the artificial heart and the left ventricular assist devices are extensions of earlier work in the development of the heart-lung machine for open heart surgery. These machines were developed both to pump blood and to oxygenate it during the short (1 to 3 h) period typically needed for repairing a cardiac defect. Because the lungs are not replaced in the artificial heart program, all that is needed is a "simple pump."

In many patients, an episode of coronary artery blockage damages the left ventricle. The left ventricle, which is the pump for the entire body, can be revascularized by coronary artery bypass but often requires time to heal. As the body must be served by the ventricle right after surgery, there can be no rest period. Many patients require temporary assistance, which may be supplied by a left ventricular assist device (LVAD) (Norman 1975). The development of the left ventricular assist device was led by Dr. John C. Norman and colleagues (Norman 1975; Norman and Huffman 1974). These devices provide partial or total support of the circulation. It was found that most patients improved in myocardial function after 96 h, so the devices could be withdrawn when the patient's own heart had sufficiently recovered.

The LVAD, whose trials continue, is based on an initial design by Dr. William Bernhard of the Children's Hospital Medical Center in Boston in collaboration with the engineers of the Thermo-Electron Corporation (Bernhard and La Farge 1969; Bernard et al. 1970). It is air-powered and has two one-way valves (Figure 3.11). The inlet tube is sewn directly into the apex of the left ventricle, replacing a core of myocardium that is removed to make room for the device. The inlet tube is made of pyrolyte carbon, which is durable and does not induce a rejection episode by the heart tissue. The inlet tube is coupled to a series of tubes flexible enough to permit optimum positioning of the LVAD in either the thoracic or abdominal cavity. When the LVAD is removed, the inlet tube is left in place in the apex of the left ventricle and the tubing disconnected, thereby minimizing the trauma to the heart tissues. The LVAD pumping chamber consists of a flexible bladder that deforms to displace a stroke volume of up to 75 milliliters (ml). The pumping chamber is in turn connected to an outflow tube sewn into the side of the aorta as it passes through either the thoracic or abdominal cavity. The aortic connection is designed for complete removal when the LVAD is no longer needed by the patient.

Recently it has been reported that 38 patients received support from the LVAD in a carefully controlled study conducted by Dr. Norman at the Texas Heart Institute. All patients were judged to be beyond help with more conventional therapy. Most of these patients eventually died from their underlying diseases but some have survived. All were shown to have benefited from the use of the device in the sense that their cardiac output was significantly augmented and in those who survived, they owed their lives to the use of this device. Clinical trials continue with improved materials and better understanding of the somewhat limited role of these devices (Pierce et al. 1981).

The LVAD has also been investigated and developed by the Stanford University team headed by Dr. Philip E. Oyler who works in conjunction with the bio-

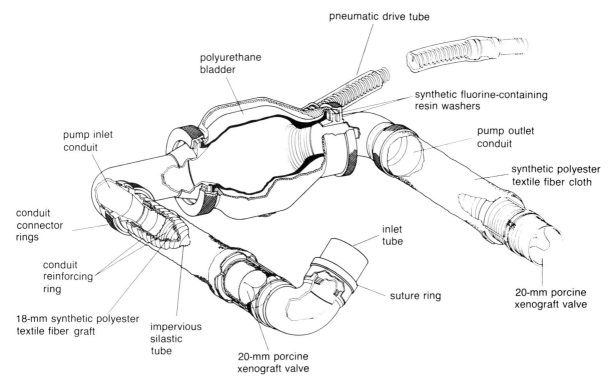

pneumatic drive tube

polyurethane
bladder

synthetic fluorine-containing
resin washers

pump inlet
conduit

pump outlet
conduit

synthetic polyester
textile fiber cloth

conduit
connector
rings

inlet
tube

conduit
reinforcing
ring

suture ring

20-mm porcine
xenograft valve

18-mm synthetic polyester
textile fiber graft

impervious
silastic
tube

20-mm porcine
xenograft valve

Figure 3.11   Design of Model X left ventricular assist device,
now in use and to be clinically tested (from Bronzino, JD:
Technology for Patient Care, St. Louis: C. V. Mosby, 1977).

medical engineering team of the Novacor Medical Research Corporation of Oak-
land, California (1985). Their device, which has Food and Drug Administration
(FDA) approval for experimental use, has already been used in a prototype form in
a human subject. The Stanford LVAD is a two-component system consisting of an
implantable pump and an electronic controller. The pump consists of a seamless
polyurethane bladder that is compressed by two plates. The inflow tube is connected
to the apex of the left ventricle and the outflow tube into the descending aorta. The
device is electrically powered, so that the bulky pneumatic tubing needed for the
Texas device is unnecessary.

In the prototype device that has already been used in one patient, the power
source was external, as was the control mechanism. The control mechanism is designed to sense the heart's own rhythm and directs the pump to function in a coordinated fashion. In the planned new Novacor LVAD, the power supply and electronic controller would be battery-powered and implanted in the patient. The
engineers are developing a microprocessor-based unit to control the pump unit just
as the pacemaker does the heart rhythm.

The power source for the projected Novacor LVAD will do what the prior
units could not do: give the patient the ability to move about freely without a bulky
power console. The unit consists of two induction coils. The secondary coil is im-

planted under the skin and completely encircles the patient's waist. It is connected to implanted rechargable batteries that power the pump. The primary coil is worn outside the skin like a belt above the secondary coil and connects to either the battery pack during ambulatory activity or to a 110-volt (V) source for major charging. Work with the LVAD is continuing to overcome the remaining problems of clot formation and materials fatigue, and this avenue of research promises much for the future.

The second and more highly publicized effort has been in the development and use of the total artificial heart. These devices are designed to replace the damaged heart completely and to support the circulation permanently. Unlike the LVAD, with which the patient's own heart can recover and the support device can be removed, the artificial heart is implanted in place of the patient's own heart, which is then discarded. The only alternative available at this point would be a heart transplant.

T. Akutsu and W. J. Kolff performed in 1957 the first animal heart replacement at the Cleveland Clinic (Kolff et al. 1975; Kolff 1975). That animal survived for only 90 min but started an era of research. In 1963, the National Advisory Heart Council gave priority to this type of research, as well as the necessary federal funding. Areas of concentration included materials, driving mechanisms, and control systems (Kusserow 1958; Lindgren 1965; Norman 1975a; Roe 1969).

In 1969 enough progress had been made that Dr. Denton Cooley of the Texas Heart Institute in Houston implanted an artificial heart into a patient awaiting heart transplantation whose own heart had failed. This revolutionary device sustained the patient for 64 h, until a suitable donor heart could be found and the heart transplant could take place. This type of temporary artifiical heart was again used in a similar circumstance by Dr. Cooley in 1981 for 54 h. Both of these uses were described as temporary. The work of Dr. William C. DeVries and Dr. Robert K. Jarvik, supported by Dr. W. J. Kolff at the University of Utah initially and now at the Humana Heart Institute in Louisville, Kentucky, has led to the use of a permanent artificial heart (DeVries et al. 1984).

The artificial heart used by this group, the Jarvik-7, consists of two pneumatically powered spherical ventricles with attached atria and great vessels that are sewn to the remnants of the patient's own atria, aorta, and pulmonary artery. Air is pulsed into the ventricular air chambers, which compress the blood-filled ventricles. These chambers, which contact the blood, are constructed of polyurethane and have a stroke volume of 100 mL. The first heart used in Utah had four tilting-disk valves of pyrolytic-carbon and of the Bjork-Shiley design (Shiley Laboratories); the subsequent device used in Kentucky utilized the monostrut Medtronic-Hall valve, which was considered more durable. The connections to the atria are made of Dacron felt and to the great vessels, Dacron vascular prosthetic graft. The air drive lines are of reinforced polyurethane tubing encased at the skin level in Dacron velour to enhance tissue ingrowth to secure the lines during patient movement more effectively.

The air drive unit allows for the different pressures and frequencies needed for the artificial left and right ventricles. In practice, the unit has typically been set to deliver up to 7 liters (L) of blood flow per minute from each ventricle. The *ejection fraction,* or percentage of blood emptied from the ventricle with each beat, is usually about 65 percent. A higher ejection fraction is possible but may cause damage to the blood.

During the first clinical use of the Jarvik-7 heart, one of the artificial valves suffered a break in one of its support struts, and the patient returned to the operating room, where Dr. DeVries replaced the entire left artificial heart. This operation was facilitated by a modular concept with quick connect-disconnect coupling.

The pneumatic drive unit is controlled electrically and is backed up by rechargeable batteries that allow the unit to continue to function even if regular electricity fails. A second, small portable drive unit has been used in Kentucky. This portable unit allows the patient to have considerable mobility for up to 4 h, the safe limit for the current unit's batteries.

While the implantation of the Jarvik-7 heart continues in Louisville, the design team of Symbion, the firm in Salt Lake City headed by Dr. Robert Jarvik, works on the successor model, the Jarvik-8. The redesign is addressing the major problems of the Jarvik-7: clotting, size, durability, and "mass" production (Lavin 1985).

The clotting problem can be approached two ways. The first is to use anticoagulants as already discussed, but this practice makes the patient susceptible to bleeding at other sites in the body. The second is to use materials that are less thrombogenic (are less likely to stimulate clot formation). This approach is the subject of much research in materials for implantation and is by no means a problem with an easy solution. The development of new, less reactive, more durable materials will be one of the keys to future of the artificial heart program.

The size of the Jarvik-7 artificial heart has limited its use to adults weighing at least 150 lb. Its shape, determined by engineering considerations, requires atrial cuffs of a relatively large size. The Jarvik-8 heart will have three sizes, the smallest suitable for a person of about 100 lb. This new size will allow the use of the artificial heart for the first time in women and smaller men. There are still no plans for an artificial heart for children.

The future of the artificial heart program depends on the success of the current trials in Louisville and on the production of the heart in numbers sufficient for demand. The Jarvik-7 model is a hand-built device unsuitable for production in large numbers. The Jarvik-8 will be produced in an almost assembly-line fashion to overcome the problems of quality control that hand-built individual components often have. The new production method will make sufficient numbers of artificial hearts available as more implantation teams are trained in its use. Plans are now being developed to train teams in ten centers around the country to select the patients, implant the artificial hearts, and provide the needed postoperative patient care.

Both the total artificial heart and the LVAD face similar engineering problems. Materials for their construction must be durable as they are truly life-sustaining. Their mechanisms must safely pump blood but should not damage the delicate cellular elements of the red blood cells. Most importantly, these devices should allow for a reasonable and tolerable lifestyle. Blood can be protected by nonocclusive pumps and anticoagulants, but the patient's own long-term responses to such devices must be borne in mind at all times. Further development should address the engineering aspects not only for function but also for their impact on lifestyle.

The future of the biomedical engineer in the treatment of patients with cardiovascular disease will emphasize both the prevention of disease and the treatment of exisiting problems. Prevention of cardiovascular disease calls for better education of the entire population, especially the young. The bioengineer can assist by developing low-cost, reliable fitness monitors that will tell individuals at play and at work the level at which they are performing. These devices could be worn like wristwatches and could monitor heart rate and rhythm, blood gases, and metabolic level. They could be preset to monitor a day or a week at a time and could at the desired intervals tell individuals how much work the heart has done and how many calories were used and in what manner. The technology needed for such a device already exists; only its application is wanting.

The treatment of cardiovascular disease will be the forte of evolving teams of physicians, surgeons, and biomedical engineers. The diagnosis will be based on accurate monitoring and prompt interpretation of all cardiovascular parameters, often by computer to assist in timely diagnosis. The therapy for patients with disease will still largely be medication, but as better devices and materials become widely available, the goal of full restoration of a normal lifestyle could be accomplished. Power sources to drive artificial hearts and pacemakers will be improved, so that replacement for reasons of power depletion will not longer be a factor. Materials will become more durable and will not cause adverse body reactions; component failure will be an oddity, rather than a commonplace. It is likely that heart disease, our now leading killer, could follow the trail of diseases such as measles and diphtheria, becoming an easily treatable problem of the past.

REFERENCES

Akutsu, T. 1975. Artificial heart: Total replacement and partial support. New York: American Elsevier.

Akutsu, T., and Kloff, W. J. 1958. Permanent substitutes for valves and hearts. *Trans Am Soc Artif Intern Organs* 4: 230–232.

American Heart Association. 1984. *Heart facts, 1984*. Dallas: American Heart Association.

Allen, P., and Lillehei, C. W. 1957. Use of induced cardiac arrest in open heart surgery: Results in 70 patients. *Minn Med* 40: 672–676.

An artificial heart that doesn't beat, 1974. *JAMA* 227:735.

Bernhard, W. F., and LaFarge, C. G. 1969. Development and evolution of a left ventricular aortic assist device. In Hastings, F. W. (ed.) *Artificial heart program conference, 1969*. Washington, D.C.: GPO.

Bernhard, W. F., LaFarge, C. G., Husain, M., Yamamura, N. and Robinson, T. D. 1970. Physiologic observations during partial and total left heart bypass. *J Thorac Cardiovasc Surg* 60: 807.

Bjork, V. O. 1984. The Development of the Bjork-Shiley Artificial Heart Valve. *Clin Cardiol* 7: 3–5.

Bryson, F. E. 1974. Countdown for the artificial heart. Machine Design 46: 34–42.

Callahan, J. A., and Bahn, R. C. 1974. Cardiac care unit. In Ray, C. D. (ed.) *Medical engineering*. Chicago: Year Book.

Chardack, W. M., Gage, A. A., and Greatbatch, W. 1960. A transistorized self-contained implantable pacemaker for the long term correction of complete heart block. *Surgery* 48:643–654.

DeSilva, R. A., Graboys, T. B., Podrid, P. J., and Lown, B. 1980. Cardioversion and defibrillation. *Am Heart J* 100: 881–895.

DeVries, W. C., Anderson, J. L., Joyce, L. D., Anderson, F. L., Hammond, E. H., Jarvik, R. K., and Kolff, W. J. 1984. Clinical use of the total artificial heart, *N Engl J Med* 310: 273–278.

Falk, R. H., Zoll, P. M., and Zoll, R. H. 1983. Safety and efficacy of noninvasive cardiac packing, *N Engl J Med* 309: 1166–1168.

Feldman, C. L., Singer, P. J., and Hubelbank, M. 1972. An on-line eight patient heart rhythm monitor. Presented at the International Congress of Cybernetics and Systems, September 1972.

Furnam, S. 1983. Newer modes of cardiac pacing. *Mod Concepts Cardiovasc Dis* 52: 1–10.

Geddes, L. A., and Hamlin, R. 1983. The first human heart defibrillation. *Am J Cardiol* 52: 403–405.

Goldenheim, D. D., and Kazemi, H. 1984. Cardiopulmonary monitoring of critically ill patients. *N Engl J Med* 311: 717–720, 776–780.

Gott, V. L., and Klopp, E. H. 1974. Cardiovascular prosthetics and mechanical assistance. In Ray, C. D. (ed.) *Medical Engineering*. Chicago: Year Book.

Green, H. L., Briller, S. A., Hieb, G. E., Parker, B., and Webb, G. N. 1983. Optimal resources for electrical equipment in critical care areas. *Circulation,* 68: 469A–477A.

Harmison, L. T. 1972. The totally implantable artificial heart, DHEW, Publication No. NIH 74–191, Washington, D.C.: GPO.

Hays, C. V. 1964. The development of the heart pacemaker. *Rose Technic Magazine.* pp. 10, 32–33.

Hershgold, E. J., Kwan-Gett, C. S., Kawai, J., and Rowley, K. 1972. Hemostasis, coagulation and the total artificial heart. *Trans Am Soc Artif Intern Organs* 18: 181–185.

Holcomb, W. G., Glenn, W. L., and Sato, G. 1969. A demand radiofrequency cardiac pacemaker. *Med Biol Eng* 7: 493–499.

Huffman, F. N., Hagen, K. G., Whalen, R. L., Fuqua, J. M., and Norman, J. C. 1974. Intracorporeal heart dissipation from a radioisotope-powered artificial heart. *Cardiovasc Dis Bull Tex Heart Inst* 1: 343–368.

Hyman, A. S. 1932. Resuscitation of the stopped heart by cardiac surgery. II. Experimental use of an artificial pacemaker. *Arch Intern Med* 50: 283–305.

Inter-Society Commission for Heart Disease Resources. 1983. *ICHD code, Circulation* 68(1): 224A–244A.

Judson, J. P., Glenn, W. L., and Holcomb, W. G. 1967. Cardiac of pacemakers: Principles and practices. *J Surg Rev* 7: 527–544.

Kantrowitz, A. F., Gradel, O., and Akutsu, T. 1965. The auxiliary ventricle. IEEE International Conv. Record, p. 12.

Karselis, T. 1973. *Descriptive medical electronics and instrumentation.* Thorofare, N.J.: Slack.

Kerber, R. E., Jensen, S. R., Gascho, J. A., Grayzel, J., Hoyt, R., and Kennedy, J. 1983. Determinants of defibrillation: Prospective analysis of 183 patients. *Am J Cardiol* 53: 739–749.

Kirkendall, W. M., Feinleib, M., Freis, E. D., and Mark, A. L. 1980. Recommendations for human blood pressure determination by sphygmomanometeters. *Circulation* 66: 1146A–1155A.

Kolff, J., Olsen, D. B., and Kolff, W. J. 1975. The mechanical heart on the medical horizon. *Cardiovasc Dis Bull Tex Heart Inst* 2: 265–272.

Kolff, W. J. 1975. Update on aritifical organs. *Cardiovasc Dis Bull Tex Heart Inst* 2: 273–284.

Kusserow, B. K. 1958. A permanently indwelling intracorporeal blood pump to substitute for cardiac function. *Trans Am Soc Artif Intern Organs* 4: 227–230.

Lavin, J. H. 1985. Almost here: The Jarvik-8. *Cardio World News* 1: 22–23.

LV assist systems progressing toward full portable device. 1985. *Cardiol World News* 1: 14.

Lindgren, N. 1965. The artificial heart—exemplar of medical engineering enterprise. *IEEE Spectrum* 2: 67–83.

Ludmer, P. L., and Goldschlager, N. 1984. Cardiac pacing in the 1980's. *N Engl J Med* 311: 1671–1680.

McGoon, D.C. 1982. Long term effects of prosthetic materials. *Am J Cardiol* 50:621–630.

Mirowski, M., Reid, P. R., Mower, M. M., Watkins, L., Gott, V. L., Schauble, J. F., Langer, A., Heilman, M. S., Kolenik, S. A., Fischell, R. E., and Weisfeldt, M. L. 1980. Termination of malignant ventricular arrhythmias with an implanted automatic defibrillator in human beings. *N Engl J Med* 303: 322–324.

Norman, J. C. 1975. The artificial heart: Perspectives, prospects, and problems of a high applied technology. *Cardiovasc Dis Bull Tex Heart Inst* 2: 259–264.

Norman, J. C. 1975. An intracorporeal (abdominal) left ventricular assist device XXII: Precis and state of the art. *Cardiovas Dis Bull Tex Heart Inst* 2: 425–437.

Norman, J. C., and Huffman, F. N. 1974. Nuclear-fueled circulatory support systems III. In Russek, H. I. (ed) *Cardiovascular disease: New concepts in diagnoses and therapy.* Baltimore: University Park.

Nose, Y., and Levin, S. N. (eds.). 1970. Advances in biomedical engineering and modern physics, vol. 3, Cardiac engineering. New York: Interscience.

Pierce, W. S., Parr, G. U. S., Myers, J. L., Dae, W. E., Jr., Bull, A. P., and Waldhausen, J. A. 1981. Ventricular-assist pumping in patients with cardiogenic shock after cardiac operations. *N Engl J Med* 305: 1606–1610.

Roe, B. 1969. Whole-body perfusion with heart-lung machines. In Burford, T. H., and Ferguson, T. B., (eds.) *Cardiovascular surgery: Current practice,* vol. 1, St. Louis: Mosby.

Sadove, M. S., Albrecht, R. F., and Schumer, W. 1974. Monitoring. In *MED equipment buyers guide.* Pittsburgh: Medical Electronics & Data.

Sutton, R., Perrins, J., and Citron, P. 1980. Physiological cardiac pacing, *PACE,* 3: 207–219.

Tacker, W. A., Galioto, F. M., Jr., Giuliani, E., Geddes, L. A., and McNamara, D. G. 1974. Energy dose for human transchest electrical defibrillation. *N Engl J Med* 290: 214–215.

Thevenet, R. P., Hodges, C., and Lillehei, C. W. 1958. The use of a myocardial electrode inserted percutaneously for control of complete atrioventricular block by an artificial pacemaker. *Dis Chest* 34: 621–631.

Thibault, G. E., Mulley, A. G., Barnett, G. O., Goldstein, R. L., Reder, V. A., Sherman, E. L., and Skinner, E. R. 1980. Medical intensive care: Indications, interventions, and outcomes. *N Eng J Med* 302: 938–942.

Thomas, H. E. 1974. *Handbook of biomedical instrumentation and measurement.* Reston, Va.: Reston.

Weirich, W. L., Gott, V. L., and Lillehei, C. W. 1957. The treatment of complete heart block by the combined use of a myocardial electrode and an artificial pacemaker. *Surg Forum* 8: 360–363.

CHAPTER 4

Pulmonary Assist and Measurement Devices

Robert Howard

Director
Biomedical Engineering
Children's Hospital National Medical Center
Washington, D.C.

INTRODUCTION

As functioning units, the lung and heart are usually considered a single complex organ, but because these organs contain essentially two compartments—one for blood, one for air—the tests conducted to evaluate heart function or pulmonary ventilation are usually separate. To provide a measure of the lung's important function of supplying tissue cells with enough oxygen and removing excess carbon dioxide, it is necessary to understand some of the fundamental physiologic concepts that are responsible for normal respiratory function. This understanding will make it apparent that the types of criteria that enable health professionals to determine the relative status of the pulmonary system are quite familiar to the engineer. The physiological variables of major importance, such as partial pressure of the gases present, lung volumes, and gas and fluid flow, have all been measured easily in many physical systems. The technology to monitor them is available. However, in the clinical setting it is extremely important to determine the parameters of importance, measure them accurately, and then present the results in a manner that the clinician can easily interpret. Only by providing an opportunity for clinically oriented engineering professionals to interact with health professionals can these conditions be met.

PULMONARY PHYSIOLOGY

The air we breathe (inspiration) travels through a treelike arrangement of bronchial passages that end in minute sacs called *alveoli*. A gaseous exchange, of oxygen for some of the blood's carbon dioxide, takes place at the alveolar surface, which consists of a mesh of fine blood capillaries. For this exchange to occur, the partial pressure of oxygen (P_{O_2}) in the alveoli must be higher than in the venous blood of the alveolar capillaries, and the partial pressure of carbon dioxide (P_{CO_2}) in the alveoli must also be less than in venous blood.

The gases present in the lungs are oxygen, carbon dioxide, nitrogen, and water vapor. Their partial pressures are normally 104, 40, 549, and 47 mmHg, respectively. These pressures represent average values for resting healthy humans at sea level, and the sum of all the partial pressures must equal the total pressure at sea level (760 mmHg). To meet the demands of the body, feedback mechanisms regulate ventilation to keep the partial pressures at or near these levels. Thus alveolar gas is comparable to a compartment of gas lying between atmospheric air and alveolar capillary blood. Oxygen and carbon dioxide are continuously exchanged with the blood flowing through the alveolar capillaries. The cyclic process of ventilation—the inspiration of fresh air followed by the expiration of some alveolar gas—supplies oxygen and removes carbon dioxide.

This gaseous exchange occurs in a surprisingly short period of time (less than 0.3) because the capillary network has so many branches that it offers remarkably little resistance to the blood. In fact, the 80 milliliters (mL) of blood that enters the lung from the right ventricle during each heartbeat is already returning to the left atrium by the time the heart is ready to experience its next contraction. This 80-mL volume of blood, however, is distributed over approximately 50 to 100 square meters (m^2) of respiratory surface in 300 million alveoli and terminal bronchioles.

Viewing the lungs as an entire unit illustrates that the lungs form elastic sacs within the air-tight barrel (thorax) of the chest. The thorax is bounded by the ribs and the diaphragm, and any movement of these two boundaries usually alters the volume of the lungs. The normal breathing cycle in humans is accomplished by the active contraction of the inspiratory muscles, which enlarges the thorax. This enlargement lowers intrathoracic and intrapleural pressure even further, pulls on the lungs, and enlarges the alveoli, alveolar ducts, and bronchioles, expanding the alveolar gas and decreasing its pressure below atmospheric. As a result, air at atmospheric pressure flows easily into the nose, mouth, and trachea.

Tidal volume (or total ventilation) is normally considered to be the volume of air entering the nose and mouth with each breath (or each minute) at rest, but it can be much larger. On the other hand, *alveolar ventilation* is the useful volume of fresh air that actually enters the alveoli during this time and is therefore obviously always less than total ventilation. The extent of this difference in volume depends primarily on the *anatomical dead space*, the 150- to 160-mL internal volume of the conducting airway passages. The term *dead* is quite appropriate, since no gas exchange occurs across the thick walls of the trachea, bronchi, and bronchioles. Since normal tidal volume is usully about 500 mL of air per breath, one can easily calculate that because of the presence of this dead space, about 340 to 350 mL actually penetrates the alveoli and becomes involved in the gas exchange process.

The lungs always contain some gas; that is, there is always a specific volume present. Residual volume, for example, is the amount of gas remaining at the end of maximal expiration. In addition, some volume of gas can be added to the normal inspiratory or expiratory cycle. For example, *inspiratory reserve volume* is the maximum volume of gas that can be inspired from the end of inspiration position, whereas *expiratory reserve volume* is the maximum amount expired from the end of expiration position. Since the lungs are elastic, they are capable of processing much larger volumes of air; hence the term *lung capacity* (or *compliance*) has been used to define specific inspiratory or expiratory events. All these events represent the storage capability of the lungs. Consider the following terms as a guideline (Comroe 1965; West 1974):

1 *Total lung capacity* (TLC): the amount of gas contained in the lung at the end of maximal inspiration

2 *Forced vital capacity* (FVC): the maximal volume of gas that can be forcefully expelled after maximal inspiration

3 *Inspiratory capacity* (IC): the maximal volume of gas that can be inspired from the resting expiratory level

4 *Functional residual capacity* (FRC): the volume of gas remaining after a normal expiration

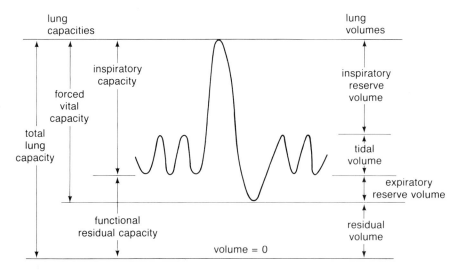

Figure 4.1   Lung volumes and lung capacities.

These volumes and specific capacities represent characteristics that enable one to quantify the status of the pulmonary system.

As Figure 4.1 illustrates, each of the lung capacities comprises two or more lung volumes. With these characteristics defined, it has been possible to design tests that will provide the clinician with information required to diagnose the nature of respiratory dysfunction. These tests provide clues that enable the physician to determine whether a physiological condition is causing inadequate air flow (for example, when air passages are physically blocked by mucus or by bronchoconstriction), inadequate gas exchange (for instance, when the alveoli are affected, as in emphysema), or inadequate blood supply.

These deficiencies may occur singly or in any combination. In addition, some of these conditions affect the total quantity of air, as well as the distribution of the air we may breathe. Others may affect the frequency of breathing and even blood pressure and chemistry. Thus, to establish a complete diagnostic protocol for determining the presence or absence of these conditions, it is necessary to conduct a number of tests (Ray 1974) to investigate the status of both the air and blood components of the system.

THE PULMONARY FUNCTION LABORATORY

The purpose of a pulmonary function laboratory is to obtain clinically useful data from patients with respiratory dysfunction. The pulmonary function tests (PFTs) within this laboratory fulfill a variety of functions. Besides quantifying a patient's breathing deficiency, they are also useful in diagnosing different types of pulmonary diseases. Also, long-term monitoring (repeat testing every few months) helps in determining a patient's response to therapy. With the increasing incidence of lung disease, screening tests of pulmonary function are becoming a routine part of the yearly physical. In addition, many surgical patients undergo presurgery screening PFTs to determine whether the presence of lung disease increases the risk of surgery (Hodgkin 1984). The increased awareness of the usefulness of these tests is partially attributable to the fact that high technology has simplified many tests that previously were complicated research tools. As a result trained technologists in a clinically oriented laboratory can now administer them easily.

Although PFTs can provide important information about a patient's condition, the limitations of these tests must be considered. First, they are nonspecific in that they cannot determine which portion of the lungs is diseased, only that the disease is present. Second, PFTs must be considered along with the medical history, physical examination, x-ray examination, and other diagnostic procedures to permit a complete evaluation. Finally, the major drawback to some PFTs is that they require full patient cooperation and for this reason have not been conducted on critically ill patients. However, in recent years, instrumentation and procedures to measure pulmonary parameters on critically ill patients at the bedside have been developed. These procedures do not require cooperation and can even be performed on the unconscious patient. Further refinement of this instrumentation, including the miniaturization of the breathing circuits, has allowed pulmonary function measurements to be performed in the intensive care nursery with newborn infants weighing as little as 5 lb. (Galioto 1984).

As a result of the technology explosion, the role of the pulmonary laboratory has continued to expand. Since the tests and measurements conducted in this facility are extremely technical, biomedical engineers have become involved not only in the measurement of the parameters of pulmonary function, but also in their interpretation. The biomedical engineer has also been instrumental in the development of new procedures and the application of existing procedures to new patient populations such as the critically ill adult and the premature infant. As these procedures are refined, they can be administered routinely at the bedside and in many instances will play a significant role in the day-to-day treatment of the critically ill patient.

To develop a better understanding of what actually occurs within the pulmonary laboratory, let us consider some of the most widely used PFTs: spirometry, body plethysmography, and diffusing capacity.

Spirometry

The simplest PFT is the spirometry maneuver. In this test, the patient inhales to total lung capacity (TLC) and exhales forcefully to residual volume. Figure 4.2 shows the instrument used for this test, the spirometer. The patient exhales into a

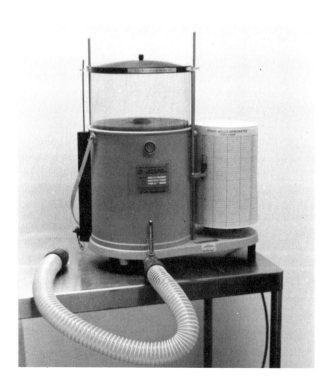

Figure 4.2 Typical water-seal spirometer (courtesy of Children's Hospital National Medical Center, Washington, D.C.).

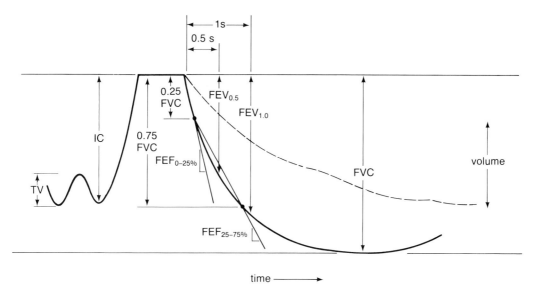

Figure 4.3 Typical spirometry tracing obtained during testing: inspiratory capacity (IC), tidal volume (TV), forced vital capacity (FVC), forced expiratory volume (FEV), and forced expiratory flows. Dashed line represents a patient with obstructive lung disease; solid line represents a normal healthy individual.

displacement bell chamber that sits on a water seal. As the bell rises, a pen coupled to the bell chamber inscribes a tracing on a rotating drum. The spirometer offers very little resistance to breathing; therefore, the shape of the spirometry curve is purely a function of the patient's lung compliance, chest compliance, and airway resistance. Also, over a large range of the expiration, the expired flow is independent of the expiratory effort. At high lung volumes a rise in intrapleural pressure results in greater expiratory flows. However, at mild lung volumes and low lung volumes the expiratory flow is constant (independent of effort) after a certain intrapleural pressure is reached.

Measurements made from the spirometry curve can determine the degree of a patient's ventilatory obstruction (Ruppel 1975). In addition to forced vital capacity (FVC), forced expiratory volumes (FEV) and forced expiratory flows (FEF) can be determined. The FEV indicates the volume that has been exhaled from TLC for a particular time interval. For example, $FEV_{0.5}$ is the volume exhaled during the first half second of the forced expiration, and $FEV_{1.0}$ is the volume exhaled during the first second of expiration; these are graphically represented in Figure 4.3. Note that the more severe the ventilatory obstruction, the lower the timed volumes ($FEV_{0.5}$ and $FEV_{1.0}$). The FEF is a measure of the average flow (volume/time) over specified portions of the spirometry curve and is represented by the slope of a straight line drawn between volume levels. The average flow over the first quarter of the forced expiration is the $FEF_{0-25\%}$, whereas the average flow over the middle 50 percent of the FVC is the $FEF_{25-75\%}$. These values are obtained directly from the spirometry curves. The less steep curves of obstructed patients would result in lower values, of $FEF_{0-25\%}$ and $FEF_{25-75\%}$.

Usually, one compares the measured values of FVC, $FEV_{0.5}$, $FEV_{1.0}$, $FEF_{0-25\%}$, and $FEF_{25-75\%}$ to normal values, which are predicted on the basis of the patient's sex, age, and height. Equations for normal values are available from statistical analysis of data obtained from a normal population. Test results are then interpreted as a percentage of normal.

Another way of presenting a spirometry curve is as a flow-volume curve; Figure 4.4 represents typical flow-volume curve. The expiratory flow is plotted against the exhaled volume, indicating the maximum flow that may be reached at each degree of lung inflation. Since there is no time axis, a timer must mark the $FEV_{0.5}$ and $FEV_{1.0}$ on the tracing. To obtain these flow-volume curves in the laboratory usually the patient exhales through a *pneumotach*. The most widely used pneumotach measures a pressure drop across a flow-resistive element (Sullivan 1984). The resistance to flow is constant over the measuring range of the device; therefore, the pressure drop is proportional to the flow through the tube. This signal, which is indicative of flow, is then integrated to determine the volume of gas that has passed through the tube.

Another type of pneumotach is the heated element type. In this device, a small heated mass responds to air flow by cooling. As the element cools, a greater current is necessary to maintain a constant temperature. This current is proportional to the air flow through the tube. Again, to determine the volume that has passed through the tube, the flow signal is integrated. As with the spirometric data, data from the normal population has also been obtained for peak flow,

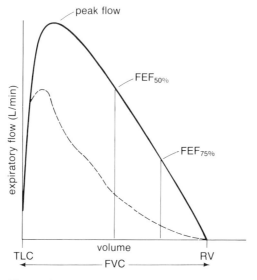

Figure 4.4   Flow-volume curve obtained from a spirometry maneuver. Solid line is a normal curve; dashed line represents a patient with obstructive lung disease.

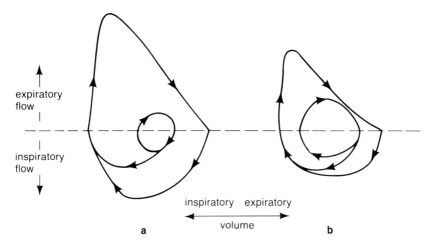

Figure 4.5 Typical flow-volume loops. (a) Normal flow-volume loop. (b) Flow-volume loop of patient with obstructive lung disease.

$FEF_{50\%}$ and $FEF_{75\%}$, which are obtained from flow-volume curves. The flow-volume loop in Figure 4.5 is a more dramatic representation of the flow-volume curve. Here the inspiratory and expiratory curves for both normal breathing and for maximal breathing are displayed. The result is a graphical representation of the patient's reserve capacity in relation to normal breathing. For example, the normal patient's tidal breathing loop is small compared to the patient's maximum breathing loop. During times of stress, this tidal breathing loop can be increased to the boundaries of the outer ventilatory loop. This increase in ventilation provides the greater gas exchange needed during the stressful situation. Compare this condition to that of the patient with obstructive lung disease. Not only is the tidal breathing loop larger than normal, but the maximal breathing loop is smaller than normal. The result is a decreased ventilatory reserve, limiting the individual's ability to move air in and out of the lungs. As the disease progresses, the outer loop becomes smaller, and the inner loop becomes larger.

The advent of microprocessor technology has simplified the job of the pulmonary technician. For example, the Spiromate AS-500 in Figure 4.6 utilizes a microcomputer to integrate the flow from the pneumotach; calculate the patient's FVC, $FEV_{1.0}$, peak expiratory flow, and $FEF_{25-75\%}$; calculate the predicted values for these parameters; and report the measured values as a percentage of the predicted values. All of this information, formerly derived by hand, is now automatically provided to the technician at the end of the test. Several manufacturers also provide PFT systems that are interfaced to a standard microcomputer or minicomputer (Figures 4.7 and 4.8). These systems are usually capable of plotting flow-volume loops as part of their report.

As previously mentioned, the primary use of spirometry is in detection of obstructive lung disease. The more severe the patient's obstructive disease, the smaller the timed volumes and measured flows during the forced expiration. Obstructive

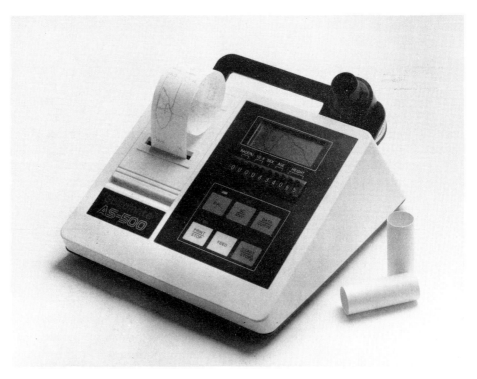

Figure 4.6   The Spiromate AS-500 computerized spirometer uses microprocessor technology (courtesy of RIKO Medical & Scientific Instrument Corp., Lake Success, N.Y.).

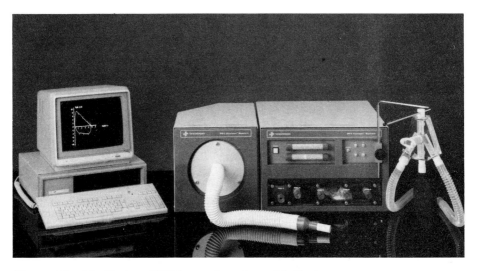

Figure 4.7   The Horizon PFT System from SensorMedics is based on the T.I. PRO microcomputer (courtesy of SensorMedics, Anaheim, Calif).

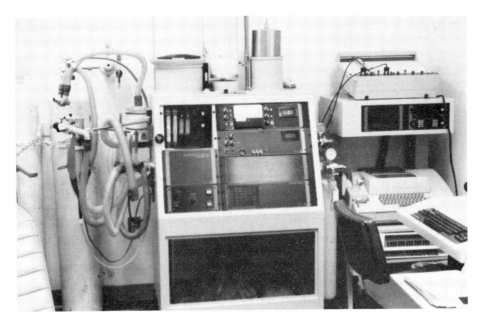

Figure 4.8   Warren E. Collins computerized PFT system
(courtesy of Children's Hospital National Medical Center,
Washington, D.C.).

lung disease results from increased resistance to flow through the airways. This
can occur in several ways:

1 Increased lung compliance (decreased elastic recoil) results in early airway
   closure because of decreased driving pressure during expiration.

2 Decreased airway diameters caused by bronchospasm or the presence of secretions increases the airway's resistance to air flow.

3 Partial blockage of a large airway by a tumor decreases airway diameter and
   causes turbulent flow.

Body Plethysmography

Spirometry has its limitations, however. It can measure only ventilated volumes. It
cannot measure lung capacities that contain the residual volume. Measurements of
TLC, FRC, and RV have diagnostic value in defining lung overdistention or re-
strictive pulmonary disease; the body plethysmograph can determine these absolute lung volumes. Figure 4.9 represents a typical body plethysmograph. The patient is put in an air-tight enclosure and breathes through a pneumotach. The flow
signal through the pneumotach is integrated and recorded as tidal breathing. At
the end of a normal expiration (at FRC) an electronically operated shutter occludes the tube through which the patient is breathing. At this time the patient
pants lightly against the occluded airway. While the patient is performing the pant-

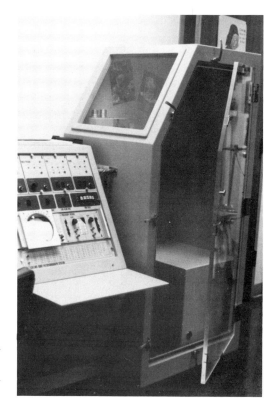

Figure 4.9 Warren E. Collins body plethysmograph (courtesy of Children's Hospital National Medical Center, Washington, D.C.).

ing maneuver, the resulting volume and pressure changes in the patient's chest are measured and displayed on an XY oscilloscope. The slope of this volume-pressure curve is then used to calculate the FRC, or the volume of air trapped in the patient's lungs (DuBois 1956a).

The body plethysmograph can also measure the airway resistance of a patient. The airway resistance maneuvers (DuBois et al. 1956b) are combined with lung volume maneuvers into one procedure. While in the air-tight enclosure the patient first breathes through a pneumotach and then performs the panting maneuver against the occluded airway. While the individual is breathing through the pneumotach, a relationship between the flow through the pneumotach and the degree of lung inflation is measured. Then, while the patient pants against the closed airway, the ratio of intrathoracic pressure to lung inflation is described. Combining these two relationships allows the patient's airway resistance (the ratio of alveolar pressure to air flow) to be calculated.

Airway resistance is generally measured and reported during inspiration and is increased in patients with asthma, bronchitis, and upper respiratory tract infections. However, in patients with pure emphysema, inspiratory airway resistance is normal, since the causes of increased expiratory airway resistance are decreased driving pressures and the resulting airway collapse phenomena. Airway resistance may also be used to determine the response of obstructed patients to bronchodilator medications.

Diffusing Capacity

So far, the mechanical components of air flow through the lungs have been discussed. Another important parameter is the *diffusing capacity* of the lung, the rate at which oxygen or carbon dioxide travel from the alveoli to the blood (or vice versa for carbon dioxide) in the pulmonary capillaries. Diffusion of gas across a barrier is directly related to the surface area of the barrier and inversely related to the thickness. Also, diffusion is directly proportional to the solubility of the gas in the barrier material and inversely related to the molecular weight of the gas.

Lung diffusing capacity (D_L) is usually determined for carbon monoxide but can be related to oxygen diffusion. The popular method of measuring carbon monoxide diffusion utilizes a rebreathing technique (Sackner et al. 1975) in which the patient rebreathes rapidly in and out of a bag for approximately 30 s. Figure 4.10 illustrates the test apparatus. The patient begins breathing from a bag containing a known volume of gas consisting of 0.3 to 0.5 percent carbon monoxide made with heavy oxygen, 0.3 to 0.5 percent acetylene, 5 percent helium, 21 percent oxygen, and a balance of nitrogen. As the patient rebreathes the gas mixture in the bag, a modified Perkin-Elmer mass spectrometer (Figure 4.11) continuously analyzes it during both inspiration and expiration. During the rebreathing procedure the carbon monoxide disappears from the patient-bag system; the rate at which this occurs is a function of the lung diffusing capacity. The helium is inert and insoluble in lung tissue and blood and equilibrates quickly in unobstructed patients, indicating the dilution level of the test gas. Acetylene, on the other hand, is soluble

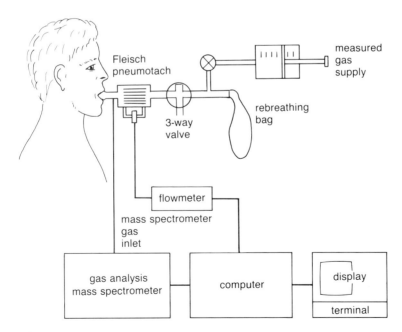

Figure 4.10 Typical system configuration for the measurement of rebreathing pulmonary diffusing capacity.

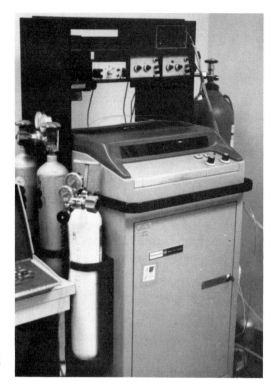

Figure 4.11 Perkin-Elmer MGA-
1100 mass spectrometer (courtesy of
Children's Hospital National Medical
Center, Washington, D.C.).

in the blood and is used to determine the blood flow through the pulmonary capillaries.

Decreased lung diffusing capacity can occur from the thickening of the alveolar membrane or the capillary membrane as well as the presence of interstitial
fluid from edema. All of these abnormalities increase the barrier thickness and
cause a decrease in diffusing capacity. In addition, a characteristic of specific lung
diseases is impaired lung diffusing capacity. For example, fibrotic lung tissue exhibits a decreased permeability to gas transfer, whereas pulmonary emphysema results in the loss of diffussion surface area.

RESPIRATORY THERAPY

With the increasing incidence of respiratory and cardiopulmonary diseases, the
technical specialty of respiratory therapy has evolved (Leggitt 1984). As hospitals
see increasing numbers of patients with these diseases, and as new instrumentation
and treatment modalities continually develop, the hospital's physicians and nurses
rely on the assistance of the respiratory therapist, a highly skilled technical specialist (Burford 1984). These individials undergo training that includes anatomy and
physiology (with emphasis on cardiopulmonary disorders and treatments); the
fundamentals of physics, air flow dynamics, chemistry, and pharmacology; and

the operating principles of the instrumentation used in their routine treatment of patients.

At least 20 percent of the patients seen at a general hospital require respiratory treatment or support (Egan 1977). Therefore, every general hospital has some form of respiratory therapy coverage. Typical services provided by a respiratory therapy department include the following:

1 Administration of oxygen to patients who cannot maintain adequate oxygen levels in their blood when breathing air

2 Administration of humidified air or oxygen to alleviate a variety of respiratory symptoms and to maintain adequate moisture levels in the patient's airways

3 Administration of bronchodilator medication in aerosol form to reverse breathing difficulty resulting from airway obstruction caused by bronchitis, bronchospasm, or excessive secretions in the airways

4 Performance of chest physical therapy, or postural drainage, to break up and remove secretions and mucus from the lungs (usually performed in conjunction with bronchodilator therapy)

5 Development of pulmonary rehabilitation programs for disabled patients, including training in breathing exercises and providing supplemental oxygen to allow ambulation

6 Performance of pulmonary function testing (many hospitals include the pulmonary function laboratory within the respiratory therapy department)

7 Mechanical ventilation of patients who are unable to breathe without assistance

Accomplishing these tasks requires a wide variety of instrumentation. For example, when patients are mechanically ventilated, the air they receive is blended with oxygen to deliver the prescribed oxygen level. This gas is then heated to body temperature and 100 percent humidified before being delivered to patients. At the same time, patients may be receiving aerosol medication through the ventilator circuit. Also, to provide an optimal response of patients' physiologic systems, ventilator controls must be set properly for tidal volume, breath rate, airway pressure limits, and the ratio of inspiratory time to expiratory time (I/E ratio). Patient response is determined by monitoring such physiological parameters as arterial blood gases, mean airway pressure, heart rate, arterial and central venous blood pressures, and cardiac output (Taylor 1978).

One of the most complex pieces of equipment the therapist uses is the ventilator. There are three categories of ventilators, the negative pressure ventilator, the positive pressure ventilator, and the high-frequency jet ventilator (Egan 1977; McPherson 1977; Chatburn 1984). The negative pressure ventilator forces air into the patient's lungs by creating a negative pressure around the patient's chest. This negative external pressure forces the expansion of the thoracic cavity, and air rushes into the stretched lungs (Figure 4.12). The negative pressure ventilator has been called a *tank ventilator* and the "iron lung" because of its physical characteristics (Figure 4.13). It was used extensively in the fifties to support polio victims and still has limited use, for example,

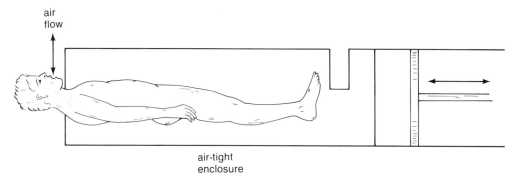

Figure 4.12 Negative pressure ventilator.

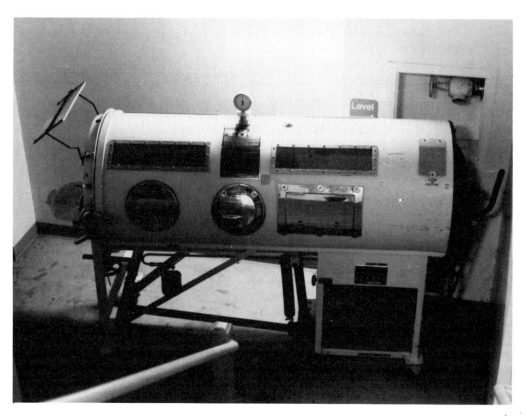

Figure 4.13 Negative pressure tank ventilator, or "iron lung" (courtesy of Children's Hospital National Medical Center, Washington, D.C.).

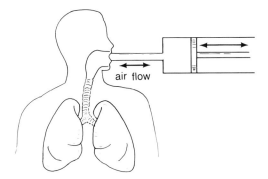

Figure 4.14 Positive pressure ventilator.

to ventilate patients suffering from neuromuscular diseases who cannot perform the muscular maneuvers required to expand their chest. These patients usually have normal lungs and do not require airway suctioning to remove secretions. Therefore, eliminating the need to intubate the patient and eliminating positive airway pressure spares the lung tissues and airways the trauma usually associated with these therapies (Alderson 1984). The major drawback to the negative pressure ventilator is that it greatly limits access to the patient.

The positive pressure device achieves ventilation by applying high-pressure gas at the entrance to the patient's lungs. The gas then flows down the pressure gradient and into the patient (Figure 4.14). With both the negative pressure and positive pressure ventilators, the pressure gradient must be sufficient to overcome the resistive and compliant forces of the lungs and thorax.

The high-frequency jet ventilator is still considered a research tool. This device delivers very rapid, low-volume bursts of air to the lungs. The delivery of oxygen to the lungs and the removal of carbon dioxide are accomplished primarily by molecular diffusion rather than by convection (Figure 4.15). The advantage of using the jet ventilator is the overall reduction of positive pressure in the airways and minimization of barotrauma to the lungs (Chatburn 1984).

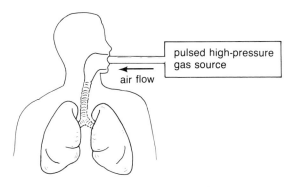

Figure 4.15 High-frequency jet ventilator.

The positive pressure ventilator is by far the most widely used; this type of ventilator, however, requires that the patient be intubated (a tube is inserted into the trachea and the other end is attached to the ventilator breathing circuit). It provides the greatest degree of flexibility in ventilating the patient and allows total access to the patient, who is not enclosed as with the tank ventilator. A wide variety of positive pressure ventilators are available, with many features common to all. For example, most units provide for oxygen delivery from 21 to 100 percent, safety features such as high-pressure and low-pressure alarms, patient disconnect alarms, and power-loss alarms. The alarms are both audible and visual, to alert the staff of a problem quickly. Other common control features allow the therapist to set the tidal volume, the breath rate and I/E ratio, the maximum airway pressure limit, and the baseline pressure (end expiratory pressure).

Most positive pressure ventilators operate in either of two modes, or in some instances, in a combination of the two modes. The first is the *control mode*, or *time cycle mode.* In this mode the ventilator is in total control and breathes for patients at fixed time intervals determined by the control settings. Patients are not allowed to breathe on their own. The second mode is the *assist mode,* or the *patient cycled mode.* Here, patients can initiate a breath by inhaling from the ventilator circuit. The ventilator senses the negative pressure from the maneuver, and breath cycle begins. In this mode, the ventilator is still breathing for the patient, but the patient initiates the breath cycle. Many ventilators operate in an assist/control mode in which a patient can initiate the breath cycle. However, if the patient does not trigger the ventilator within a specified time interval, the ventilator initiates the breath.

Once a ventilator breath is initiated, a method for controlling the inspiratory phase of the cycle is needed. Otherwise, air could be forced into the patient until the lungs ruptured. Several methods control or limit, the inspiratory phase. If the inspiration is terminated when a predetermined airway pressure is reached, the ventilator is pressure-limited. If the inspiratory phase ends after a specific volume is delivered, it is *volume-limited.* And if the inspiratory cycle is determined strictly by timing, the unit is said to be time-limited. Usually, a time-limited or volume-limited ventilator also provides pressure limiting as a safety feature.

Ventilators can be powered either electrically or pneumatically. Typically, pneumatically powered units require a source of compressed air or oxygen at a pressure of 35 to 55 pounds per square inch (psi) to function properly. Electrically powered ventilators deliver pressurized gas with a small rotary compressor or with a motorized piston. Also, independent of the power source, a ventilator can be controlled either electronically or pneumatically. Those ventilators developed most recently incorporate microprocessor control.

The Sechrist IV100 Infant/Pediatric Ventilator in Figure 4.16 is time-cycled and pneumatically powered. An 8085A microprocessor assists its fluidic control system. This unit ventilates the patient by providing a continuous flow through the breathing circuit. Closing and opening the exhalation valve (Figure 4.17) alternately routes this flow to the patient and vents it to the atmosphere. Closing the exhalation valve forces the gas into the patient's lungs. When the exhalation valve is open the patient's exhaled gases leave the circuit along with the continuous gas flow.

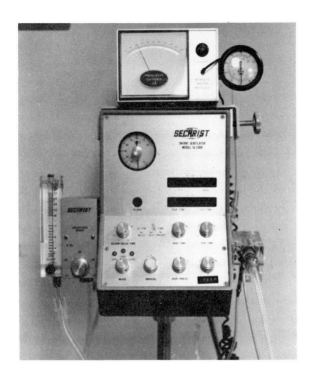

Figure 4.16 Sechrist IV100 infant/
pediatric ventilator (courtesy of
Children's Hospital National Medical
Center, Washington, D.C.).

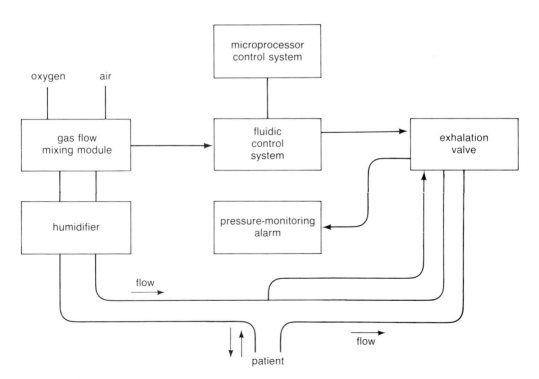

Figure 4.17 Control circuit for Sechrist IV100 infant/
pediatric ventilator (obtained from Sechrist Industries, Inc.,
Anaheim, Calif.).

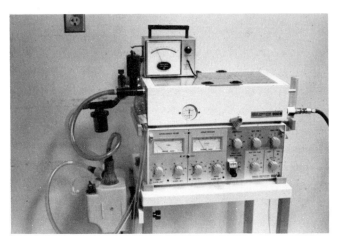

Figure 4.18   Siemens Servo 900B
ventilator with heated humidifier and
oxygen monitor (courtesy of
Children's Hospital National Medical
Center, Washington, D.C.).

Figure 4.18 shows the Siemens Servo 900B ventilator. This unit is pneumatically powered and electronically controlled. Air is delivered to the patient from a spring-loaded bellows (Figure 4.19). The electronic control module monitors the airway pressure and the inspiratory and expiratory flows and operates the inspiratory and expiratory valves on the basis of these readings. The Servo 900B can operate in the control mode, the assist mode, or the assist/control mode, with pressure-limiting capability.

The Bourns Bear 1 adult volume ventilator (Figure 4.20) is a pneumatically powered, electronically controlled device that can be used in control mode, assist mode, or assist/control mode and may be time-, volume-, or pressure-limited. The pneumatic circuit shown in Figure 4.21 is quite complex; this unit incorporates an air compressor for use when external compressed air is not available. It also includes a smaller air compressor to operate a nebulizer circuit.

The ventilators described here are representative of those that are currently available. These units are generally used with auxiliary equipment such as humidifiers, oxygen monitors, and airway pressure monitors. Also, each of the ventilators requires an external source of compressed air or oxygen to function. For this reason, these units are normally used only in hospitals. Recent concern about escalating hospital costs, however, has spurred the development of small, low-cost portable ventilators for home use (Giovannoni 1984). The LP4 ventilator (Figure 4.22) is one of these ventilators; the unit is electrically powered and electronically controlled. A motorized piston alternately draws air in from the atmosphere and then pushes it into the patient. This ventilator can be used in the control or assist mode and can be volume- or pressure-limited. An internal battery provides power when the unit is unplugged, and a larger external battery can be used. The small size of the ventilator and the battery capability make this unit very portable, as it can be easily mounted on a wheelchair. The practice of treating chronic ventilator

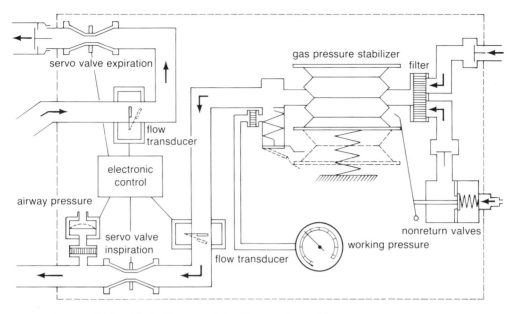

Figure 4.19   Block diagram of the Siemens Servo 900B ventilator (obtained from Siemens-Elema Ventilator Systems, Elk Grove Village, Ill.).

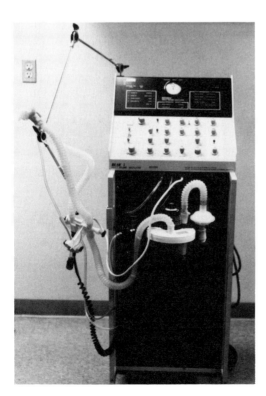

Figure 4.20   Bourns Bear 1 adult volume ventilator with heated cascade humidifier (courtesy of Children's Hospital National Medical Center, Washington, D.C.).

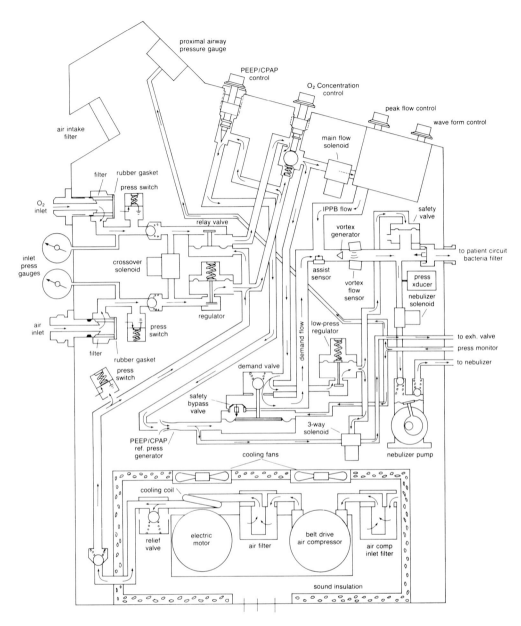

Figure 4.21   Pneumatic circuit of the Bourns Bear 1
ventilator (obtained from Bear Medical Systems, Inc.,
Riverside, Ca.).

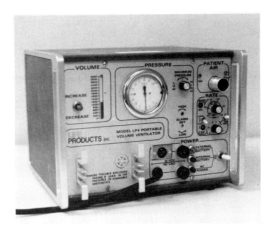

Figure 4.22 Life Products LP4 portable ventilator (courtesy of Children's Hospital National Medical Center, Washington, D.C.).

patients at home has been gaining popularity; however, it does involve a high degree of coordination of the hospital, the physician, the respiratory therapist, and the patient's family.

RESPIRATORY INTENSIVE CARE

The respiratory intensive care unit (RICU) is a special-care nursing unit used to treat patients suffering from acute respiratory insufficiency. These patients' lungs cannot provide adequate gas exchange with the blood without respiratory support. The patients' acute condition usually results from a chronic pulmonary disorder, but it may be caused by a severe respiratory infection in a normally healthy individual. In general, individuals with these disorders are placed in the medical intensive care unit (MICU). Whether in the RICU or the MICU, many of these patients require the use of positive pressure ventilators at some time during their hospitalization. Although ventilator therapy benefits gas exchange, it can have serious adverse effects on other physiological systems (Concepcion 1984; Montenegro 1984).

During a spontaneous inspiration as the chest expands, it produces a negative pressure in the thorax. In addition to causing air to flow into the lungs, this negative pressure increases the flow of venous blood back to the heart. When a patient is mechanically ventilated with positive pressure, however, the intrathoracic pressure is positive during inspiration. This positive pressure impedes the venous return to the heart and causes an increase in the pulmonary vascular resistance (PVR), resulting in a decreased cardiac output. Other complications that result from mechanical ventilation include fluid retention, acid-base imbalance, and pulmonary barotrauma (rupture of the lung tissue). To treat the respiratory disease optimally and to minimize these complications, monitoring not only the ventilatory parameters, but also such hemodynamic parameters as arterial pressure, central venous pressure, cardiac output, and arterial blood gases (Osgood 1984) is necessary.

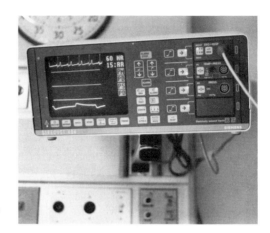

Figure 4.23 Siemens 404 modular physiologic monitor will accept four physiologic parameter cartridges (courtesy of Children's Hospital National Medical Center, Washington, D.C.).

The basic physiological monitoring in the RICU is no different from that in a MICU or in a surgical intensive care unit (SICU). It includes heart rate monitoring, respiration monitoring using impedance pneumography, temperature monitoring, and usually monitoring of two or three invasive blood pressures. Most of the physiological monitoring systems used today provide this capability, with the new generation of monitors incorporating microprocessors. The use of microprocessors enhances the operation of the monitor and provides for future versatility. The Siemens 404 monitor (Figure 4.23), for example, utilizes microprocessor technology. Updates in monitoring techniques can be incorporated simply by replacing the memory chips in the monitor. Also, the modularity of this system accommodates new physiological cartridges as they are developed.

Recent advances in instrumentation have emphasized noninvasive monitoring. Eliminating the need to enter the patient's body minimizes the risk of complications such as infection or embolism formation. Significant advances have been made in the noninvasive measurement of arterial blood gases. Arterial PO_2 and PCO_2 can be measured with an electrode on the skin surface (Hill 1982). Since the measurement is indirect it is technically an approximation of the arterial PO_2 and PCO_2; however, under the proper conditions, the measurements correlate well with the arterial blood gas measurements (Shoemaker 1981; Hazinski 1982). The transcutaneous PO_2 and PCO_2 monitor in Figure 4.24, manufactured by Sensormedics, uses microprocessor techology to simplify calibrations, to stabilize the transducer circuit, and to store and plot the measured values for up to 8 hours (h). This system consists of up to eight remote shuttles that are maintained by one base station. The battery-powered shuttle is placed at the bedside to monitor transcutaneous PO_2 and PCO_2 for 8 h, when it is returned to the base station. There, within a half hour, the battery is recharged, the shuttle is recalibrated, and the last 8 h of data collected is hard-copied in a graphical format.

Two other noninvasive monitors are also available for estimating the oxygenation and the CO_2 levels of the patient's blood. The Nellcor pulse oximeter (Figure 4.25) measures the oxygen saturation of the hemoglobin in the blood. The disposable transducer consists of a bandaid containing two light-emitting diodes and a photodiode that is placed on the finger. The amount of light that is absorbed as it

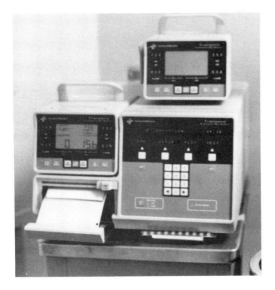

Figure 4.24 Sensormedics transcutaneous P_{O_2} and P_{CO_2} monitoring system, showing two shuttles and one base station. The shuttle on the left is connected to the station for a battery charge and a sensor calibration (courtesy of Children's Hospital National Medical Center, Washington, D.C.).

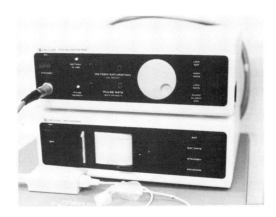

Figure 4.25 Nellcor pulse oximeter for finger measurements of oxygen saturation (courtesy of Children's Hospital National Medical Center, Washington, D.C.).

passes through the finger determines the measured O_2 saturation. The Siemens CO_2 monitor in Figure 4.26 measures the carbon dioxide level in the patient's exhaled gases to estimate the arterial P_{CO_2}. It is attachable to a ventilator circuit and is useful in determining ventilator settings. The sensor is placed in line with the breathing circuit, and infrared radiation is passed through the exhaled gas as it flows through the tube. The amount of infrared absorbed by the gas is proportional to the amount of CO_2 present in the sample (Hill 1982).

Arterial blood gas measurements are important in the treatment of respiratory disease, particularly for ventilator patients, because they indicate how well oxygen is being supplied to, and carbon dioxide removed from, the blood. The noninvasive monitoring devices described, used properly, minimize the number of arterial blood samples that must be drawn and provide continuous monitoring and important trend information with hard-copy recording.

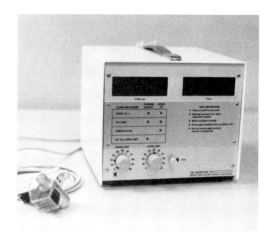

Figure 4.26 Siemens Model 130 infrared CO_2 monitor (courtesy of Children's Hospital National Medical Center, Washington, D.C.).

Another device that has received wide application is the automatic noninvasive blood pressure monitor (Figure 4.27), which monitors arterial blood pressure without cannulation of the patient. A cuff that is automatically inflated and deflated by the monitor at specified time intervals is placed on the patient's arm. During cuff deflation the monitor identifies and amplifies the pressure perturbations in the artery resulting from the restricted pulsatile flow. Identifying the cuff pressures at which these perturbations start and stop as the cuff deflates determines the systolic and diastolic pressures (Hill 1982). Advantages of the automatic blood pressure monitor over the manual method of measurement are that it is more consistent and is not affected by the subjectivity associated with an individual's hearing and technique, particularly when the pressures to be measured are low.

The technology exhibited by these "stand-alone" monitors is becoming routine in many ICUs. As it is refined, these functions will be incorporated into the bedside physiological monitors. For example, the Siemens 404 monitor in Figure 4.23 already has a cartridge for performing infrared CO_2 analysis of expired gases; another cartridge interfaces to the Siemens Servo 900B ventilator (Figure 4.18) to

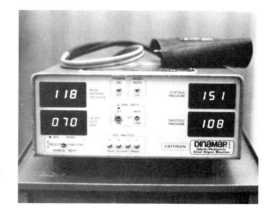

Figure 4.27 Dinamap adult/ pediatric vital signs monitor for noninvasive monitoring of arterial blood pressure (courtesy of Children's Hospital National Medical Center, Washington, D.C.).

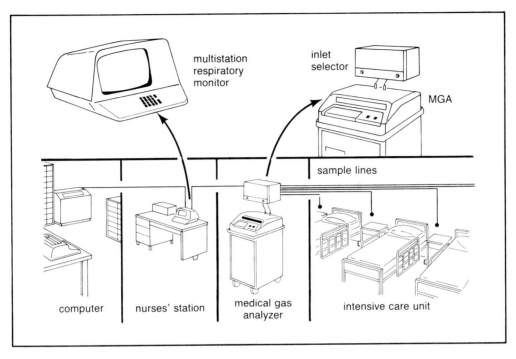

Figure 4.28   Perkin-Elmer RMS-III respiratory monitoring
system (obtained from Perkin-Elmer Corp., Pomona, Calif.).

provide tidal volume and airway pressure measurements. Other manufacturers are
already incorporating transcutaneous PO_2 and noninvasive blood pressure functions into their bedside monitors.

One monitoring system designed primarily for the RICU, is the computerized respiratory gas analysis system, one example being the Perkin-Elmer RMS–III
(Figure 4.28). The heart of this system is a mass spectrometer for measuring the inspired and expired O_2, CO_2, and N_2 gas concentrations for up to 16 patients. Sampling entails computer-controlled sequencing of an automatic valving system. To
supplement the gas analysis, a pneumotach and a pressure transducer can be incorporated at each bedside with their outputs tied to the computer. Now, in addition
to the inspired and expired gas concentrations, such parameters as tidal volume,
minute ventilation, peak airway pressure, mean airway pressure, and breath rate
can be measured. Further, lung mechanics measurements of compliance and airway resistance can be determined at the bedside for each patient. Other capabilities
include the calculation of oxygen consumption (the amount of O_2 used each minute by the patient) and carbon dioxide production (the amount of CO_2 exhaled
each minute by the patient), metabolic parameters that are useful in determining
nutritional needs. This type of respiratory monitoring system will meet many of
the needs of the RICU. It must, of course, be used in conjunction with physiological monitors for heart rate, blood pressures, and body temperature. The computer
control of the system minimizes the staff interaction with the hardware while providing extensive information pertaining to the patient's respiratory status.

With the availability of high technology to the medical field continuing to increase, it is important to remember that the primary goal is good patient care. As the technology explosion continues we must differentiate between instrumentation that simply exploits technology and instrumentation that has a valid and useful place in patient care.

EXTRACORPOREAL MEMBRANE OXYGENATION

As indicated previously, positive pressure ventilation may have adverse effects on other physiological systems. It can also produce permanent lung damage resulting from the prolonged use of high positive pressures. Consequently, an alternative therapy was developed in the early 1970s (Bartlett 1977). This therapy utilized the technology developed for heart/lung bypass during open heart surgery. The procedure requires that blood be removed from the patient, passed through an artificial lung for oxygenation and removal of carbon dioxide, warmed to body temperature in a heat exchanger, and then returned to the patient. As blood is pumped through the circuit, this artificial organ system replaces the functions of the lungs and the heart. The procedure has been well defined and successful for short-term use, that is, for the several hours required for open heart surgery but needed further refinement to make it suitable for long-term cardiopulmonary support. Initial attempts at long-term support resulted in excessive damage to the blood cells in the bubbler oxygenator. The development of the silicone membrane lung minimized the damage to blood cells, and long-term cardiopulmonary support became viable. In this artificial lung, the blood is separated from the oxygen source by a thin silicone membrane (Zapol et al. 1977). As the blood flows through the membrane lung, the gases diffuse across the membrane. Following the partial pressure gradient, the blood is oxygenated and the carbon dioxide is removed. With the use of the membrane lung, the procedure is now referred to as *extracorporeal membrane oxygenation*, or ECMO.

Initially, ECMO was used with both adults and children in cardiopulmonary failure. Early criteria required that the patient have reversible cardiopulmonary disease and be unresponsive to conventional positive pressure ventilation and drug therapies. ECMO did not alter the probability of survival in adult patients (Zapol et al. 1979), possibly because of underlying sepsis that not only limited their response to conventional ventilator therapy, but also limited their response to ECMO (Browdie 1977). The most dramatic results have been obtained with newborn infants with reversible pulmonary disease (German 1980; Hardesty 1981; Kirkpatrick 1983).

Typical disease states that benefit from ECMO are meconium aspiration syndrome (MAS) and persistent fetal circulation (PFC). When the fetus inhales its first stool just prior to birth, MAS results; this foreign matter in the lungs severely impedes ventilation and gas exchange. Pulmonary hypertension causes PFC. To bypass the increased pulmonary vascular resistance, blood flows through the ductus, the pathway for fetal circulation that normally closes at birth. Blood following this route bypasses the lungs and therefore does not undergo gas exchange. In addition, PFC may develop after the surgical repair of congenital diaphragmatic hernia. With both MAS and PFC, reversible disease traumatizes the infant's lungs. Conventional ventilator therapy with high oxygen concentrations and high positive pressure further traumatizes the diseased lungs, causing permanent lung damage. However ECMO therapy oxygenates the patient's blood outside the body, eliminating the need for pulmonary ventilation. While on ECMO, the patient's lungs are allowed to rest and heal themselves. During this time, ventilator settings are decreased to minimum settings to maintain open airways and to aid in the removal of secretions. Within 2 to 3 days the lungs have healed, and the patient is weaned from the ECMO system. Typically, an infant placed on ECMO has less than 20 percent chance of survival with conventional therapy. An infant who survived with conventional therapy would most likely have a chronic pulmonary disability. In contrast, current survival rates for ECMO infants are about 75 percent, and most of these patients leave the hospital as normal, healthy infants.

These results are quite dramatic, but one must remember that significant risk is involved in the procedure. Complications such as intracranial hemorrhage, embolism formation, and sepsis can result in death. Also, excessive bleeding may result from using anticoagulants in the system. The success of ECMO therapy can be attributed to the development of strict entrance criteria for the patient. To qualify for ECMO therapy, the infant must have reversible lung disease and must demonstrate little or no response to high oxygen positive pressure ventilation for a specified time period. Also the infant must not have been on ventilator therapy long enough to sustain permanent lung damage. Therefore, the patient must be identified early after birth, and a timely decision to initiate ECMO must be made. Infants with sepsis, damage to the central nervous system, or other debilitating conditions are not considered for ECMO therapy because the presence of additional medical complications guarantees failure.

The success of ECMO therapy requires the development of a highly trained team of specialists (Wetmore 1979). Typically the "ECMO team" includes surgeons, neonatologists, perfusionists, and trained nurse specialists. The biomedical engineer is also an important member of this team. Initiation of an ECMO program requires a significant amount of time to develop the methodology, test it in the laboratory, and train the team to handle any problem that may develop, whether medical or equipment-related.

Since no "ECMO system" is commercially available, each system is developed to meet the specific medical, environmental, and financial needs of each program. The biomedical engineer's task is to take the basic building blocks and integrate them into a workable system. Figure 4.29 shows a typical ECMO circuit. It consists of a rotary pump to push blood through the external circuit and into the patient, a membrane oxygenator for gas exchange, a heat exchanger and heater to warm the blood to body temperature, and a flowmeter to measure the blood flow through the circuit. The venous cannula empties into a small reservoir before entering the pump head. Since the venous blood flow is determined only by a hydrostatic pressure gradient, servoregulation for the pump is necessary. If the venous return cannot keep up with the pump flow, the blood in the reservoir decreases. The servomechanism (dubbed *venous return monitor* at Children's Hospital) then shuts off the pump until the reservoir is filled. This eliminates the possibility of the pump's pulling a negative pressure on the venous side of the circuit.

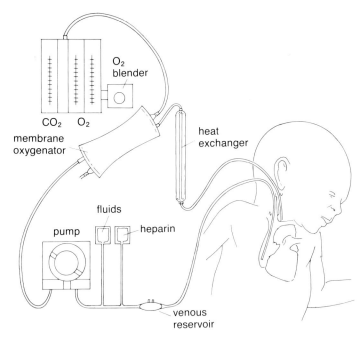

Figure 4.29   ECMO circuit for infants (courtesy of Children's Medical Center, Washington, D.C.).

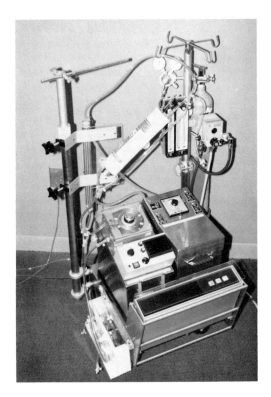

Figure 4.30   ECMO system used at Children's Hospital National Medical Center. (courtesy of Children's Hospital National Medical Center, Washington, D.C.).

The ECMO system developed and used at Children's Hospital National Medical Center is shown in Figure 4.30. At this time approximately ten medical centers in the United States have active ECMO programs. Because of the demonstrated success with ECMO, many medical centers are now looking at it as a viable program. In addition to the development of new ECMO centers, research to refine current ECMO technology and to apply it to new medical situations continues. This provides a challenging opportunity to the biomedical engineer to solve complex problems through the application of basic physical principles.

REFERENCES

Alderson, S. H., and Warren, R. H. 1984. Ventilatory management of muscular dystrophy patients following spinal fusion. *Respir Care* 29:829–832.

Bartlett, R. H., Gazzaniga, A. B., Fong, S. W., Jeffries, M. R., Roohk, H. V., and Haiduc, N. 1977. Extracorporeal membrane oxygenator support for cardiopulmonary failure: Experience in 28 cases. *J. Thorac Cardiovasc Surg* 73(3):375–386.

Browdie, D. A., Deane, R., Shinozaki, T., Morgan, J., DeMeules, J. E., Coffin, L. H., and Davis, J. H. 1977. Adult respiratory distress syndrome (ARDS), sepsis, and extracorporeal membrane oxygenation (ECMO). *J Trauma*, 17(8):579–586.

Burford, J. G., and George, R. B. 1984. Some recent advances in respiratory therapy. *Respir Ther* 14(3):17–28.

Chatburn, R. L. 1984. High frequency ventilation: A report on a state of the art symposium, *Respir Care* 29:839–849.

Comroe, J. H., Jr. 1965. *Physiology of Respiration*. Chicago: Year Book.

Concepcion, I. 1984. Ventilatory support in ARDS. *Respir Ther* 14(1):53–61.

DuBois, A. B., Botelho, S. Y., Bedell, G. N., Marshall, R., and Comroe, J. H., Jr. 1956. A rapid plethysmographic method for measuring thoracic gas volume. *J Clin Invest* 35:322–326.

DuBois, A. B., Botelho, S. Y., and Comroe, J. H., Jr. 1956. A new method for measuring airway resistance in man using a body plethysmograph. *J Clin Invest* 35:327–335.

Egan, D. F. 1977. *Fundamentals of respiratory therapy,* (3d ed.). St. Louis: Mosby.

Galioto, F. M., Jr., Brudno, S., Rivera, O., and Howard, R. P. 1984. Use of the rebreathing method in differential diagnosis of congenital heart disease and persistent fetal circulation. *J Cardiol* 54:1305–1309.

German, J. C., Worcester, C., Gazzaniga, A. B., Huxtable, R. F., Amlie, R. N., Brahmbhatt, N., and Bartlett, R. H. 1980. Technical aspects in the management of the meconium aspiration syndrome with extracorporeal circulation. *J Pediatr Surg* 15(4):378–383.

Giovannoni, R. 1984. Chronic ventilator care: From hospital to home, *Respir Ther* 14(4):29–33.

Gray, B. N. 1975. Pulmonary function testing. *Med Electron Data* 36:33–37.

Hardesty, R. L., Griffith, B. P., Debski, R. F., Jeffries, M. R., and Borovetz, H. S. 1981. Extracorporeal membrane oxygenation: Successful treatment of persistent fetal circulation following repair of congenital diaphragmatic hernia. *J Thorac Cardiovasc Surg* 81(4):556–563.

Hazinski, T. A., and Severinghaus, J. W 1982. Transcutaneous analysis of arterial P_{CO_2}. *Med Instrum* 16(3):150–153.

Hill, D. W., and Dolan, A. M. 1982. *Intensive care instrumentation,* (2d ed.). New York: Grune and Stratton.

Hodgkin, J. E. 1984. Preoperative assessment of respiratory function. *Respir Care* 29:496–503.

Kirkpatrick, B. V., Krummel, T. M., Mueller, D. G., Ormazabal, M. A., Greenfield, L. J., and Salzberg, A. M. 1983. Use of extracorporeal membrane oxygenation for respiratory failure in term infants. *Pediatrics*, 72(6):872–876.

Leggitt, M. S. 1984. Facility report: Respiratory therapy department at Hartford Hospital. *Respir Ther* 14(3):43–46.

McPherson, S. P. 1977. *Respiratory therapy equipment*. St. Louis: Mosby.

Montenegro, H. D. 1984. Complications of mechanical ventilation. *Respir Ther* 14(5):20–27.

Osgood, C. F., Watson, M. H., Slaughter, M. S., and McIntyre, N. R. 1984. Hemodynamic monitoring in respiratory care. *Respir Care* 29:25–34, 1984.

Pulmonary terms and symbols: A report of the ACCP-ATS Joint Committee on Pulmonary Nomenclature. 1975. Chest 67:583–593.

Ray, C. 1974. Instrumentation for pulmonary function. In *Medical Engineering*. Chicago: Year Book.

Ruppel, G. 1975. *Manual of pulmonary function testing*. St. Louis: Mosby.

Sackner, M. A., Greeneltch, D., Helman, M. S., Epstein, S., and Atlins, N. 1975. Diffusing capacity, membrane diffusing capacity, capillary blood volume, pulmonary tissue volume, and cardiac output measured by a rebreathing technique. *Am Rev Respir Dis* 3:157–165.

Shoemaker, W. C., and Vidyasagar, D. (eds.). 1981. Transcutaneous O_2 and CO_2 monitoring of the adult and neonate. *Crit Care Med* (symposium issue) 9(10):689–760.

Sullivan, W. J., Peters, G. M., and Enright, P. L. 1984. Pneumotachographs: Theory and clinical application. *Respir Care* 29:736–749.

Taylor, J. P. 1978. *Manual of respiratory therapy*, (2d. ed.). St. Louis: Mosby.

West, J. B. 1974. *Respiratory physiology - the essentials*. Baltimore: Williams and Wilkins.

Wetmore, N. E., Bartlett, R. H., Gazzaniga, A. B., and Haiduc, N. J. 1979. Extracorporeal membrane oxygenation (ECMO): A team approach in critical care and life support research. *Heart Lung* 8(2):288–295.

Zapol, W. M., Snider, M. T., Hill, J. D., Fallat, R. J., Bartlett, R. H., Edmunds, L. H., Morris, A. H., Pierce, E. C., II, Thomas, A. N., Proctor, H. J., Drinker, P. A., Pratt, P. C, Bagniewski, A., and Miller, R. G., Jr. 1979. Extracorporeal membrane oxygenation in severe acute respiratory failure: A randomized prospective study. *JAMA* 242(20):2193–2196.

Zapol, W. M., Snider, M. T., and Schneider, R. C. 1977. Extracorporeal membrane oxygenation for acute respiratory failure. *Anesthesiology* 46(4):272–285.

CHAPTER 5

Neurophysiological Measurements

George V. Kondraske, Ph.D.

The University of Texas at Arlington
Arlington, Texas

INTRODUCTION

One by one, the mysteries that underlie the function of the human nervous system, especially the brain, are beginning to be unraveled. After many years of intense interest and significant research efforts, progress in deciphering some of the complex communication mechanisms involved in many aspects of brain function, such as memory, consciousness, imaging, and voluntary and involuntary control of all body functions, is being made. Recently, progress has been directly related to the development of sophisticated probes and analytical tools and the vision of astute scientists and engineers willing to take advantage of such technological innovations.

Of particular note, the digital computer has provided the processing and storage capabilities necessary to reduce masses of information to interpretable forms. The digital systems that permit computerized axial tomography (CAT) scans and facilitate measurement of evoked responses (discussed in a later section) emplify the many computer-based systems that have had dramatic clinical impact in neurology in recent years. In the research laboratory, the impact of computers has been just as dramatic, enabling researchers to monitor long-term experiments and to compute parameters that relate neurophysiological events and neuroanatomy to behavior, locomotion, and processing of sensory stimuli.

In spite of all the progress to date, however, researchers have only begun to understand the neurological puzzle. Many brain mechanisms still remain beyond our understanding. In the future, advances will depend on the formation and interactions of multidisciplinary teams of physiologists, psychologists, biochemists, clinicians, and biomedical engineers. The efforts of these teams will focus on the development of better measurement systems and their clinical application.

The purpose of this chapter is to present the neurophysiological measurements that are available. However, understanding the devices and analytic techniques that provide these neurological measures requires a knowledge of the anatomical and physiological concepts relevant to measurements within the nervous system. Because clearly a complete treatment of this material would constitute volumes of text, this chapter will highlight and summarize activity within the nervous system.

BASIC NEUROANATOMY AND NEUROPHYSIOLOGY

This chapter uses a top-down, systems-level approach to familiarize the reader with the subsystems, anatomical components, communication pathways, and functions of the human nervous system. This perspective, in some ways, parallels the chronological order in which neurological research has progressed: from a coarse realization of the role of the brain to more detailed understanding of events that occur at the cellular level.

Overview of Primary Structures

The nervous system has traditionally been studied as two subsystems: the central nervous system (CNS) and the peripheral nervous system (PNS). The brain and spinal cord are the major components of the CNS. Although the CNS exhibits anatomical bilateral symmetry, functional asymmetries exist within it. Most notable is right-left brain activity as it differs among individuals in a manner that has been termed *cognitive style* (Doktor and Bloom 1977; Schadke and Potvin, 1981), which has attracted recent interest. In addition, a number of crossovers occur whereby function is represented on the side of the brain opposite to the body side where the function actually takes place. Such functions are said to be *contralateral,* as opposed to those that are *ipsilateral,* in which brain and body side correspond.

In a general sense, the brain is the processor and storage unit (memory) of the nervous system, and the spinal cord is a communication vehicle between the brain and a large part of the PNS. However, the spinal cord also contains sites that serve as local processors involved in reflex control of neuromuscular activities, as well as in functions that are not yet defined. These distributed processors operate independently from the brain but can be overridden by it (influenced from above) to handle situations beyond the capability of local processors.

The PNS consists of several distinct subsystems, with associated components categorized by the functions that they implement. Collections of *afferent nerves* (those that carry input information to the brain) relay information from skin (tactile) and other peripheral sensors to the brain via the spinal cord in most cases, and through direct connections (*cranial nerves*) in others. This is called the *somatic sensory nervous system.* Motor neurons, or *efferent fibers* (those that carry information from the CNS to the periphery), in the CNS and PNS control muscle activity in response to somatic sensory input. The *visual* and *auditory pathways* implement the functions of vision and hearing, providing information to the brain from complex transducers: the eyes and ears.

Another PNS division, the *autonomic nervous system,* translates emotional responses to control smooth muscle tissue (in blood vessels and parts of the digestive tract), glandular secretions, and heart muscle. The autonomic nervous system is further divided into the so-called sympathetic and parasympathetic nervous systems. The former (commonly referred to as "fight or flight" system) readies the body in threatening situations by speeding up heart rate, initiating secretions of some glands, and inhibiting functions of lesser importance. The partially complementary parasympathetic system tends to slow the heart and controls contraction of, and secretions within, the stomach.

With regard to nervous system measurements, primary interest has focused on recording the spontaneous electrical activity and the electrical activity resulting from external stimuli of the brain over time, via the *electroencephalogram.* Numerous studies have related specific recorded electrical events to functions and clinical abnormalities (anatomical, physiological, or behavioral). In recent years, electrical activity emanating from the spinal cord has received increased interest, especially during delicate spinal surgery procedures. *Nerve conduction velocities* and *relative neural activity* in the PNS are measured via electrical means for clinical assessment of physiological abnormalities. These measurements represent the average electrical activity of many cells, spontaneously or synchronously, as in *evoked responses,* generated by individual electrical activities. *Single cell recordings* of electrical activity, although not performed clinically, have been important research tools for understanding principles of nerve cell (*neuron*) function and are playing a greater role in unlocking the details of operation in CNS functional subsystems, for example, in the initiation and refinement of sensory-motor activities. Further anatomical and physiological background is now presented to illustrate these types of neurological measurements.

Central Nervous System

The human brain

The human brain can be divided organizationally into three general regions: the brainstem, cerebellum, and cerebral cortex (see Figure 5.1).

The *brainstem* is actually an extension and elaboration of the spinal cord. This section of the brain evolved first and includes a structure (*medulla*) that contains the centers that control regulatory systems necessary for life support, such as respiration and heart rate maintenance and temperature regulation. In addition, all sensory pathways find their way into the brainstem (via a structure known as the *pons*), thereby permitting the integration of complex input patterns within its

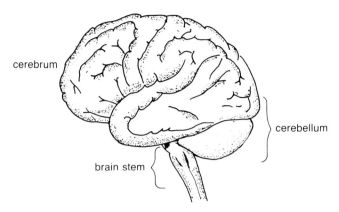

Figure 5.1 Major regions of the human brain (modified from Bronzino JD: *Technology for Patient Care,* St. Louis: C. V. Mosby, 1977).

domain. The pons is like a relay station for spinal motor neurons and auditory signals, mediating some interaction between these functional subsystems. The pons also contains *nuclei* (dense collections of neurons) of the cranial nerves associated with sensation from the face and control of facial musculature.

Higher up the brainstem, posterior to the pons, is a special mass of brain tissue called the *cerebellum.* This fascinating signal processor is crucial to maintaining balance and executing finely coordinated, smooth movements. Although the cerebellum does not initiate a movement, it serves to modify motor neuron activity continuously during complex motions. This provides the necessary fine-tuning in response to sensory afferent inputs that results in effortless and smooth motions that would otherwise be labored and jerky.

The *thalamus* acts as the primary collection point for all sensory information (visual, auditory, and somatosensory) that eventually reaches the complex outer layer of the brain, known as the *cortex.* Some form of integration and translation of this information most likely occurs, although details of such interactions are not well known.

Surrounding the thalamus and receiving sensory signals from it, the *recticular activating system* (RAS) has the function of arousing the cortex to pay attention to and process sensory inputs. Evidence indicates that this system, which is modulated by neurohormonal factors, controls sleep patterns. When active, the RAS keeps an individual awake and alert.

These brainstem and midbrain structures, and their positions in relation to the cortex, are illustrated in Figure 5.2.

The highest-level and most voluminous portion of the brain, called the *cerebrum,* consists of right and left cerebral hemispheres. The *cerebral cortex* forms the surface layer of each hemisphere. Compared to most mammals, it is so large in humans that it becomes a covering that surrounds and hides most of the other regions of the brain. Wrinkled and folded, containing ridges (*gyri*) and valleys (*sulci*), the cerebral tissue is literally squeezed into the limited space allocated to it.

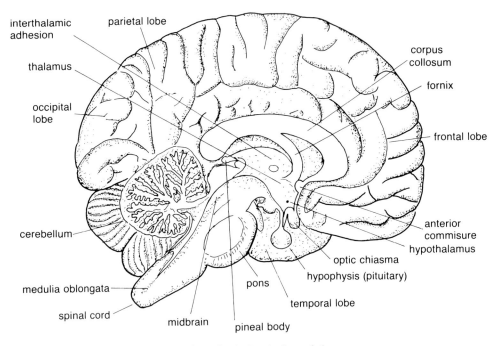

Figure 5.2   Cross-sectional (sagittal plane) view of the human brain (after Evans WF: *Anatomy and Physiology, The Basic Principles,* Englewood Cliffs, N.J.: Prentice-Hall, 1971).

Although the overall operation of this complex structure is not completely understood, sections of the cerebral cortex can be identified in terms of their anatomical locations and corresponding functional significance (Figure 5.3):

1 The *occipital lobe,* or *primary visual cortex,* at the back of the head.

2 The *temporal lobe,* occupying the lower middle side region of each hemisphere and containing the *primary auditory cortex.*

3 The *parietal lobe,* bound by the occipital lobe posteriorly and a prominent sulcus running right to left (*central fissure*) anteriorly. The parietal lobe comprises somewhat distinct areas: one responsible for receiving sensory signals from each body site (the *postcentral gyrus,* behind the central fissure, also referred to as the *somatosensory cortex*) and a more anterior region related to higher-order, discriminatory sensory perception (such as the ability to identify different objects by shape when they are placed in the palm of the hand) and proprioception (one's own awareness of body and limb positions in space).

4 The *frontal lobe,* the part of the right and left hemispheres anterior to the central fissure. Just anterior to the central fissure is the *precentral gyrus,* or *primary motor cortex,* which generates coarse neural control of motor neurons in the ventral region of the spinal cord. Note that the proximity of this area to the somatosensory cortex implies that significant integration of sen-

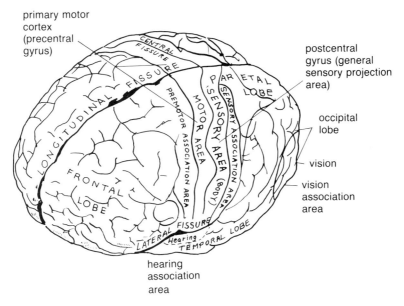

primary motor
cortex
(precentral
gyrus)

postcentral
gyrus (general
sensory projection
area)

occipital
lobe

vision

vision
association
area

hearing
association
area

Figure 5.3 The cerebrum (after McNaught AB and
Collander R: *Illustrated Physiology, 3d ed.* Edinburgh:
Churchill Livingstone, 1975).

sory information, along with voluntary thought processes, occurs at this level to
influence initiation of motor activities. More complex motor activities
(speech, for example) require greater orchestration, which occurs in the next
most anterior area, the *premotor cortex.* It has been suggested that the most
anterior and lowest (inferior) part of the frontal lobe are associated with behavioral patterns and functions that are considered to be primary intellectual
in nature. However, this association has not yet been proved.

The attentive reader may notice that every square centimeter of the brain has not
been labeled functionally. Remaining regions are often called *association* areas;
some have suggested that these regions are involved in integrating information
from other areas to modify other neuronal processes. Figure 5.3 illustrates the distribution of functional areas over the cortex.

In addition to the topological relationships between general functions and
specific areas of the cortex, mapping also occurs within these areas. For example,
quadrants of the visual field map onto different regions of the visual cortex of the
occipital lobe. Such relationships have been worked out in great detail for the somatosensory cortex and motor cortex, where mapping occurs between mediolat-
eral cortical position and body site. Highly innervated body sites such as the hand
are represented over disproportionately large cortical areas, as Figure 5.4 indicates. Such a drawing, mapping body site to cortical topography, is known as a *ho-
munculus.*

The brain mass is composed of billions of nerve cells, whose general anatomical structure is described in the discussion of the PNS. In the brain, two types

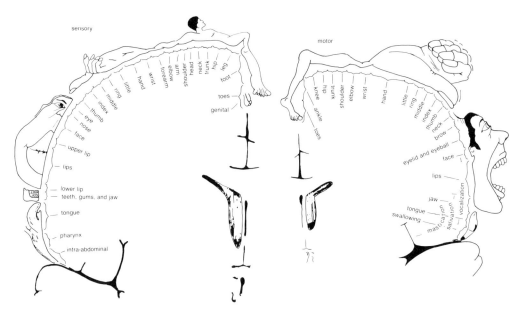

Figure 5.4 Mapping of body sites to regions of the cortex is graphically illustrated via sensory and motor homunculi (after Evans WF: *Anatomy and Physiology, The Basic Principles,* Englewood Cliffs: Prentice-Hall, 1971).

of cell collections exist, termed *white* and *gray matter* because of their appearance. Gray matter comprises cell bodies and the relatively small nerve fibers of these cells; white matter contains certain cells with long connecting fibers that are covered with the fatty substance *myelin*. Excellent treatments of the various types of nerve cell structures within the brain are available (Mountcastle 1980; Guyton, 1981).

Spinal cord

Although the spinal cord can be thought of as the communication channel (for sensory inputs and motor control of smooth and skeletal muscles) between the brain and peripheral body sites, evidence indicates that extensive processing takes place within this structure as well. For example, there are approximately 375,000 nerve cell bodies interspersed between sensory inputs and motor outputs at the canine seventh lumbar spinal cord segment (Gelfan 1963). Their presence alone suggests complex processing capabilities.

For the present purpose, the spinal cord can be discussed in terms of sensory inputs, motor outputs, *interneurons* (neurons between input and outputs), and function-oriented *tracts*. The spinal cord gives rise to afferent and efferent nerve fibers that enter and leave the cord at each spinal level, through intervertebral *foramina* (holes) on each side of the spinal column. Motor neurons (efferents) leave the cord from the *ventral horn* (most anterior) of the cord to innervate skeletal muscles, and sensory inputs enter via *spinal ganglia* through dorsal (most poste-

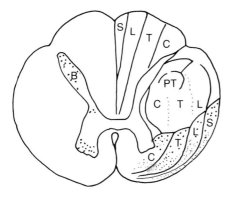

Figure 5.5 The cell groups of dorsal horn and arrangement of spinothalamic and other tracts in cervical region of the spinal cord (after Walker AE, *Arch Neurol and Psychiat*, vol. 43: p. 284, 1940).

rior) spinal cord roots. They join to form PNS nerve trunks (total of 31 right-left pairs) that exit at cervical, thoracic, lumbar, and sacral spinal levels to innervate specific body sites.

The interneurons are known to play an active role in sensory-motor function, transforming incoming signals into new patterns required to achieve the desired motor activity. These transformations can occur as a result of the properties of individual interneurons, as well as through circuits between interneurons. Interneurons exhibit different types of functions (Henneman 1980):

1 Amplifiers of discharge rate and intensity by cascading cells
2 Controlled gates in a sort of variable gain control circuit
3 Signal inverters that are excitatory to inhibitory signals and vice versa
4 Terminal common pathways for excitation or inhibition

A cross section through the spinal cord at a given level reveals that distinct regions, known as *tracts* (Figure 5.5), exist. Topographic mappings to body sites also occur within some of these tracts. In addition, tracts are often organized according to function: the spinothalamic tract carries afferent pain and temperature sensory fibers, and the pyramidal tract contains descending motor efferent fibers.

Peripheral Nervous System

Nerves, such as the nerve trunks emanating from the spinal cord, contain bundles of individual afferent and efferent *nerve fibers.* Each fiber is either an *axon* (transmitting fiber of a nerve cell) or *dendrite* (input fiber of a nerve cell).

A neuron, or nerve cell, is the basic anatomical and functional unit of the PNS, as well as the CNS. Each neuron consists of a *soma* (cell body), at least one but possibly more dendrites, and a single long axon that can be almost 1 meter (m) in length.

The site where the axon joins the soma is known as the *axon hillock*. At this point action potentials, the most discrete form of neuronal electrical activity, are usually generated. Nerve fibers are *myelinated* (covered with a fatty insulator) or unmyelinated. *Nodes of Ranvier* interrupt the *myelin sheath* at fixed intervals in

Table 5.1   The 12 cranial nerves

Number	Name*	Number	Name*
I	Olfactory (S)	VII	Facial (M, S)
II	Optic (S)	VIII	Auditory (S)
III	Motor oculi (M)	IX	Glossopharyngeal (S)
IV	Trochlear (M)	X	Pneumogastric or vagus (M, S)
V	Trifacial (S, M)	XI	Spinal accessory (M)
VI	Abducent (M)	XII	Hypoglossal (M)

*S: sensory; M: motor.

some fibers, facilitating greater conduction velocities for the propagation of neu-rological signals through a process known as *saltatory* conduction (Brinley 1980). Evidence of the importance of myelination are the severe functional deficits (spas-ticity, loss of movement control, tremors, sensory loss) associated with neurologi-cal disorders known as *demyelinating diseases* (such as multiple sclerosis).

A particular pathway may include several neurons, for example, in a reflex arc in which afferent information resulting from a tendon tap makes its way through the spinal cord and in turn generates a motor neuron response action. The site where portions of two nerve cells come into close contact with each other is called a *synapse* (Nastuk 1980). Through a chemical transmission process, action potentials propagate across a small gap between neurons (*synaptic cleft*), allowing the formation of multiple neuron pathways and the complex neuronal communi-cation network.

Peripheral nerves branch out from the spinal column and usually undergo further branching to innervate tactile sensory receptors of the skin, sensory organs associated with muscles (stretch and position sensors such as *Golgi tendon organs* and *muscle spindles*), and motor units that control muscular contraction. The 12 total cranial nerves (Table 5.1), named numerically and also according to function or anatomical destination, primarily form the peripheral nervous system of the

Table 5.2   Some major peripheral nerves and body sites innervated

Nerve	Sites
Circumflex	Shoulder
Subscapular	Shoulder
Median ⎫	Arm, elbow, forearm,
Ulnar ⎬	wrist, hand
Radial ⎭	
Obturator	Hip, thigh
Anterior crural	Hip, thigh (front), knee
External popliteal or peroneal	Knee, lower leg
Great sciatic	Thigh (back), lower leg, foot
Tibial	Lower leg, ankle, foot

head. However, it is noted that two cranial nerves (X and XI) actually descend into the thorax. Table 5.2 lists some major peripheral nerves and the muscles or body sites that they innervate.

ORIGIN AND CHARACTERISTICS OF NERVOUS SYSTEM POTENTIALS

All nervous system electrical potentials arise from chemical activities that mediate the generation or conduction of nerve impulses. It is indeed fortunate that these chemical events are ionic in nature, since the charge distributions generated give rise, through charge separations and the process of ohmic conduction, to measurable electrical signals.

Single Unit Potentials: The Action Potential

Nerve cells, as well as muscle cells, possess the characteristic of *excitability.* There is a natural tendency to achieve equilibrium between the inner and outer ion concentrations (as well as electrical charge) of these cells. The primary ions are sodium (Na^+), potassium (K^+), and chloride (Cl^-). Excitable cell membranes allow ready passage of potassium and chloride ions but block sodium ions. To counteract the high positive concentration of sodium ions outside the cells, additional positive potassium ions enter. However, because of the resultant potassium ion concentration imbalance, the positive sodium ion charge cannot be completely offset. This results in a *resting transmembrane potential* for the cell, with the inside negative (-60 to -100 millivolts [mV]) with respect to the extracellular fluid space.

If ionic flow or other types of energy (mechanical, heat, and so on, as in the case of special cells such as mechanoreceptors in the skin) perturb the membrane of excitable cells, the membrane lets some sodium ions enter the cell, initiating a "snowball effect" known as *depolarization.* This results from the rush of sodium ions into the cells and the attempt of slower-moving potassium ions to leave the cell (to eliminate the potassium ion concentration imbalance caused by high extracellular sodium concentration prior to excitation). Over a short period of time (about 1 millisecond [ms]), the cell potential changes from -60 to -100 mV to $+20$ to $+30$ mV.

After this time a new equilibrium state is reached, and a *repolarization* process is started by means of an active cell membrane process known as the *sodium pump.* This pump is important, since after depolarization the cell membrane is no longer permeable to sodium ions, which must be moved out of the cell to restore the original resting membrane potential status. This cycle of depolarization and repolarization constitutes the temporal event referred to as an *action potential,* the basic nerve impulse (Figure 5.6). Some important characteristics of action potentials are the following:

1 The action potential is an *all-or-none* phenomenon: given a stimulus that depolarizes the cell membrane beyond a threshold value, the action potential proceeds through its cycle.

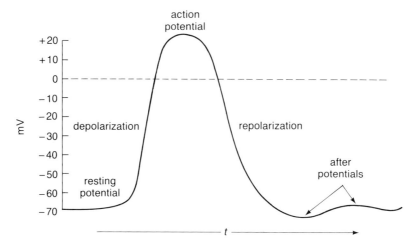

Figure 5.6   Time course of potential change across the membrane of excitable cells illustrating the action potential (after Cromwell/Weibel/Pfeifer, *Biomedical Instrumentation and Measurement,* 2nd Ed., © 1980, p. 52. Reprinted by permission of Prentice-Hall, Englewood Cliffs, N.J.).

2 The action potential *propagates* along nerve fibers at a constant velocity (with different constant velocities depending on type and size of fiber) by causing depolarization of regions adjacent to a given action potential start point.

3 An *absolute refractory period* exists during the first phase of an action potential. During this time, external stimuli cannot elicit a membrane response, regardless of their intensity.

4 Following the absolute refractory period is the *relative refractory period,* when only an *intense suprathreshold stimulus* can initiate a membrane response.

5 Refractory periods limit the firing rate of fibers to a maximum of about 1000 times per second.

Volume Conductor Potentials

It is impractical to attempt to obtain general information about nervous system function and integrity only from the measurement of single action potentials. As will be seen, such measurements require invasive techniques, specialized instruments, and skillful execution. For many clinical purposes, results would be equivocal. More commonly, clinicians observe or measure the average activity of many individual action potentials. The net electrical activity is electrically *conducted* to surface body sites, such as the scalp. At these sites, electrodes can be placed with relative ease to monitor resulting surface potentials that correspond to the overall activity within the *volume* from which the activity emanates.

Through experimental studies of cause and effect, surface potentials resulting from electric fields within volume conductors have been categorized according to temporal, amplitude, and spatial patterns. The primary sources of volume conductor potentials are nerves consisting of multiple fibers (usually in the PNS) and neurons.

Multiunit recordings

When making surface measurements in the periphery, one is usually attempting to obtain a measurement from a major nerve. Since each nerve is composed of more than one fiber, such measurements are termed *multiunit* recordings. Because of the presence of electrically active musculature, which generates signals (or noise artifacts when one is interested in neuronal activity) that can equal or exceed the amplitude of surface measured nerve impulses, peripheral measurements sometimes require special techniques to minimize the effects of these artifacts.

The electroencephalogram

The ongoing or *spontaneous* neuronal activity within the skull gives rise to scalp surface potentials that, when recorded over time, produce a tracing known as the *electroencephalogram* (EEG). Researchers have attempted to determine precise relationships between the sources of electrical activity and surface electrodes by using a mathematical, three-layer volume conductor model (Rush and Driscoll 1969; Paicer et al. 1967). However, such meritorious efforts have provided less useful information than have less rigorous studies that focus on the meaning, as opposed to the origin, of complex EEG patterns.

Caton (1875) published the initial account of the recording of the spontaneous electrical activity of the brain from the cerebral cortex of an experimental animal. The amplitude of these electrical oscillations was so low that Caton's discovery is all the more incredible because it preceded the availability of suitable electronic amplifiers by 50 yr. In 1924, Hans Berger, of the University of Jena in Austria, carried out the first human EEG recordings, using electrical metal strips pasted to the scalps of his subjects as electrodes and a sensitive galvanometer as the recording instrument. Berger was able to measure the irregular, relatively small electrical potentials coming from the brain. By studying the successive positions of the moving element of the galvanometer recorded on a continuous roll of paper, Berger observed the resultant patterns in these brain waves as they varied with time. From 1924 to 1938, he laid the foundation for many of the present applications of electroencephalography. Berger noted that these brain waves were not entirely random but instead displayed certain periodicities and regularities. For example, he observed that although these brain waves were slow in sleep and states of depressed function, they were faster during waking behavior. He suggested, quite correctly, that the brain's activity changed in a consistent and recognizable pattern when the general status of the subject changed, as a change from a relaxed to an alert state.

Berger also concluded that certain pathological conditions could greatly affect brain waves, after noting the marked increase in the amplitude of these brain

Table 5.3   EEG breakdown into patterns according to frequency bands

Designation	Frequency* Range (Hz)	Other Characteristics	Conditions
Delta	0–3.5	—	Sleep, infancy, brain disorders
Theta	3.5–8	Infrequent occurrence	Mostly in adolescents; during stress in adults
Alpha	8–13	Very rhythmic	Awake; quiet and restful thought
Beta	13–50	More irregular Two types (beta I, II)	Tension; beta I disappears during intense mental activity; beta II is elicited by mental activity

*Band cutoff frequencies are approximate only: exact cutoff frequencies are subject to controversy.

waves brought about by convulsive seizures. However, in spite of the insights provided by these studies, Berger's original paper (Berger 1929) did not excite much attention, and his efforts were largely ignored until similar investigations were carried out and verified by British investigators.

Not until Adrian and Mathews (1934) published their classic paper verifying Berger's findings were the reality of human brain waves accepted and EEG studies put on a firmly established basis. One of their primary contributions was the identification of certain rhythms in the EEG, regular oscillations at approximately 10 Hz, from the occipital lobes of the cerebral cortex. Investigating the response of this activity (later known as *alpha activity*) to light and other stimuli, they found that this alpha rhythm in the EEG disappeared when the brain displayed any type of attention or alertness or focused on objects in the visual field.

Since the most distinctive characteristic of EEG patterns appears to be frequency content, different bands in addition to the alpha waves described have been defined. These are commonly referred to by other Greek letter names and are summarized in Table 5.3.

Evoked responses

Normal EEGs provide an indication of the spontaneous or background electrical activity of the brain. Taking into account the location of scalp electrodes, they provide an indication of the *state of the brain* under certain global conditions (eyes open or closed; asleep or awake; normal activity or seizure in progress). Indeed, typical time records of the EEG appear to be somewhat random, although specific patterns become apparent even to the untrained eye at times (Figure 5.7).

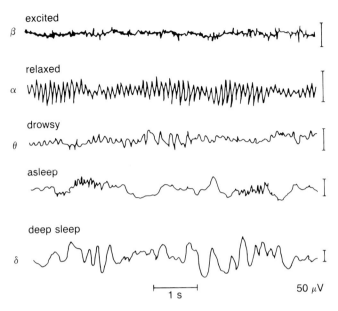

Figure 5.7 Electroencephalographic records during excitement, relaxation, and varying degrees of sleep (after Jasper HH, in Penfield and Erickson (Eds), *Epilepsy and Cerebral Localization,* Springfield, Ill.: Charles C Thomas, 1941)

However, even a relatively dramatic external stimulus, such as a flash of light into the eyes, results in only a small contribution to the net sum of background electrical activity present in scalp recordings over the occipital lobe. Although it is reasonable to assume that some change should occur (and it does), seeing it is another matter.

One can imagine flying over New York City on a clear night, observing the incredible number of light sources below. Assume that you have remote control of just one of those lights and are alternately turning it off and on, while trying to find the corresponding change in the lighted area below. In fact, you might be able to find your light under such conditions because the background would be relatively constant. Now assume that the situation is further complicated so that all other light sources are randomly flashing; this condition more closely approximates the EEG phenomena. If you take a series of photographs of all these flashing lights and control the situation so that your light (the signal) is always on when you take each photograph, it is likely that certain background lights (the noise) will be on in some photographs and off in others. After many photographs, the average contribution of your light (always on) will be large compared to the average effect of each other source (which may be on or off). Thus, an average of the light at each point in the photographs should yield one very bright point that can be identified easily.

In 1947, Dawson used similar principles to detect cerebral action potentials that occurred in response to electrical stimulation of a peripheral nerve in a human

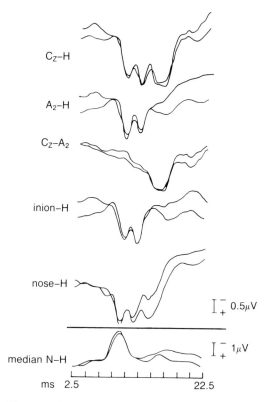

Figure 5.8   Evoked potentials to right median nerve
stimulation (after Cracco RQ and Cracco JB: Somatosensory
evoked potentials in man: far field potentials.
Electroencephalogr and Clin Neurophysiol, 41:460–466,
1976).

subject (Dawson 1947). Such potentials are known as *evoked responses,* since their
occurrence depends on a specific stimulus. In the experiment, Dawson displayed
an EEG trace on an oscilloscope and superimposed a number of tracings on a single photograph under typical background conditions (no presence of dramatic
stimuli), and also with the presence of periodic electrical nerve stimulation. In the
latter case, EEG tracings were synchronized, so that each stimulus triggered recordings. Because the random EEG activity averaged to zero over a large number
of recordings, and the change due to stimulation averaged in a reinforcing way,
Dawson demonstrated that a reproducible EEG change occurred at a fixed time
after the nerve stimulation. The important measured parameter in this evoked response is the time between stimulus and response, as Figure 5.8 indicates. The type
of evoked response that Dawson recorded is called a *somatosensory evoked response* (SER), since it was elicited by direct stimulation of a peripheral nerve of the
somatic sensory system. Other common types of evoked responses that are now
routinely measured include *brain stem* (because of the location of nuclei chiefly responsible for observed response peaks), or *auditory evoked responses* (BSER) and
visual evoked responses (VER). Evoked responses are also commonly referred to
as *evoked potentials* (EP).

This section has introduced several primary types of measurable neurophysiological electrical events:

1 The single unit action potential

2 Multiunit potentials in the peripheral nerves

3 Spontaneous EEG potentials

4 Evoked potentials

The next section discusses instrumentation and methods for measuring these potentials.

MEASUREMENT TECHNIQUES AND SYSTEMS

Single Cell and Multiunit Recordings

As pointed out previously, single neuron recordings require not only special equipment, but also a greater than average level of skill. Single action potentials can be recorded *intracellularly*, by using a microelectrode that must penetrate the cell membrane. The less daring can observe action potentials *extracellularly*, with the microelectrode located just outside the membrane.

A basic principle of measurement is that the measurement technique should not in any way affect the measurement itself. Since this ideal is difficult to realize in single cell measurements, effects should be minimized at least. Therefore, intracellular microelectrodes must be as small as $\mu 0.05$ m in diameter, and usually no longer than 1.0 μm, so that electrode penetration does not damage the cell. Microelectrodes must also be strong enough to withstand forces encountered during penetration of the cell membrane. Since the electrode body must pass through the extracellular electrolyte fluid that serves as the reference for intracellular potential measurement, the electrode body must be electrically insulated. Designers faced with these criteria have created microelectrodes of two general types:

1 Fine wire or metallic microelectrodes constructed from a strong metal (stainless steel, tungsten) needle or wire, less than 1 μm in diameter, that has been treated to etch a very fine tip. The body is insulated with a varnish of synthetic polymer (Figure 5.9) up to the tip.

2 Glass or micropipet electrodes formed by quickly pulling apart a glass micropipet having a small base capillary that has been heated to soften the glass to form a fine tip at the point of breakage. Thus, the entire body is made of glass, which is an excellent electrical insulator. The capillary is filled with an electrolyte in electrical contact with a wire electrode at the body end and with intracellular fluid when the tip is inserted into the cell (Figure 5.10).

Table 5.4 summarizes important microelectric characteristics. Generally, microelectrodes require amplifiers with very high input impedances to avoid distorting the measured event. For some applications, glass micropipet electrodes can have too low a frequency response (less than 2 to 3 kilohertz [kHz]) due their dominant low pass characteristic.

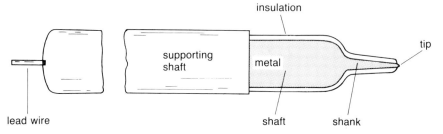

Figure 5.9   Structure of metal microelectrode for
intracellular recordings (after Neuman MR: Biopotential
electrodes, in Webster JG (ed.), *Medical Instrumentation:
Application and Design.* Boston: Houghton, Mifflin, 1978).

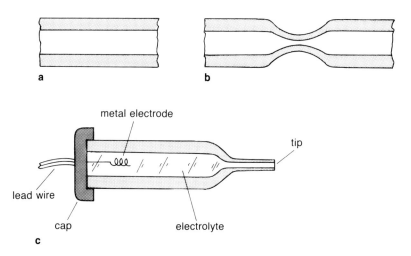

Figure 5.10   Glass micropipet electrode filled with an
electrolytic solution. (a) Section of a fine-bore glass capillary.
(b) Capillary narrowed through heating and stretching.
(c) Final structure of glass-pipet microelectrode (after Neuman
MR: Biopotential electrodes, in Webster JG (ed.), *Medical
Instrumentation: Application and Design.* Boston: Houghton
Mifflin, 1978).

Extracellular recordings employ larger-diameter (10 μm) electrodes of similar construction. Because of the larger diameter, however, impedances are generally lower. Details of fabrication, characteristics, and use of microelectrodes are available elsewhere (Phillip 1973; Neuman 1978; Cobbold 1974; Ferris 1974; Geddes 1972).

Both intracellular and extracellular recordings require a reference electrode. In intracellular recordings, an extracellular electrode placed near the cell is used so that the *transmembrane potential* is measured. Extracellular recordings can use two closely spaced electrodes for *bipolar* recordings (such as along an axon), or the reference can be at an indifferent and distant location. In the latter case, measurements are *unipolar,* since it is clear which electrode serves as the reference.

Table 5.4 Microelectrode characteristics

Type	Impedance*	Frequency Transfer Characteristic
Metal	10–100 MΩ, frequency-dependent, resistive and capacitive	High pass if input impedance of amplifier is too low ($<10^{10}$)
Glass micropipet	1–100 MΩ, primarily resistive	Low pass, with long time constant; needs compensation for recording fast events

*Increases as tip diameter decreases.

Amplifiers for single cell and multiunit recordings require input impedances as high as 10^{10} ohms (Ω), voltage gains of about 50 to 10,000 (assuming actual potentials of 10 μV to 100 μV), and a flat frequency response up to 10 kHz. A *differential instrumentation amplifier* (Figure 5.11) with high common mode rejection ratio to reduce interference from other electrical sources that both the signal and reference leads may sense is desirable. Chart recorders can record limited information such as relative firing frequency. An oscilloscope with storage capability or a computerized data acquisition system is useful for recording single action potentials. A typical laboratory setup is shown in schematic form in Figure 5.12. If one is interested in recording only high-frequency events, such as *spiking* (described later), a high pass characteristic (cutoff of 1 to 10 Hz) is suggested, and sometimes required, to remove effects of electrode drift or half cell direct current (dc) potential differences associated with the electrodes.

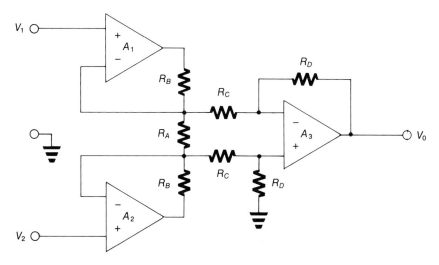

Figure 5.11 Schematic diagram of instrumentation amplifier.

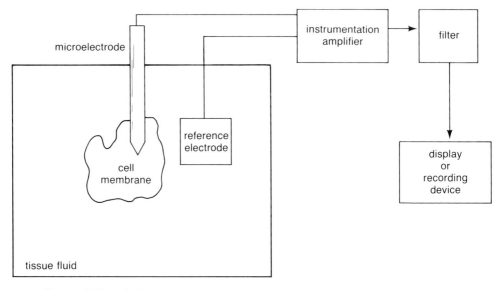

Figure 5.12   Typical instrumentation arrangement for intracellular single-cell recording.

As indicated, for many nerve fibers the level of excitation is related to the frequency of firing. Thus, the excitation is communicated via frequency modulation, which is in turn related to factors such as load on a muscle, pain, or touch. Because of this information coding scheme, scientists often record the firing rate. In research involving single cell recordings (Towe 1973), the firing is often converted to an audio signal (clicks) to help researchers monitor activity with greater laboratory freedom. Circuitry (a frequency-to-voltage converter) (Stout 1976) often provides a voltage that is a direct indicator of firing rate and therefore nerve activity. Figure 5.13 illustrates typical records.

A common clinical multiunit measurement is the determination of nerve conduction velocities. Surface stimulation of a given peripheral nerve at a selected site along its length may generate an evoked response. Stimulation resulting in synchronous depolarization generates a local multiunit action potential that propagates along the nerve through the saltatory conduction process. By measuring the time t_p the action potential requires to propagate to a recording site at a distance d_s centimeters from the stimulation site, the conduction velocity can be determined from

$$\text{conduction velocity (m/s)} = \frac{d_s \text{ (cm)}}{t_p \text{ (ms)} \times 10.0}$$

Commercially available devices contain stimulation, recording, and automated signal processing components so that the conduction velocity is directly displayed. A hand-held stimulation/recording head, containing electrode pairs at a fixed (and therefore known) separation, provides convenient and noninvasive surface measurements. Figure 5.14 is a simplified block diagram of the internal design of such a device.

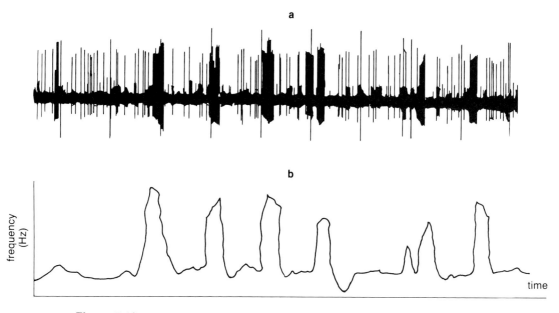

Figure 5.13 (a) Single cell activity in voltage versus time. (b) Cell firings per unit time converted to a voltage that can be monitored.

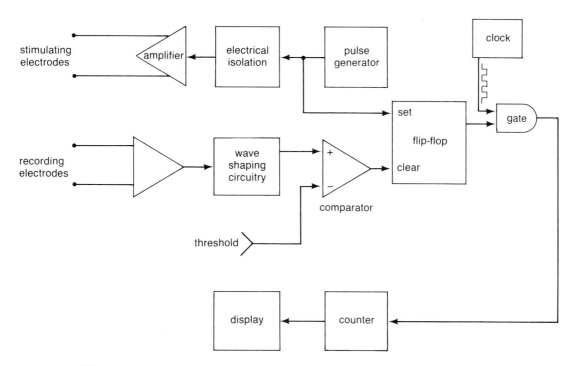

Figure 5.14 Block diagram of instrumentation for measurement of nerve conduction velocity

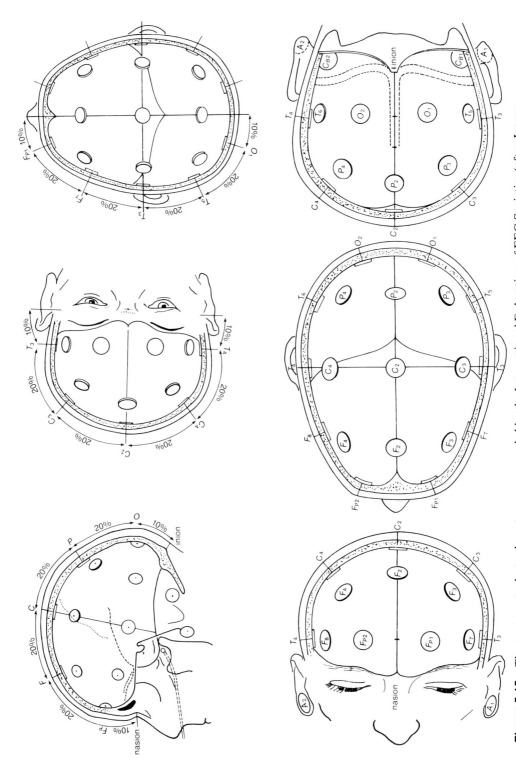

Figure 5.15 The ten-twenty electrode system recommended by the International Federation of EEG Societies (after Jasper HH: The ten-twenty electrode system of the International Federation in Electroencephalography and Clinical Neurophysiology. *EE6 Journal*, 10:371–375, 1958).

Electroencephalography Techniques

Scalp recordings of spontaneous neuronal activity of the brain, identified as the EEG, allow measurement of potential changes over time (brain waves) between a signal electrode and a reference electrode. Compared to other biopotentials, such as the electrocardiogram, the EEG is extremely difficult for an untrained observer to interpret. As might be expected, partially as a result of the spatial mapping of functions onto different regions of the brain, correspondingly different waveforms are visible, depending on electrode placement. Recognizing that some standardization was necessary for comparison of research as well as clinical EEG records, the International Federation in Electroencephalography and Clinical Neurophysiology adopted the *10-20 electrode placement system* (Jasper 1958) shown in Figure 5.15. The system is so named because it divides the linear distances between temples (right-left) and between the masion and inion (fore-aft), across the top of the head, into two 10 percent and four 20 percent regions. The points of intersection formed by drawing perpendicular lines to the anterior-posterior and

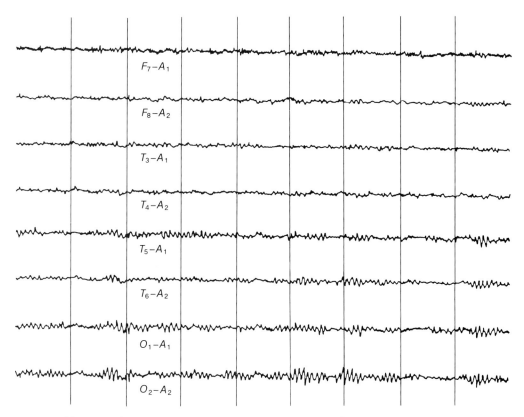

Figure 5.16   Typical human electroencephalogram (after Cromwell/Weibel/Pfeifer, *Biomedical Instrumentation and Measurement,* 2nd Ed. © 1980. Reprinted by permission of Prentice-Hall, Englewood Cliffs, N.J.).

right-left lines at each 10 or 20 percent demarcation represent the standard electrode placement sites. Each site is designated with a standard label for easy reporting purposes (C_z, P_3, and so forth). Figure 5.16 depicts a typical multichannel EEG, with each trace identified by corresponding electrode pair. Note that each channel uses an ear electrode (right or left) as the reference.

Instrumentation required for EEG recordings can be simple or elaborate (Niedermeyer and da Silva 1982). Although the discussion presented in this section is for a single channel system it can be extended to simultaneous multichannel recordings simply by multiplying the hardware by the number of channels required. In cases that do not require true simultaneous recordings, special electrode selector panels can minimize hardware requirements. The general EEG system consists of electrodes, amplifiers (with appropriate filters), and a recording device.

Commonly used scalp electrodes consist of Ag–AgCl disks, 1 to 3 mm in diameter, with a very flexible long lead that can be plugged into an amplifier. Although it is desirable to obtain a low impedence contact at the electrode-skin interface (less than 10 kΩ), this objective is confounded by hair, the time necessary to apply all electrodes for a "full head" recording, and the difficulty of mechanically stabilizing the electrodes. Conductive electrode paste helps obtain low impedance and keep electrodes in place. A type of cement (collodion) is used to fix small patches of gauze over electrodes for mechanical stability, and leads are usually taped to the subject to provide some strain relief. Slight abrasion of the skin is sometimes used to obtain better electrode impedances, but this can cause irritation and sometimes infection (as well as pain in sensitive subjects).

For long-term recordings, as in seizure monitoring, electrodes present major problems. Needle electrodes, which must be inserted into the tissue between the surface of the scalp and skull, are sometimes useful. However, the danger of infection increases significantly. Electrodes with self-contained miniature amplifiers are somewhat more tolerant because they provide a low impedance source to interconnecting leads, but they are expensive. Despite numerous attempts to simplify the electode application process and to guarantee long-term stability, none has been widely accepted.

Instruments are available for measuring impedance between electrode pairs. The procedure is recommended strongly as good practice, since high impedance leads to distortions that may be difficult to separate from actual EEG signals. In fact, electrode impedance monitors are built into some commercial devices for recording EEGs. Standard dc ohmmeters should not be used, since they apply a polarizing current that causes build-up of noisy electrode potential at the skin-electrode interface. Commercial devices apply a known-amplitude sinusoidal voltage (typically 1 kHz) to an electrode pair circuit and measure root mean square (rms) current, which is directly related to the magnitude of the impedance. General information regarding electrodes is presented elsewhere (Webster 1978; Geddes 1972).

From carefully applied electrodes, signal amplitudes of 1 to 10 μV can be obtained. Considerable amplification (gain = 10^6) is required to bring these levels up to an acceptable level for input to recording devices. Because of long electrode leads and the common electrically noisy environment where recordings take place, differential amplifiers with inherently high input impedance and high common mode rejection ratios are essential for high-quality EEG recordings.

In some facilities, special electrically shielded rooms minimize environmental electrical noise, particularly 60-Hz alternating current (ac) line noise. As will be seen, much of the information of interest in the EEG lies in frequency bands less than 40 Hz, so that low pass filters in the amplifier can be switched in to attenuate 60-Hz noise sharply.

Recording short-duration events, such as in BSER recordings, requires a higher-frequency response. For this reason, low pass filters usually have switch selectable cutoff frequencies. For attenuating ac noise when the low pass cutoff is greater than 60 Hz, many EEG amplifiers have notch filters that attenuate only frequencies in a narrow band centered around 60 Hz. Since important signal information may also be attenuated, notch filtering should be used only as a last resort; one should try to identify and eliminate the source of interference instead.

In trying to identify 60 Hz sources to eliminate or minimize their effect, it is sometimes useful to use a dummy source, such as a fixes resistor attached to the electrodes. Usually a 100-kΩ resistor is used. This arrangement essentially provides a model for all aspects of the test situation, except that no EEG signal is present. Thus, the amplifier output represents only contributions from interfering sources. If noise can be reduced to an acceptable level (at least a factor of 10 less than EEG signals) under this condition, one is likely to obtain uncontaminated EEG records since interelectrode impedances should be much lower.

Different types of recording instruments obtain a temporary or permanent record of the EEG. The most common recording device is a pen or chart recorder (usually multichannel) that is an integral part of most commercially available EEG instruments. The bandwidth of interest in clinical EEGs is relatively low (less than 40 Hz) and therefore within the frequency response capabilities of these devices. Recordings are on a long sheet of continuous paper (from a folded stack), fed past the moving pen at one of several selectable constant speeds. The paper speed translates into distance per unit time or cycles per unit time, to allow EEG interpreters to identify different frequency components or patterns within the EEG. Paper speed is selected according to the monitoring situation at hand: slow speeds (10 mm/s) for observing the spiking characteristically associated with seizures and faster speeds (up to 120 mm/s) for the presence or absence of individual frequency bands in the EEG.

In addition to (or instead of) a pen recorder, the EEG may be recorded on a multichannel *frequency modulated* (FM) analog tape recorder. During such recordings, a visual output device such as an oscilloscope or video display usually displays the EEG with each of N channels switch-selected for display. This nonpermanent display is necessary or at least desirable to allow visual qualitative monitoring of recorded signals, so that corrective action (reapplying electrodes and so on) can take place immediately if necessary.

Sophisticated FM cassette recording and playback systems allow clinicians to review long EEG recordings over a greatly reduced time, compared to that required to flip through stacks of paper or observe recordings as they occur in real time. Such systems take advantage of *time compression* schemes, whereby a signal recorded at one speed (speed of the tape moving past the recording head of the cassette drive) is played back at a different, faster speed. The ratio of playback to recording speed is known, so the appropriate correction factor can be applied to played-back data to generate a properly scaled video display. A standard ratio of 60:1 is often used. Thus, a trained clinician can review each minute of real-time EEG in 1 s. The display appears to be scrolled at a high rate horizontally across the display screen. Features of these instruments allow the clinician to freeze a segment of EEG on the display and to slow down or accelerate tape speed from the standard playback rate as needed. A time mark channel is usually displayed as one of the traces as a convenient reference (vertical "tick mark" displayed at periodic intervals across the screen).

Computers can also be recording devices, digitizing (converting to digital form) one or several amplified EEG channels at a fixed rate. In such *sampled data systems* (Roden 1979), each channel is repeatedly sampled at a fixed time interval (*sample* interval) and this sample is converted into a binary number representation by an *analog-to-digital (A/D) converter*. The A/D converter is interfaced to a computer system so that each sample can be saved in the computer's memory. A set of such samples, acquired at a sufficient sampling rate (at least two times the highest frequency component in the sampled signal), is sufficient to represent all the information in the waveform. To ensure that the signal is band-limited, a low pass filter with a cutoff frequency equal to the highest frequency of interest is used. Since physically realizable filters do not have ideal characteristics, the sampling rate is usually greater than two times the filter's cutoff frequency.

Computer recordings are only practical for short-term recordings or for situations in which the EEG is immediately processed. This limitation is primarily due to storage requirements. For example, a typical sampling rate of 128 Hz yields 128 new samples per second that require storage. For an 8-channel recording, 1,024 samples are acquired per second. A 10-min recording period yields 614,400 data points. Assuming 8-bit *resolution* per sample, over 0.5 megabyte (MB) of storage is required to save the complete recording. This is roughly equivalent to the storage capacity of an entire floppy disk.

Processing can consist of compression for more efficient storage (with associated loss of total information content), as in data record or *epoch* averaging associated with evoked responses, or feature extraction and subsequent pattern recognition, as in automated spike detection in seizure monitoring.

Advanced EEG Systems

Advanced EEG systems that take advantage of the power of the computer have become available in recent years or are near commercial availability. One such system is the brain electrical activity mapping (BEAM) system (Duffy 1981, 1982), first developed at Harvard University around 1975 and now being marketed by Braintech, Inc. From a montage of 20 scalp EEG electrodes, the individually measured surface activities are computer-processed to obtain a color display spatially mapping electrical activity to a top-down planar representation of the scalp (Figure 5.17). Different colors represent different frequency bands when monitoring rest-

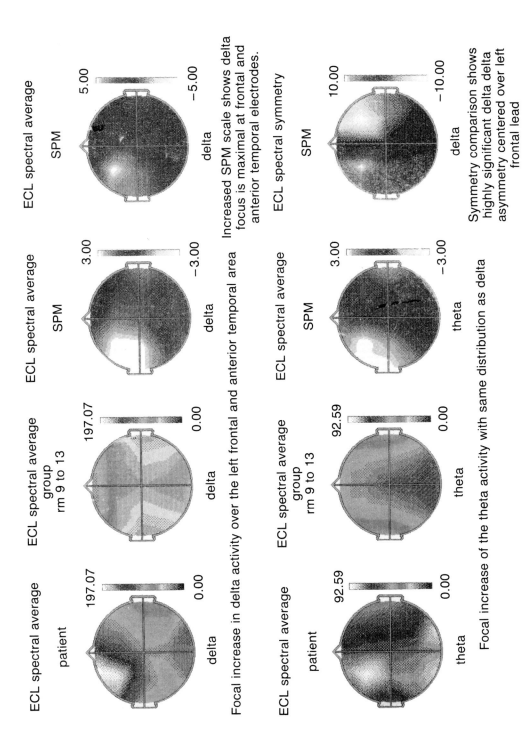

Figure 5.17 Typical output from BEAM machine scans (courtesy of Braintech, Inc, Maryland).

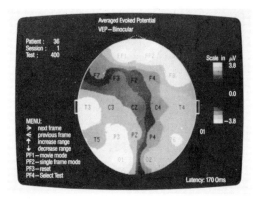
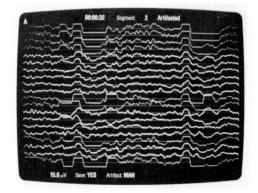
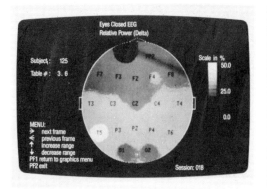
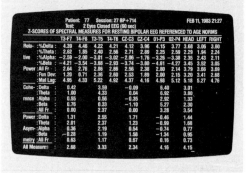

Figure 5.18 Different neurophysiological measurements
from the computerized brain scan system analyser (BSA)
(courtesy of Cadwell Laboratories, Kennewick Washington).

ing EEG signals. The system can also map evoked potentials, with different colors
representing different response amplitudes in relation to appropriate norms.

Another sophisticated system, the brain state analyzer (BSA) is based on
neurometrics (John et al. 1977, 1982). It is anticipated that the BSA system will be
available soon through Cordis Corporation in Miami, Florida. In addition to sophisticated acquisition and display capabilities, this system is based on a detailed
data base of statistical characteristics of EEG patterns associated with various
brain disorders. Signal processing extracts characteristic features from multielec-
trode recordings and parameter values obtained from patterns that can be compared to those that distinguish specific dysfunctions or conditions. Figure 5.18
shows typical output displays provided by the BSA.

For many applications, both the BEAM and BSA systems require adequate
reference data bases, which currently are considered to be small. As use increases,
the size of data bases will undoubtedly grow. However, it is difficult to ensure that
only good-quality data, representative of a given population, enter such data
bases. Strict screening procedures are essential to maximize data base integrity,
which is imperative to the success and realization of the full potential of these new
assessment tools.

Evoked Response Recording Techniques

Independent of the *modality* (somatosensory, auditory, or visual) selected, measurement of evoked responses requires the following instrument components:

1. An EEG system (electrodes, amplifiers, and display device)
2. A computer equipped with an A/D converter (usually multichannel)
3. An appropriate computer-triggerable and controllable stimulus source for the modality selected
4. A visual display (and optionally, a hard copy device such as a plotter) interfaced to the computer system

Figure 5.19 is a block diagram of the general arrangement. As indicated, each modality requires different stimulus sources. Somatosensory evoked response measurement uses a controlled electrical shock pulse applied via surface electrodes at constant current to a peripheral nerve (usually the median nerves), while auditory and visual evoked responses are elicited with click and flash or pattern reversals (Figure 5.20), respectively. Pulse trains have also been used for somatosensory evoked responses (Namerow et al. 1974). In each case, the measured response de-

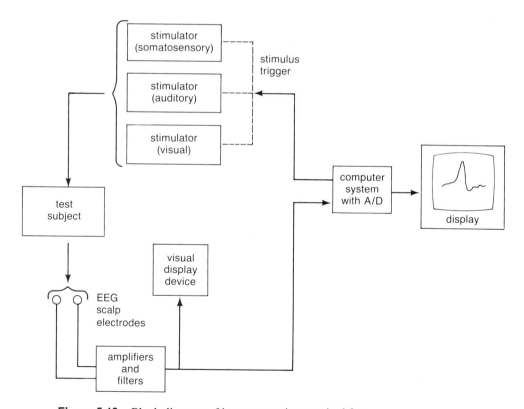

Figure 5.19   Block diagram of instrumentation required for measurement and recording of evoked potentials.

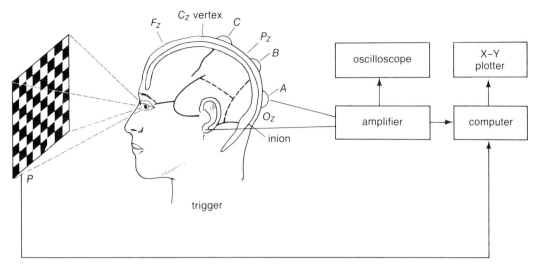

Figure 5.20   Schematic diagram of electrode locations and electronic equipment for recording human VEP (after Sokol S: Visually evoked potentials: Theory, techniques, and clinical applications. *Survey of Ophthalmology,* July–August, 278–304, 1976).

pends upon stimulus characteristics (magnitude and duration of electrical shock pulse or number of pulses per train, click intensity in decibels, flash intensity and spatial distribution, and pattern content and reversal rate).

In a typical setup, either the computer generates a stimulus trigger signal at a programmed, fixed rate to indicate the beginning of an averaging cycle, or the stimulus source contains a pulse generator that in turn triggers the computer to begin a signal averaging trial. Regardless of the implementation scheme, synchronization of the averaging data acquisition cycle to stimulus occurrence is essential to obtaining a meaningful result.

After each stimulus occurs, the desired EEG channels (containing random EEG activity as well as the desired evoked response) are digitized for a relatively short time period. This time must be long enough to record characteristic peaks that occur in typical evoked responses. These peaks have been associated with the electrical activity emanating from specific neuroanatomical structures (such as brain stem nuclei) that occurs after the action potential propagates from the stimulus input site (peripheral nerve, ear, or eye) to the peak generating site. The time between stimulus and response peak (or peaks, as will be seen for BSER) is known as the *latency time.* Normal subjects exhibit amazingly consistent latency times for a given modality, provided that test conditions are constant, but latencies vary considerably across modalities (refer to Table 5.5). The time that expires before a new stimulus can be generated must be greater than the latency time of the last peak that is to be observed. Thus, latency time (plus an arbitrary reasonable safety factor) determines the maximum stimulus repetition rate possible.

Table 5.5 Normal latency times for various evoked response modalities

Modality	Stimulus	Latency (ms)	Response Duration (ms)	Digitization Rate (Hz)	Notes
Visual	Light flash Reversing checkerboard pattern	100–150	50–75	1,000	Observed over occipital lobe
Auditory					Recorded over mastoid
Early		15–75	60	6,000–10,000	First 6 peaks (all positive)
Middle	Audible clicks	9–45	35		2 positive, 3 negative peaks
Late		50–1000	950	2,000	2 positive, 2 negative peaks
Somatosensory	Electrical shock	10–20	300	500–2,000	Depends on peripheral stimulation site Observed over contralateral parietal lobe

Digitization rate depends on the frequency content of the response contained with the recorded EEG. Since the nature of the response varies with modality, different rates are recommended for each modality (Table 5.5).

To combine the EEG records digitized after each stimulus to produce the final waveform, different averaging processes can be used. From these waveforms, evoked response peaks can be observed and latency times can be measured. Each digitized record contains a fixed number of points, each representing a sample of the EEG at a given poststimulus time. Since time averaging is desired, one can save a large number of such records, add together points from all records that represent a given point in time, and divide by the total number of data records to arrive at the averaged response for a given time segment. This process is repeated for each time segment (sample) in the data records. The result is a new record, with a number of points equal to that in each of the previous records, that contains samples of the desired averaged waveform (Figure 5.21). In practice, averaging a fairly large number of data records is necessary to obtain a result from which peaks can be easily identified. There is really a tradeoff between the time required to obtain a set of data records (K times the interstimulus time interval) and the quality of the average produced. In general, the signal (response) to noise (background EEG) ratio improves by a factor equal to the square root of the number of EEG records averaged. It may be feasible for an individual to sit quietly while subjected to auditory click stimuli at a 10-Hz rate for about 100 s to yield 1,024 separate records. However, to acquire the same number of records for flash VER would require 1,024 s, or approximately 17 min. Fortunately, responses that are most difficult to extract from

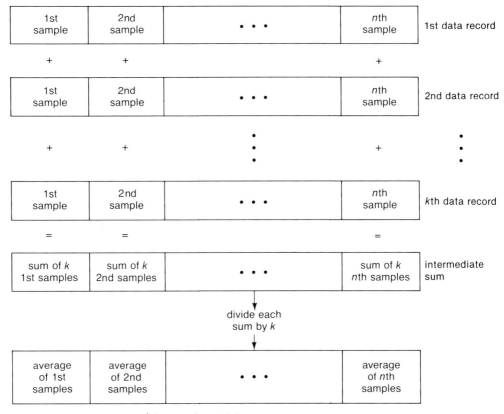

data record containing average response

Figure 5.21   Illustration of signal averaging operation on digitalized EEG waveforms to determine average evoked response.

background EEG and, therefore, those that absolutely require a large number of records to compute the average, also allows relatively rapid stimulus repetition rates. Thus, reasonably good flash VEP records can be obtained from averaging as few as 32 data records.

Because a large number of records may be required (more than 1,024), the averaging technique described is not always applied. Storing a large number of records requires considerable core computer memory. In addition, arithmetic overflow can easily occur from adding a large number of sample points. To bypass such implementation problems, intermediate averages (for example, after 16 records have been acquired) are sometimes computed. Each intermediate record so produced is then averaged with subsequent intermediate records. This represents a modified average, but good results can be obtained. The number of records used to compute the intermediate average is usually 2^n, since the division process is reduced to an arithmetic shift of each binary sum for these cases (each shift to the right is equivalent to dividing by 2).

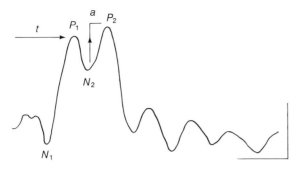

Figure 5.22 Flash-elicited visual evoked potential (after Sokol S: Visually evoked potentials: Theory, techniques, and clinical applications. *Survey of Ophthalmology,* July–August, 278–304, 1976).

As indicated previously, an accurate time base is necessary for implementing an evoked response test system. This is usually achieved with a programmable real-time clock that serves as one of the peripheral devices interfaced to the computer system. This time base is needed to control stimulus repetition rate and the digitization sample interval accurately, so that measurement of latency times, based on the latter, will also be accurate.

Computer power has also been exploited in evoked potential systems. In early systems, a technician converted distance measurements from a display screen and a subjective impression of where a peak occurred (peaks are not always well defined) to latency times. Some researchers have attempted to process the averaged waveform and thereby automate the procedure of extracting latency times (Aunon 1978; Billings 1981; Callaway, Halliday, and Herning, 1983).

Since the point on a waveform that defines the peak is controversial, a number of proposed processing algorithms have been tried. No single approach has been widely accepted. Commercial ER systems compromise by allowing technicians to use the skilled judgment they acquire through extensive experience to identify the location of a peak visually (yet still subjectively). Technicians can easily move a spot (*cursor*) about the screen with a hand-operated control to specific sites on the displayed waveform. When the cursor is over a site determined to be a peak, the technician presses a button and displays, records, or prints the amplitude and latency for the selected peak with appropriate labels. Figures 5.22, 5.23, 5.24, and 5.25 illustrate the types of waveforms that are obtained from flash VER, pattern reversal VER, and auditory evoked responses. Refer to Figure 5.8 for a typical somatosensory evoked response.

CLINICAL APPLICATIONS

Although many clinical applications of neurophysiological measurement techniques have been discussed in previous sections, it is worthwhile to expand and highlight a few of these. As already noted, single unit recordings are primarily

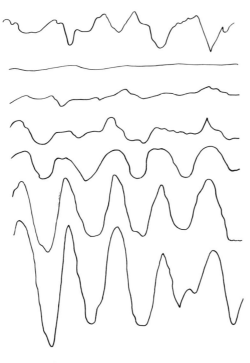

Figure 5.23   Pattern reversal visual evoked potentials obtained with a checkerboard stimulus (after Sokol S: Visually evoked potentials: Theory, techniques, and clinical applications. *Survey of Ophthalmology,* July–August, 278–304, 1976).

made in research rather than applications (Philips 1973; Towe 1973); they therefore are not discussed here. Thus, of the various measurement variables presented, nerve conduction velocities, the EEG, and evoked responses find the most widespread clinical application.

Nerve Conduction Velocities

Nerve conduction velocity measurements are made at peripheral body sites when neuromuscular dysfunction indicates a potential problem. In the case in which correlation and dysfunction and injury are not correlated, the clinician often desires to locate the source of the problem whether it is neurological or muscular, and if it is neurological, to determine whether the problem lies in the peripheral or central nervous system. One aspect of peripheral nervous system integrity can be determined from nerve conduction velocity measurements.

Conduction velocity in a motor nerve that has been injured and is undergoing the process of regeneration is generally reduced. The appearance of abnormal conduction velocities in afferent sensory nerve fibers has been useful diagnostically (Buchthal and Rosenfalck 1966; Painatal 1973; Hume and Cant 1978).

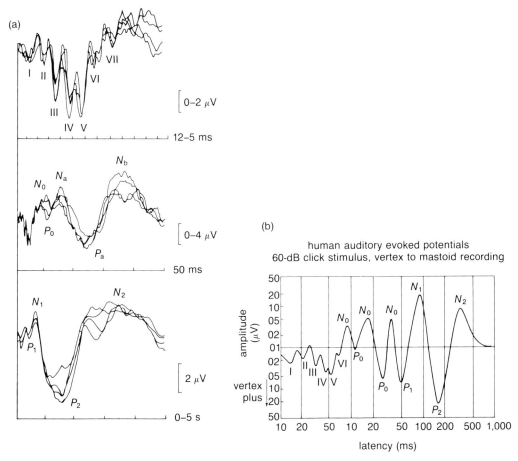

Figure 5.24 Waveforms obtained from auditory evoked responses (after Picton TW, Hillyard SA, Krausz HI, and Galambos: Human Auditory Evoked Potentials: Evaluation of Components. *Electroencephalogr and Clin Neurophys,* 36:179–190, 1974).

EEG Applications

Three areas in which the EEG is found in active use are in seizure diagnosis and monitoring (for therapy evaluation) (Gotman et al. 1982; Whisler et al. 1982), diagnosis and characterization of sleep disorders (Niedermeyer and da Silva 1982; Reynolds et al. 1983), and determination of brain death (Walker 1981). An increasing clinical application that may be implemented away from the clinic (in the home) uses EEG measurements as part of certain biofeedback techniques (Bronzino 1977). Overviews are included to familiarize readers with the scope of EEG applications.

In seizure or epileptic monitoring, goals include localizing the brain site of abnormal electrical activity (referred to as the *focus*) and defining the nature of ac-

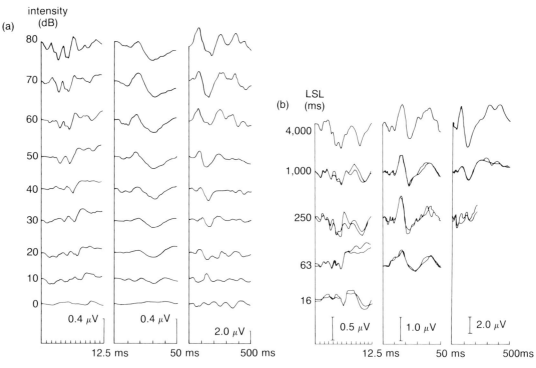

Figure 5.25   Waveforms obtained from auditory evoked responses (after Picton TW, Hillyard SA, Krausz HI, and Galambos: Human Auditory Evoked Potentials: Evaluation of Components. *Electroencephalogr and Clin Neurophys,* 36:179–190, 1974).

tivity that occurs during the event. In a given patient, these parameters can change over time, depending on adequacy of antiepilepsy medication and the natural development of the disorder. Therefore, periodic monitoring, often prescribed because of exacerbation of symptoms, has become an important clinical tool.

Although some more subtle abnormal electrical activity may be detected when the patient is not experiencing a seizure, it is most informative for initial diagnosis and follow-up monitoring to record electrical activity during a seizure. In many patients seizures seem to occur at random intervals, often with relatively long (weeks to months) quiet episodes between short periods (seconds) of abnormal activity. Because of these factors, specialized instrumentation setups and devices have been developed to allow continuous, long-term EEG monitoring. Portable FM analog cassette recorders worn by patients as they move about freely are sometimes used. Tapes can be processed at high speeds by using the time compression approach described previously. For subtle abnormalities, visual inspection of recordings is usually required. For identification of more intense abnormal epochs that are somewhat easier to detect, computer-based processing can screen hours or days of EEG records to locate the short epochs of interest. Then, visual inspection of only portions of the records is necessary to extract the desired clinical information, which is saved to document the patient's status. Electromyographic artifacts and maintenance of good electrode impedances can make such long-term monitoring efforts difficult, and special digital signal processing algorithms are often used to distinguish artifacts from true seizure activity during automated screening.

Seizures have been characterized according to type, and EEG records are usually important to make this diagnosis. Epileptic seizures that involve the majority of the brain are said to be *generalized,* as opposed to those that are restricted to a given region of the brain, termed *partial* seizures. Generalized epilepsies are also categorized according to type: (1) the more intense, or *grand mal* seizures, in which abnormal discharges begin in the portion of the recticular activating system near the brain stem and can spread throughout the cortex; and (2) *petit mal* seizures, which may exhibit observable patient characteristics very similar to those of grand mal seizures. In petit mal seizures, the attack may be very short, characterized by an intense uncontrollable movement of the head or arms (myoclonic type), or the patient may lose consciousness (absence type) and experience muscular twitching.

To determine the focus of a partial seizure, one must instrument many scalp sites with electrodes. Noting the spread of abnormal electrical activity with respect to recording sites allows estimates of the brain site involved. The problem amounts to a vector type analysis of an electrical dipole within the volume conductor that is being monitored.

Focused abnormal electrical activity may not be intense or diffuse enough, or in a critical brain area, so that an actual epileptic episode results, although the activity can increase the probability of such attacks. Surgical procedures are sometimes warranted, in part because of EEG findings, in which the focus is excised to prevent epileptic seizures due to tumors or otherwise diseased brain tissue.

Since the EEG has been studied to determine the normal progression of brain activity during sleep, it is also used diagnostically to determine different types of sleep disorders. Another application is in determining whether a patient's primary complaint (such as "always tired") results from a sleep disorder or some other condition. For these cases, patients are wired for EEG and sleep in special laboratories equipped to monitor other physiological variables, as well as EEG, continuously.

During progression of the sleep state, shifts occur in an individual's EEG characteristics from the alpha rhythm associated with relaxation to lower-frequency, larger-amplitude waveforms. In intermediate sleep depths, this slowed activity is periodically interrupted by *sleep spindles,* which are short duration bursts of alpha rhythms. Sleep is generally characterized by a more synchronous (and therefore higher-voltage) brain electrical activity. However, during rapid eye movement (REM) sleep, periods of electrical activity that more closely resemble the lower-voltage, asynchronous activity of the awake state occur. Dreaming has been associated with REM sleep; it is interesting to note that newborns spend a large percentage of their sleep time in the REM state, a percentage that progressively decreases as they grow to adulthood. In very deep sleep states, the EEG exhibits slow, large-amplitude delta waves.

Deviations from these normal sleep EEG patterns provide an estimate of the percentage of time that a subject spends in good-quality restful sleep stages, as opposed to interrupted or light sleep stages. Determining the time of the change in progression from light to deep sleep from EEG variables and correlating this event with changes in other physiological variables monitored may indicate the underlying causes of sleep disorders (lack of sufficient oxygen, cardiac arrythmias, and so on).

With the increased ability to sustain life by artificial means in recent years, defining death has become correspondingly more difficult and important. Although institutional policies and state laws vary because of the controversial nature of the subject, the absence of any or certain types of brain electrical activity is now commonly sufficient criterion to declare a patient to be brain dead. Ethical issues are further complicated by the rapid development of transplant technologies, since the majority of commonly sought organs must be obtained in situations where timing is crucial. In these cases, the EEG provides documented evidence to justify declaring a patient to be brain dead so that organ donation procedures can begin while the useful organs are still suitable for transplant use.

With the advent of inexpensive sophisticated electronic devices, biofeedback has become popular in many clinical arenas. The frequency breakdown of normal EEG presented earlier illustrates that certain normal awake states that are considered to be more desirable (relaxed versus tense or stressed) can be identified by monitoring the EEG. Special biofeedback devices have been developed to convert the type of EEG activity into audio or visual displays so that more pleasing feedback, low-pitch sounds, or displays with softer colors are associated with relaxed states. These devices can be used therapeutically to train patients to control their bodies (and minds) so that they can correlate feelings that can be perceived without biofeedback instrumentation with different states. By doing so, patients may be able to carry over these associations into everyday life and take necessary corrective action to improve their quality of life or decrease the likelihood of more serious medical problems such as hypertension and cardiovascular disease.

Evoked Potential Applications

Comprehensive reviews of evoked potential clinical applications have been presented (Courjon et al. 1982; Desmedt 1980). The basic information provided is the amplitude and latency of characteristic responses, but these measurements have many applications when interpreted in the proper clinical context under which they are obtained. Representative examples are included to illustrate the nature and scope of clinical applications.

It is generally accepted that impaired conduction across demyelinated areas in the CNS produces the symptoms of multiple sclerosis (MS) and other demyelinating diseases. It is also know that MS frequently affects the visual system. It would seem, then, that VER is well suited indeed to studying the MS patient.

An early study (Rickey et al. 1971) examined 50 patients with MS in acute exacerbation by using flash evoked responses and compared the results to age-matched normal controls. They found 40 percent of the MS patients had abnormal VER, and 6 percent of the controls were abnormal.

About the same time (Namero and Enns 1972), 20 MS patients who had a history of retrobulbar neuritis and a central visual field defect were examined. Researchers found a delay in the late peaks in all but one MS patient. The delays were largest in the patients classified as severely affected on the basis of nonneuroelectric measures.

Behrman and coworkers (Behrman et al. 1972) compared the use of flash-evoked responses to pattern-evoked responses in MS. Like others before them, they found a much greater variability of the latencies in the flash-evoked potentials. Also, because of intersubject variability of waveform, it was often difficult to compare a particular component with certainty. Pattern-evoked potentials, in comparison, had an easily recognizable major peak and a regular latency in their control population.

A large series of MS patients were tested with VER using pattern-evoked responses (Halliday et al. 1973). Ninety-six percent, or 49 of 52 clinically diagnosed MS patients (definite, probable, or possible MS), had abnormal VER.

Delicate surgical procedures, in which abnormal response might indicate that a neural area is in jeopardy and early warning can prevent extensive or further damage, also employ evoked responses. These procedures may be particularly valuable in spinal surgery, in which spinal cord evoked potentials (Yates et al. 1982) must be measured.

Symann-Louett (1977) studied a type of visual evoked response (using flashes of short words) in reading-disabled children and compared it to age-matched normal subjects (it should be noted she used flashes of short words as a stimulus, rather than the usual techniques). A significant difference was found in the VER over the left parietal region in the reading-disabled population.

Visual evoked response was used with children with Down's syndrome, who were compared to normal subjects. Normal children have an asymmetry, with late waves being larger over the right hemisphere; children having Down's syndrome have no asymmetry. The significance and specificity of this finding are unclear (Beck et al. 1975).

Auditory evoked responses are applied commonly in infants suspected of deafness (Despland and Galambos 1982). Normal responses indicate that major mechanical components of the ear and the primary auditory pathway are intact. Abnormalities in the evoked response indicate not only the presence, but also an estimate of the magnitude of hearing loss. Findings can lead to the earliest possible intervention to obtain improved prognosis.

Auditory evoked responses (AERs) largely result from stem electrical activity. In comatose patients with a toxic or metabolic cause, the auditory evoked responses were normal (or no different from those when the patient was awake) (Starr and Achor 1975). Thus, normal AER in a comatose patient is of toxi-metabolic origin or a diffuse cortical process is causing the comatose state and sparing the brain stem.

REFERENCES

Adrian, E. D., and Mathews, B. H. C. 1934. Berger rhythm: Potential changes from occipital lobes in man. *Brain* 57: 355–85.

Aunon, J. I. 1978. Computer techniques for the processing of evoked potentials. *Comput Programs Biomed* 8(3–4):243–255.

Beck, E. C., Dustman R. E., and Lewis, E. G. 1975. The use of averaged evoked potentials in evaluation of central nervous system disorders. *Int J Neurol,* 9:211–232.

Behrman, J., Halliday, A. M., and McDonald, N. I. 1972. VER to flash and pattern stimulation in patients with retrobulbar neuritis. *EEG* 33:445.

Berger, H. 1929. Uber das elektrenkaphologramm des menschen. *Arch Psychiatr Nervenkr* 87:527–570.

Billings, R. J. 1981. Automatic detection, measurement, and documentation of the visual evoked potential using a commercial microprocessor-equipped averager. *Electroencephalogr Clin Neurophysiol* 52(2):214–217.

Brinley, F. J. 1980. Excitation and conduction in nerve fibers. In Mountcastle, V.B. (ed.), *Medical physiology,* vol. 1. St. Louis: Mosby. pp. 46–81.

Bronzino, J. D. 1977. Biofeedback: Medical technology enables patients to control their bodies. In *Technology for Patient Care.* St. Louis: Mosby.

Buchsbaum, M. S., Inguar, D. H., Kessler, R., Water, R. N., Cappeletti, J., von Kamen, D. P., King, A. C., Johnson, J. C., Manning, R. G., Flynn, R. W., Mann, L. S., Bunney, W. E., and Sokoloff, L. 1982. Cerebral glucography with positron tomography. *Arch Gen Psychiatry* 39:251–259.

Buchthal, F., and Rosenfalck, A. 1966. Evoked potentials and conduction velocity in human sensory nerves. *Brain Res* (special issue) 3:1–122.

Caderas, M. et al. 1982. Sleep spindles recorded from deep cerebellar structures in man. *Clin Electroencephalogr,* 13(4):216–225.

Callaway, E., Halliday, R., and Herning, R. I. 1983. A comparison of methods for measuring event-related potentials. *Electroencephalogr Clin Neurophysiol,* 55(2):227–232.

Caton, R. 1875. The electric currents of the brain. *Br Med J,* 2:278, 1875.

Cobbold, R. S. C. 1974. *Transducers for biomedical measurements: Principles and applications.* New York: Wiley.

Courjon, J., Mauguiere, F., and Revol, M. 1982. *Clinical applications of evoked potentials in neurology.* New York: Raven.

Cracco, R. Q., and Cracco, J. B. 1976. Somatosensory evoked potentials in man: Far field potentials. *Electroencephalogr Clin Neurophysiol* 41:460–68, 1976.

Dawson, C. D. 1947. Cerebral responses to electrical stimulation of peripheral nerve in man. *J Neurol Neurosurg Psychiatry* 10:134.

Desmedt, J. E. 1980. Clinical Uses of Cerebral, Brainstem, and Spinal Somatosensory Evoked Potentials. In *Progress in Clinical Neurophysiology,* vol. 7. New York: Karger.

Despland, P. A., and Galambos, R. 1982. The brainstem auditory evoked potential is a useful tool in evaluating risk factors for hearing loss in neonatology. In Courjon, J., Mauguiere, F., and Revol. M. (eds.) *Clinical applications of evoked potentials in neurology.* New York: Raven.

Doktor, R., and Bloom, D. M. 1977. Selective lateralization of cognitive style related to occupation as determined by EEG alpha asymmetry. *Psychophysiology* 14:385–387.

Duffy, F. H. 1981. Brain electrical mapping (BEAM): Computerized access to complex brain function. *Int J Neurosci,* 13(1):55–65.

Duffy, F. H. 1982. Topographical display of evoked potentials: Clinical applications of brain electrical activity mapping (BEAM). *Ann NY Acad Sci,* 388:183–196.

Ferris, C. D. 1974. *Introduction to bioelectrodes.* New York: Plenum.

Geddes, L. A. 1972. *Electrodes and the measurement of bioelectric events.* New York: Wiley.

Gelfan, S. 1963. Neurone and synapse populations in the spinal cord: indication of role in total integration. *Nature* 198:162.

Gloor, P. 1982. Long term monitoring of the EEG: the challenge of the future. *Electroencephalogr Clin Neurophysiol* (suppl.) 36:579–583.

Gotman. 1982. Automatic recognition of epileptic seizures in the EEG. *Electroencephalogr Clin Neurophysiol* 54(5):530–540.

Guyton, A. C. 1981: *Basic human neurophysiology.* Philadelphia: Saunders.

Halliday, A. M., McDonald, W. I., and Mushin, J. 1973. Visual evoked response in diagnosis of multiple sclerosis. *Br Med J.* 4(893):661–664.

Henneman, E. 1980. Organization of the spinal cord and its reflexes. In Mountcastle, V. B. (ed.), *Medical Physiology.* St. Louis: Mosby.

Hume, A. L., and Cant, B. R. 1978. Conduction time in central somatosensory pathways in man. *Electroencephalogr Clin Neurophysiol,* 45:361–375.

Jasper, H. H. 1958. The ten-twenty electrode system of The International Federation. *Electroencephalogr Clin Neurophysiol* (app.) 10:371–75.

John, E. R., Baird, H., Fridman, J., and Bergelson, M. 1982. Normative values for brain stem auditory evoked potentials obtained by digital filtering and automatic peak detection. *Electroencephalogr Clin Neurophysiol* 54: 153–160.

John, E. R., Karmel, B. Z., Corning, W. C., Easton, P., Brown, D., Ahn, H., John, M., Harmony, T., Prichep, L., Toro, A., Gerosn, I., Bartlett, F., Thatcher, R., Kaye, H., Valdes, P., and Schwartz, E. 1977. Neurometrics. *Science* 196(4297):1393–1410.

Kuffler, S. W., and Nichols, J. G. 1976. *From Neuron to Brain,* Sunderland: Sinauer.

Mattson, R. H., et al. 1983. Closed-circuit televised videotape recording and electroencephalography in convulsive status epilepticus. *Adv Neurol* 34: 37–46.

Mountcastle, V. B. 1980. *Medical Physiology.* St. Louis: Mosby.

Namerow, N. S., Sclabass, R. J., and Enns, N. F. 1974. Somatosensory responses to stimulus trains: Normative data. *Electroencephalogr Clin Neurophysiol* 37:11–21.

Namerow, N. S., and Enns, N. F. 1972. Visual evoked responses in patients with multiple sclerosis. *J Neurol Neurosurg Psychiatry* 35:829–833.

Nastuk, N. L. 1980. Neuromuscular transmission. In Mountcastle, V. B. (ed.) *Medical Physiology,* vol. 1. St. Louis: Mosby. pp. 151–183.

Neuman, M. R. 1978. Biopotential electrodes. In Webster, J. G. (ed.) *Medical instrumentation: Application and design.* Boston: Houghton Mifflin. pp. 215–272.

Niedermeyer, E., and da Silva, F. L. 1982. *Electroencephalography: Basic principles, clinical applications, and related fields.* Baltimore: Urban and Schwarzenberg.

Paicer, P. L., Larson, S. J., and Sances, A., Jr. 1967. Theoretical evaluation of cerebral evoked potentials. *Proc Annu Conf Eng Med Biol* 14:1.

Painatal, A. S. 1973. Conduction in sensory nerve fibres. In Desmedt (ed.) *New developments in electromyography and clinical neurophysiology,* vol. 2. Basel: Karger. pp. 19–41.

Philips, M. I. 1973. *Brain unit activity during behavior.* Springfield: Thomas.

Reynolds, C. F., Spiker, D. G., Hanin, I., and Kupfer, D. J. 1983. Electroencephalographic sleep, aging, and psychopathology: new data and state of the art. *Biol Psychiatry,* 18(2):139–155.

Richey, E. T., Kooi, K. A., Tourtellotte, W. W. 1971. Visual evoked responses in multiple sclerosis. *J Neurol Neurosurg Psychiatry* 34:275–280.

Roden, M. S. 1979. *Analog and digital communication systems.* Englewood Cliffs: Prentice-Hall. Chap. 1, 6, and 7.

Rush, S., and Driscoll, D. A. 1969. EEG electrode sensitivity: An application of reciprocity. *IEEE Trans Biomed Eng,* 16:126.

Schadke, L. L., and Potvin, A. R. 1981. Cognitive style, EEG waveforms and brain levels. *Hum Systems Manage* 2:329–331.

Starr, A., and Achor, L. J. 1975. Auditory brain stem responses in neurological disease. *Arch Neurol* 32:761–768.

Stout, D. F. 1976. Demodulators and discriminators. In Kaufman, M. (ed.) *Handbook of operational amplifier circuit design.* New York: McGraw-Hill. pp. 4–7.

Symann-Louett, N., Gascon, G. G., Matsumiya, Y., and Lombroso, C. T. 1977. Waveform differences in visual evoked responses between normal and reading disabled children. *Neurology,* 27:156–159.

Towe, A. I. 1973. Sampling single neuron activity. In Thompson, R. F., and Patterson, M. M. (eds.) *Bioelectric recording techniques. Part A: Cellular processes and brain potentials.* New York: Academic Press. pp. 82–86.

Walker, A. E. 1981. Electroencephalographic findings in cerebral death. In Walker, A. E. (ed.) *Cerebral death,* (2d ed.). Baltimore: Urban and Schwarzenberg. chap. VI, pp. 65–95.

Webster, J. G. 1978. *Medical instrumentation: Application and design.* Boston: Houghton Mifflin.

Whisler, J. W., ReMine, W. J., Leppik, I. E., McLain, L. W., and Gummit, R. J. 1982. Machine detection of spike-wave activity in the EEG and its accuracy compared with visual interpretation. *Electroencephalogr Clin Neurophysiol* 54(5):541–551.

Yates, B. J., et al. 1982. Origin and properties of spinal cord field potentials. *Neurosurg* 11(3):439–450.

CHAPTER **6**

Musculoskeletal Biomechanics: Fundamental Measurements and Analysis

Roy B. Davis, III, Ph.D.

Assistant Professor of Engineering
Trinity College, Hartford, Connecticut

INTRODUCTION

The term *biomechanics* often notes that area of biomedical engineering that is concerned specifically with human biodynamics. In this context, biomechanics certainly involves the quantitative description of the kinematics, kinetics, and mechanical work and power associated with human motion. However, these topics represent only a subset of a field of study that also includes such broadly related areas as the biomechanical response of soft tissue to loading and cardiovascular dynamics, among others. In reality, therefore, the scope of activities involving biomechanics is broad.

Since one of the major tasks of biomedical engineering professionals is to develop diagnostic, therapeutic, and assessment devices that enhance the capabilities of the clinical staff in meeting the needs of their patients, it is important to review the role "biomechanical studies" play in this process. At the outset, for example, one might easily ask, Who is interested in the examination of biomechanical performance? The list of users of this technology is extensive and constantly expanding:

1 In the clinical area, the list of professionals includes orthopedists, orthotists, prosthetists, rehabilitation engineers, and therapists (physical, occupational,

recreational) all concerned with properly diagnosing and treating patients with biomechanical deficits.

2 In sports biomechanics, coaches and trainers, as well as sports equipment designers and manufacturers, are keenly interested in quantifying the limits of athletic performance.

3 In industry, human factors specialists are interested in designing appropriate workplace environments for the human worker or in implementing a growing robotic workforce.

Consequently, although clinical applications have received significant emphasis, it is important to stress that work and activity in musculoskeletal measurements are not restricted solely to the clinical setting.

In an effort to describe biomechanical measurement and analysis techniques most commonly employed today, this chapter focuses upon the differences in measurement and description and in description and assessment. The terms *measurement, description, analysis,* and *assessment* have been defined in engineering terms by Winter (1979), who stated that "any quantitative assessment of human motion must be preceded by a measurement and description phase, and if more meaningful diagnostics are needed, a biomechanical analysis is usually necessary." If we follow this definition, it can be noted that measurement provides the means of generating a quantitative description or analysis. Once this is accomplished, assessments logically follow. Figure 6.1 illustrates the process one might follow to approach problems related to the implementation and utilization of any biomechanical measurement system. For example, a clear understanding of the initial problem leads to a statement of the desired assessment capabilities (for example, if fundamental gait characteristics are understood, then assessment criteria related to gait that is not "normal" may be developed). In the planning or implementation stage, these assessment requirements lead to a quantified description and analysis process, which in turn prescribes the required biomechanical measurements. Ultimately, the utility of the system is evaluated through its use.

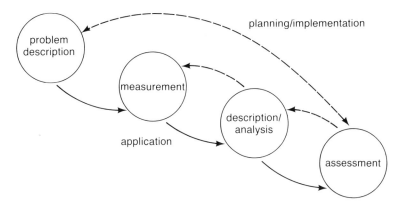

Figure 6.1   Block diagram illustrating the planning, implementation, and application of motion measurement problem solution strategies.

The material in this chapter is organized much as the problem-solving structure described is. For example, we shall initially discuss measurement parameters and techniques, then quantitative description and analysis techniques, and finally assessment strategies.

MEASUREMENT PARAMETERS, METHODS, AND SYSTEMS

Parameter Specification

A variety of physiological tests may be prescribed to assess neuromuscular performance, including the following:

1 Constrained motion
   a Upright bicycle ergometer
   b Step test
   c Treadmill
2 Unconstrained motion
   a Gait (walking)
   b Running

In each of these cases, the basis of the description and analysis of the biomechanical measurements may be Newtonian or classical mechanics or a consideration of work/power relationships. Therefore, any measurement arrangement for the preceding types of analysis must acquire or determine the following supporting parameters:

1 Displacements (linear and angular) of the body segments(s)
2 Velocities (linear and angular) of the segment(s)
3 Accelerations (linear and angular) of the segment(s)
4 External forces acting on the segment(s): ground force reactions, wind resistance, and so on
5 Mass and inertial characteristics of the segment(s)
6 Level of muscular activity

Employing the first five parameters either acquired directly or computed from acquired data, a mechanical description may be developed. Although the collection of electromyographic (EMG) data, with its foundations in the understanding of electrophysiology (see Chapter 5), receives little attention here (for detailed reviews see Winter [1979] and Astrand and Rodahl [1977]), the assessment process typically correlates EMG activity with biomechanical analysis results.

Methods and Systems

Measurement systems may be broadly categorized as either mechanical transducers attached to the test subject or electro-optical techniques. Mechanical transducer techniques employed in biomechanical data collection include the following.

Electrogoniometers

A *goniometer* measures the *relative* angle between two body segments, such as the knee angle formed between thigh and shank. Shown schematically in Figure 6.2, a goniometer is typically composed of a resistance potentiometer with a leg connected to both the shaft and base for attachment to each body segment. Advantages associated with the goniometer include a relatively low cost, simple construction, and an analog output that is readily digitized by a microprocessor-based analog-to-digital converter. The relative angle the goniometer describes, however, is less biomechanically useful than *absolute* angles, from which relative angles can be calculated. In addition, questions of whether the goniometer interferes with or constrains the motion of the limb or body segments it is monitoring arise. For additional information and illustration through application, the reader can consult the work of Lamoreux (1981), Marsolais (1981), and Perry (1981).

Accelerometers

Piezoelectric or strain gauge accelerometers attached to a body segment at a specific point allow for the measurement of *absolute* acceleration in one or three orthogonal directions simultaneously. Biomechanically, because segment motion commonly includes rotation as well as translation, the output of the triaxial transducer is significant only if combined with additional kinematic information (such as limb angular orientation) and may be misleading unless segment motion is constrained in some fashion, for example, rotation of a shank or foot segment about a fixed knee joint. In its favor, this type of transducer does measure an absolute quantity (referenced to an inertially fixed coordinate system) as opposed to a rela-

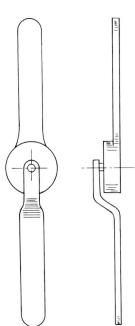

Figure 6.2   Planar electrogoniometer comprising two attachment legs, one fixed to the shaft and the other to the body of a rotational potentiometer used to acquire the relative orientation of two limb segments.

tive value (referenced to a moving coordinate system) and is useful in some applications. For additional information, refer to works by Judge (1975), Plaja and associates (1976), Smidt and coworkers (1977), and Morris (1972, 1973).

Pressure transducers

Piezoelectric or strain gauge pressure sensors are useful in the quantification of force and pressure distribution patterns on contact surfaces. Application examples include the examination of the tissue pressure distribution at contact points on orthotic devices and at the stump-socket interface on prosthetic limbs. Studies have examined socket pressures as related to particular limb designs and as a function of gait characteristics (Rae and Cockrell 1971; Davis and Burger 1985).

Force platforms

Force platforms allow for the measurement of ground force reactions that are applied to the foot (or feet) during movement. Typically, force platforms measure three orthogonal components of force (producing a force vector) and three orthogonal components of moment (used to determine the instantaneous center of contact pressure, or the point of application of the reaction force vector). For examples of force plate applications in gait analysis, the reader will find an extensive literature including work by Chao and associates (1980), Cohen and collaborators (1980), Draganich and coworkers (1980), Groh and Baumann (1976), Jarrett and associates (1980), Kairento and Hellen (1981), Lord (1981), and Stokes and coworkers (1974). In sports medicine, Grahammer (1979), Cavanaugh and Lafortune (1980), Mason and associates (1979), Williams and Cavanaugh (1980), Clark and coworkers (1980), and Coutts (1980) have contributed research.

Switches

Microswitches provide a means of monitoring displacement and observing contact patterns. For example, a "foot switch," schematically represented in Figure 6.3, allows one to determine the "heel strike" and "toe off" points in the gait cycle when attached to subject's foot (or feet). The particular design illustrated in Figure 6.3 was conceived in the Gait Analysis Laboratory at the Scottish Rite Hospital for Crippled Children (Dallas, Texas) and demonstrates an inexpensive technique for collecting fundamental stride information.

   In addition to these mechanical transducer methods, electro-optical techniques in kinematic (motions analysis) include the following:

Photographic filming

Cinemagraphic cameras (Golbranson et al. 1981; Hagy 1981; Kairento and Hellen 1981; Kunz and Kaufmann 1981) and interrupted-light (strobe light) photography (Wyss and Pollack 1980; Woltring 1980; Murray et al. 1981) record the displacement of reflective body segment markers (Figure 6.4). The marker displacement film is digitized frame by frame, and velocities and accelerations are determined by

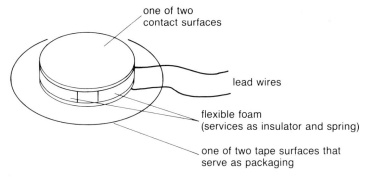

Figure 6.3 Schematic representation of the Scottish Rite foot switch design to monitor ground contact sequencing (courtesy of the Texas Scottish Rite Hospital for Crippled Children, Dallas, Texas).

numerically differentiating the displacement data (the analytical details of this process are described in a later section). The advantages of these techniques over those described later are associated with costs; while the utility of these systems is limited by the labor-intensive nature of the digitization process and the longer "turn-around" time between filming and analysis. In addition, the results of the interrupted light photography technique are subject to influence by the required lighting arrangement, that is, the strobe lighting may be distractive.

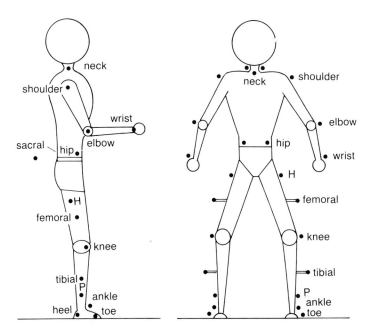

Figure 6.4 Schematic diagram illustrating the placement of a passive body segment marker system (courtesy of the Newington Children's Hospital, Newington, Connecticut).

Video recording

A technique useful in qualitative assessment of motion is video recording. This facility is particularly valuable in conjunction with a more quantitatively oriented system, that is, a system that generates a model representation of the analysis, for example, stick figures. An example of this type of application is found at Texas Scottish Rite Hospital where engineers with a special-effects (slow motion) video recording of the gait examination, along with selected EMG information (Carollo 1981). Employing the system shown in Figure 6.5, the output of frontal and lateral video cameras (Sony RSC-1050 rotary shutter) is presented on one video screen along with the desired EMG trace(s). Clinical assessment may then take the form of a frame-by-frame analysis or slow-motion playback. With this capability, the clinician has the opportunity to associate and correlate gait characteristics with muscle activity level.

Optical tracking systems

Optical tracking systems incorporate the kinematic quantification objective of the photographic filming techniques discussed, but at greatly reduced labor and time

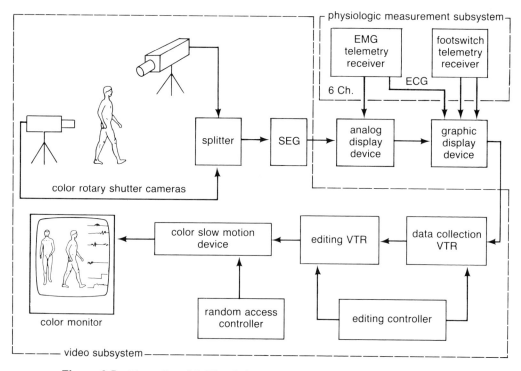

Figure 6.5 Texas Scottish Rite Gait Analysis Laboratory System schematic, illustrating the application of a dual-channel slow-motion video monitoring display (courtesy of the Texas Scottish Rite Hospital for Crippled Children, Dallas, Texas).

expenditures. All four of the particular systems described briefly next share a common operating principle: a computer-interfaced optical monitoring device(s); for example, a video camera "tracks" a system of reflective body segment markers (Figure 6.4) and stores the coordinate histories of each marker in the secondary storage device of a computer for processing.

Three examples of commercially available motion measurement systems are (1) Vicon (marketed in the United States by Oxford Metrics, Inc., Clearwater, Florida); (2) CODA-3 (marketed in the United States by Advanced Mechanical Technology, Inc., Newton, Massachusetts); and (3) Selspot II (marketed in the United States by Selective Electronic, Inc., Valdese, North Carolina). In addition, a motions analysis system designed by the United Technologies Research Center (East Hartford, Connecticut) and in use at the Newington Children's Hospital (Newington, Connecticut) will be discussed.

Vicon.   As shown in Figure 6.6, the Vicon system employs from two to seven high-stability, 625-line, 2:1 interlaced television cameras to collect up to 50 fields of data per second for determination of three-dimensional marker coordinates. Each camera is equipped with a synchronous infrared strobe (940-nanometer [nm] wavelength, 2-ms pulse duration) and a lens system equipped with a 700- to 2,800-nm bandpass filter. With this capability, the system operates fundamentally as fol-

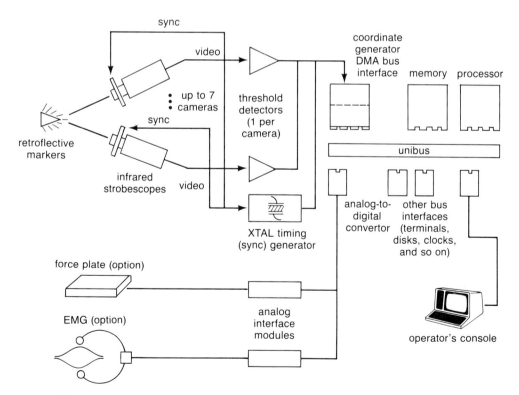

Figure 6.6   Block diagram of the Vicon motion measurement system (courtesy of Oxford Metrics, Inc., Clearwater, Florida).

lows: up to 30 of the retroreflective Scotchlite markers (either conical [19 mm by 19 mm] or cylindrical [14 mm by 12 mm]) are tracked simultaneously; a marker detector module (interfaced with each camera) converts the video pulses associated with each infrared marker reflection into digital timing signals; then a coordinate generator integrates the timing pulses from each camera and generates an array of space coordinates describing the instantaneous marker system position. The operator then has available a data file that includes not only marker coordinate history, but force plate data (ground force reactions) and EMG data. The kinematic data are sorted with the aid of the operator, labeling each coordinate marker in each frame of data. For the most part, the computer performs this data reduction process, with the operator assisting when data are incomplete: one or more markers were not in view of the camera(s) for one or more frames (referred to as *missing*

Table 6.1   Comparison of motion measurement systems

	CODA-3	Vicon	Selspot II	UTC
Motion camera/ scanning system				
Number of channels	3	2–7	1–16	3
Spatial incremental resolution				
Horizontal	$0.1z$ (600 Hz)	1:1,000	0.025% of field	1:2,000
Vertical	$0.1z^2$	1:300 (50 Hz)		1:2,000
	(z in meters)	1:600 (25 Hz)		
Accuracy	—	1:100	>99.5% of field	1:500
Number of markers	Up to 12	Up to 30	Up to 120	24
Marker type	Passive, retro-reflective	Passive, retro-reflective	Infrared LEDs	Passive, retro-reflective
Marker illumination wavelength	Color-coded	940 nm	950 nm	880 nm
Data collection rate	Up to 600 Hz	25 or 50 Hz	10-kHz maximum	30 or 60 Hz
Visual camera system				
Number of channels		Motion cameras used		3
Force measurement system				
Number of platforms		Up to 4		2
Number of force components (per platform)		3		3
Number of torque components (per platform)		3		3
Analog channels available for emg		Up to 32	Up to 32	Up to 16

markers). The system offers a variety of result display format options, including graphs, stick figures, histograms, numerical results, and planar projections of three-dimensional representations. Advantages of this system include unrestricted camera placement so that cameras may be located (and then calibrated) in an optimal arrangement for each type of experiment and videotape archiving capability of the real-time data. The operation of the system does depend to some degree upon the operator's experience in sorting the data, particularly in the sense that the operator may be viewing the motion from a nonconventional perspective, for example, a view of the motion that is not necessarily a primary plane projection (sagittal, frontal, or transverse). Table 6.1 summarizes the technical specifications associated with this system in comparison with the three other techniques.

CODA-3. The CODA-3 system is an optical scanning device, as opposed to a camera or lens-based system, such as Vicon. This device, shown schematically in Figure 6.7, employs three fan-shaped beams of white light that are swept across the field of view by three multifaceted polygonal mirrors. Light reflected by retroreflective markers (small pyramidal assembly; 14 by 14 by 10 mm, 2 grams (g); comprising four corner-mounted prisms) travels back along original light paths to photodetectors located in one of the three scanning units. The phase of returning

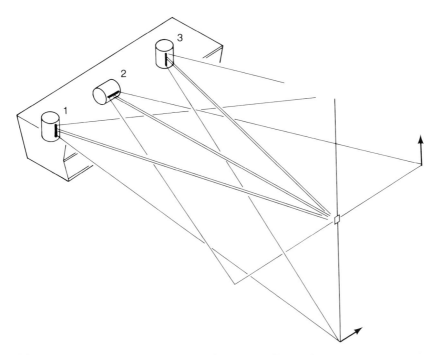

Figure 6.7 CODA-3 motion monitoring system, illustrating the arrangement of the three optical scanners (courtesy of Advanced Mechanical Technology, Inc., Newton, Massachusetts).

pulse with respect to polygon mirror rotation provides an indication of the spatial position of a marker. Shown in Figure 6.7, two scanning drums, mounted 1 m apart on a rigid chassis, scan horizontally to provide triangulation for marker distance (away from scanner) as well as a horizontal position coordinate; a third scanner, mounted between the first two, scans vertically to provide marker location in that direction. Sixteen-bit microprocessors reduce light pulse data from each scanner into xyz coordinate information while the scanning is in progress (within the scanner period of 1.67 ms, this results in a maximum sampling rate of 600 Hz). The system (which also incorporates 16 transistor-transistor logic [TTL] compatible outputs) is controlled and data are displayed on a stand-alone minicomputer. Advantages of this system are (1) that it is not lens-based and consequently is not subject to lens parallax distortion at limits of a field of view; each marker is color-coded so that interactive marker labeling by the operator after a test is performed is not necessary and (2) no calibration scheme is required (CODA-3 includes a zero set facility so that a coordinate origin may be established). The motion system is currently limited to a maximum of 12 markers at this time. Plans for this motions measurement include the incorporation of force platforms and the development of kinematic reduction software. Again, Table 6.1 summarizes the technical specifications associated with this system in comparison with the other techniques.

Selspot II. The standard Selspot II system includes one or more (up to 16) cameras, a set of infrared light-emitting diode (LED) segment markers, an administration unit that preprocesses the camera signals, and a computer for data reduction and graphical output. The heart of the Selspot camera is a photodetector sensor comprising a flat semiconducting SiTek disk coated on both sides with a light-sensitive material. The camera lens system focuses the pulses of infrared light (950-nm) from body markers on associated points on the photosensitive surface of the disk, to determine the instantaneous planar positions of that light source in space and time. Two or more cameras or photodetector units used simultaneously produce a three-dimensional coordinate history for each marker. Although this type of camera sensor affords a continuous operation, the sampling rate of the system ultimately depends upon the number of cameras employed (10 kHz maximum sampling rate, 100×10^{-6} sampling time for each three-dimensional point). The resolution of this system is 0.025 percent of the measuring range, or field of view. The system administration unit, in addition to preprocessing the camera signals, functions as an analog-to-digital data logger for electrocardiographic, electromyographic, and force plate signals. A well-developed software package includes body segment position or angle as a function of time, velocity or acceleration as a function of time, stick figure representation of the movement, and auxillary data (ECG, EMG, force plate) as a function of time.

The active marker system offers the advantage of pulse labeling the markers for identification during tracking; that is, because the light emitted from each marker is pulsed in a controlled manner, the camera(s) may record the activity of each segment marker sequentially. Affording the user this capability requires that the subject be attached to power-control cables that may be distracting. Table 6.1 summarizes further the comparative capability of this system.

Newington Children's Hospital Gait Analysis Laboratory

Figure 6.8 illustrates schematically the layout of the Gait Analysis Laboratory at the Newington Children's Hospital, Newington, Connecticut, which was designed and implemented by the United Technologies Research Center, East Hartford, Connecticut. The fundamental components of this system include the following:

1 A three-channel motion camera system (Vidicon Camera C-1000, Hamamatsu TV Co., Ltd., Hamamatsu, Japan)

2 A three-channel visual camera system

3 A 16-channel EMG telemetry system (Bio-Sentry Telemetry Model 7144, Bio-Sentry Telemetry, Inc., Torrance, California, and L & M Model 1006 Telemetry System, L & M Electronics Inc., Daly City, California)

4 A force measurement system with two force platforms (Model OR6-3 Force-Torque Dynamometer, Advanced Mechanical Technology, Inc., Newton, Massachusetts).

The subject is fitted with a set of 24 retroreflective markers that are illuminated by near-infrared LEDs located at each motion camera. The lens system of each motion camera is equipped with an optical filter that is matched to the wavelength of the energy spectra reflected from the marker system; the motion cameras detect only the reflected near-infrared light. Synchronous videorecording by the set of visual cameras allows not only film archiving for viewing at a later date, but

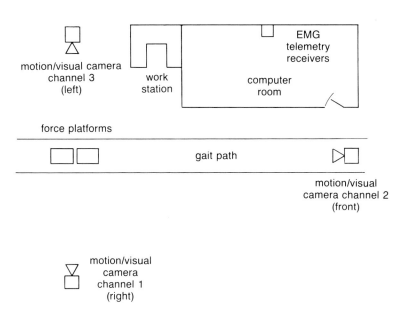

Figure 6.8 Motion Analysis Laboratory at the Newington Children's Hospital, showing the relative positions of the three motion cameras (courtesy of the Newington Children's Hospital, Newington, Connecticut).

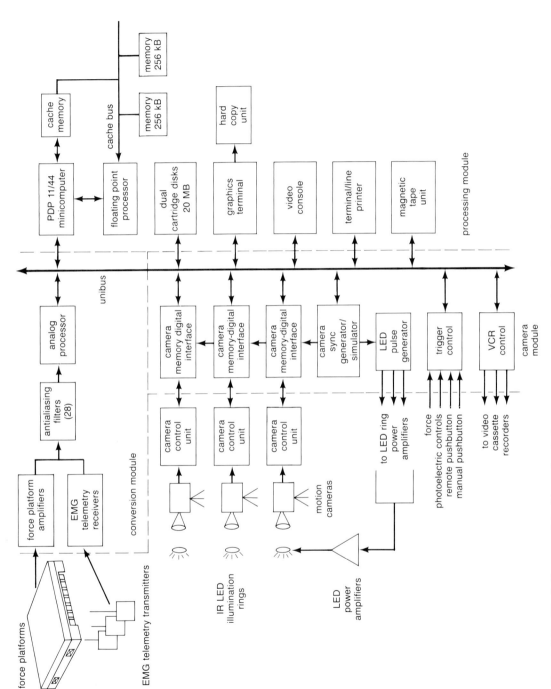

Figure 6.9 Block diagram of the biomechanical measurement system configuration at the Newington Children's Hospital (courtesy of the Newington Children's Hospital, Newington, Connecticut).

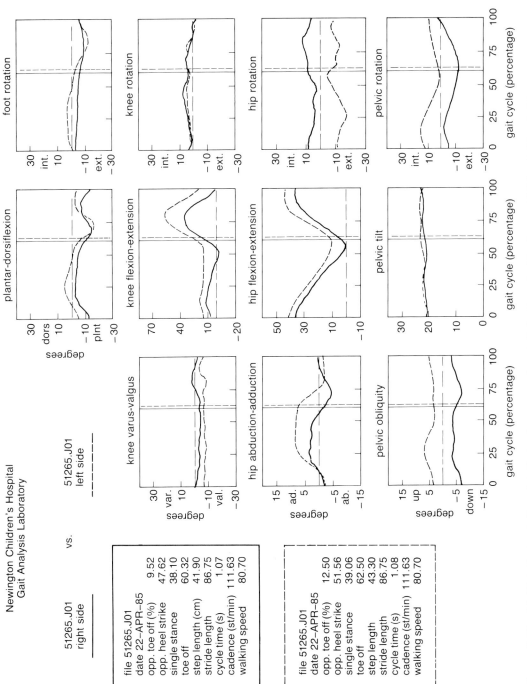

Figure 6.10   Multiple limb rotation plot display format employed clinically at the Newington Children's Hospital (courtesy of the Newington Children's Hospital, Newington, Connecticut).

also a frame-by-frame comparison with the observed motion (marker displacement) data. The supervisory computer system (shown in Figure 6.9) that collects the data from the motion cameras, force plates, and EMG system has the following basic components: (1) the camera module, which includes motion and visual camera control hardware; (2) the conversion module, which includes signal conditioning and analog-to-digital conversion hardware; and (3) the processing module, which includes the minicomputer and associated peripherals. Triggering of the system is accomplished either manually via a remote switch or automatically with a pair of microwave velocity sensors or a pair of photoelectric switches.

After data collection, marker centroids are calculated, interactive (user-assisted) marker tracking is accomplished, marker coordinate calculations are performed, instantaneous joint centers are determined, and gait display information is compiled. Figure 6.10 and 6.11 illustrate the array of display formats available to the clinician, for instance, individual segment rotation history and EMG activ-

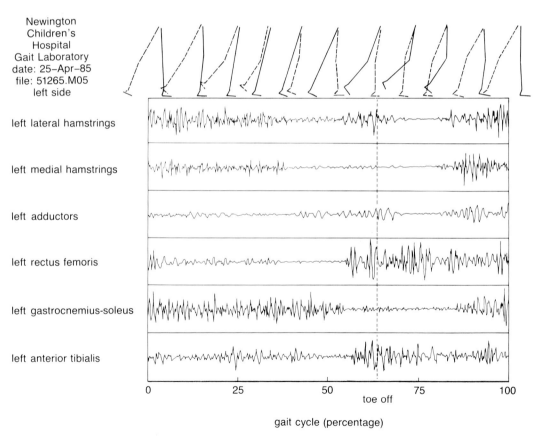

Figure 6.11   EMG/stick figure plot display correlating limb displacement with muscular activity level (courtesy of the Newington Children's Hospital, Newington, Connecticut).

ity. Energy expenditure software also examines and compares preoperative to postoperative gait performance. For additional details, the reader can consult Taylor and coworkers (1982, 1984) and Gage (1983, 1984). Again, Table 6.1 summarizes the capabilities of this particular system in comparison with the three previously described.

METHODS OF ANALYSIS

Newtonian Mechanics

Assume that one has the task of describing for assessment purposes, in as complete a fashion as possible, the biodynamics of body segment movement, including an estimation of joint forces, muscle movements, and mechanical work done during the movement (defined later). Because of these assessment specifications, a description or analysis based on Newtonian mechanics (kinematics and kinetics) is desired, that is, an analysis that employs the relationships

$$\Sigma \mathbf{F} = m\mathbf{a} \tag{1}$$

and

$$\Sigma \mathbf{M} = I\alpha \tag{2}$$

where
$\mathbf{F}$ = vector sum of the external forces acting on the segment of interest
m = mass of the segment
$\mathbf{a}$ = instantaneous linear acceleration of the segment
$\mathbf{M}$ = vector sum of the external moments acting on the segment
I = centroidal mass moment of inertia of the segment
α = instantaneous angular acceleration of the segment

Consequently, measurement techniques and systems capable of identifying the orientation (spatial position) of one or more body segments and measuring external forces, such as ground force reactions, presented in the previous section can provide appropriate biomechanical measures.

The current section demonstrates the relation of coordinate locations of body segment markers to (1) the angular displacements of the segment(s), (2) the linear and angular velocities of the segment(s), and (3) the linear and angular accelerations of the segment(s). It also provides illustrations that use equations (1) and (2) to relate external forces acting on the segment(s) (that is, the system kinetics, such as ground force reaction), and the mass and inertial characteristics of the segment(s) to the kinematics.

Kinematics

Given the two markers shown in Figure 6.12, then the instantaneous position of the markers in relation to an inertially fixed coordinate system, *xyz*, may be defined as vectors by

$$\mathbf{r}_1 = x_1\mathbf{i} + y_1\mathbf{j} + z_1\mathbf{k} \tag{3}$$

$$\mathbf{r}_2 = x_2\mathbf{i} + y_2\mathbf{j} + z_2\mathbf{k} \tag{4}$$

where

$$
\begin{aligned}
\mathbf{r}_1 &= \text{instantaneous position vector of marker 1} \\
\mathbf{r}_2 &= \text{instantaneous position vector of marker 2} \\
x_1, y_1, z_1 &= \text{instantaneous coordinates of marker 1} \\
x_2, y_2, z_2 &= \text{instantaneous coordinates of marker 2} \\
\mathbf{i}, \mathbf{j}, \mathbf{k} &= \text{orthogonal unit vectors in the x, y and z axial directions, respectively}
\end{aligned}
$$

and

$$\mathbf{r}_{2/1} = \mathbf{r}_2 - \mathbf{r}_1 \tag{5}$$

where

$$
\mathbf{r}_{2/1} = \text{position vector describing the location of marker 2 relative to marker 1}
$$

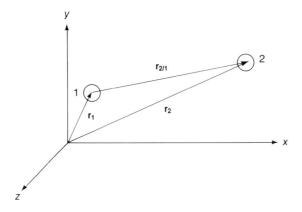

Figure 6.12 Relative position of two body segment markers, described by vector $r_{2/1}$.

or, in general, for the position of ith marker

$$\mathbf{r_i} = x_i\mathbf{i} + {}_i\mathbf{j} + z_i\mathbf{k} \quad \text{for } i = 1, n \tag{6}$$

where

n = total number of body segment markers employed in the system

Since xyz are *absolute* coordinates measured in relation to an inertially fixed coordinate system, then the linear velocity of the ith marker, $\mathbf{v_i}$, is defined as the first derivative of ith marker position vector with respect to time, or

$$\mathbf{v_i} = \frac{d\mathbf{r_i}}{dt} = \dot{x}\,\mathbf{i} + \dot{y}\mathbf{j} + \dot{z}_i\mathbf{k} \tag{7}$$

and similarly, the linear acceleration of the ith marker, $\mathbf{a_i}$, is defined as the first derivative of the ith marker velocity vector with respect to time, or

$$\mathbf{a_i} = \frac{d\mathbf{v_i}}{dt} = \dot{v}_{xi}\mathbf{i} + v_{yi}\mathbf{j} + \dot{v}_{zi}\mathbf{k} \tag{8}$$

where

v_{xi}, v_{yi}, v_{zi} = components of the linear velocity of the ith marker in the three orthogonal directions, x, y, and z, respectively

Keep in mind that $\mathbf{a_i}$ is the *instantaneous* linear acceleration of the ith marker based on the instantaneous position of the ith marker. Recall that the available data (for the ith marker) consist of one set of coordinates for every frame of data; for example, for the ith marker and jth data frame, the position vector, $\mathbf{r_i}\,|\,_j$, may be written in the following general form,

$$\mathbf{r_i}\,|\,_j = x_i\,|\,_j\mathbf{i} + y_i\,|\,_j\mathbf{j} + z_i\,|\,_j\mathbf{k} \tag{9}$$

To determine velocities and accelerations associated with the jth frame, position data from the previous $(j - 1)$ frame and the next $(j + 1)$ frame are used in the following manner. If t is defined as the time period between frames j and $j - 1$ as well as between frames j and $j + 1$, then a coordinate position, say x_{j-1} or x_{j+1}, may be defined by using Taylor's series expansions as

$$x_{j+1} = x_j + t\dot{x}_j + \left(\frac{t}{2}\right)^2 \ddot{x}_j + \ldots \tag{10}$$

and

$$x_{j-1} = x_j - t\dot{x}_j + \left(\frac{t}{2}\right)^2 \ddot{x}_j - \ldots \tag{11}$$

Subtracting equations (10) and (11) and solving for $\dot{x}_j$ and $\ddot{x}_j$ yields

$$\dot{x}_j = \frac{x_{j+1} - x_{j-1}}{2t} \tag{12}$$

and

$$\ddot{x}_j = \frac{x_{j+1} - 2x_j + x_{j-1}}{t^2} \tag{13}$$

At this point, the central difference relationships defined by equations (12) and (13) may be employed to redefine the linear velocity relationships (equation [7]) for the ith marker, jth frame as

$$\mathbf{v_i} = \frac{x_i\,|_{\,j+1} - x_i\,|_{\,j-1}}{2t}\,\mathbf{i} + \frac{y_i\,|_{\,j+1} - y_i\,|_{\,j-1}}{2t}\,\mathbf{j}$$

$$+ \frac{z_i\,|_{\,j+1} - z_i\,|_{\,j-1}}{2t}\,\mathbf{k} \tag{14}$$

and

$$\mathbf{a_i} = \frac{v_x\,|_{\,j+1} - v_x\,|_{\,j-1}}{2t}\,\mathbf{i} + \frac{v_y\,|_{\,j+1} - v_y\,|_{\,j-1}}{2t}\,\mathbf{j}$$

$$+ \frac{v_z\,|_{\,j+1} - v_z\,|_{\,j-1}}{2t}\,\mathbf{k} \tag{15}$$

or

$$\mathbf{a_i} = \frac{x_i\,|_{\,j+1} - 2x_i\,|_{\,j} + x_i\,|_{\,j-1}}{t^2}\,\mathbf{i}$$

$$+ \frac{y_i\,|_{\,j+1} - 2y_i\,|_{\,j} + y_i\,|_{\,j-1}}{t^2}\,\mathbf{j} \tag{16}$$

$$+ \frac{z_i\,|_{\,j+1} - 2z_i\,|_{\,j} + z_i\,|_{\,j-1}}{t^2}\,\mathbf{k}$$

Example 1: Given an individual flexing a forearm in the sagittal plane about a fixed elbow axis such that the coordinates presented in Table 6.2 define the wrist marker displacement with time, determine the linear velocity and acceleration vectors associated with the wrist marker displacement. Note that the data presented in Table 6.2 are representative of the type of results expected from one of the previously described motions measurement systems (with a 1/60-sampling time interval).

Table 6.2 Planar elbow flexion marker motion results: coordinates of curvilinear displacement

Frame	Time (s)	Marker Coordinates x (cm)	y
0	0.0000	35.60	0.00
1	0.0167	35.60	0.08
2	0.0333	35.59	0.62
3	0.0500	35.54	2.05
4	0.0667	35.29	4.67
5	0.0834	34.54	8.62
6	0.1000	32.82	13.80
7	0.1167	29.60	19.78
8	0.1334	24.53	25.80
9	0.1500	17.64	30.92
10	0.1667	9.46	34.32
11	0.1834	0.89	35.59
12	0.2000	−7.10	34.88
13	0.2167	−13.79	32.82
14	0.2334	−18.85	30.20
15	0.2501	−22.33	27.72
16	0.2667	−24.49	25.84
17	0.2834	−25.63	24.71
18	0.3001	−26.09	24.22
19	0.3167	−26.18	24.13

Solution: Applying equations (14) and (15) yields the desired results, as illustrated by determining the marker velocity and acceleration vectors associated with frame 8, approximately 0.13 s into flexion. Substituting marker displacement data from frames 7 and 9 into equation (14) results in the linear velocity vector components v_x and v_y for frame 8, or

$$v_x = \frac{(17.64 - 29.60)\,\text{cm}}{2(0.01667)\,\text{s}} \tag{1.1}$$

or

$$v_x = -358.7\,\text{cm/s} \tag{1.2}$$

and

$$v_y = \frac{(30.92 - 19.78)\,\text{cm}}{2(0.01667)\,\text{s}} \tag{1.3}$$

or

$$v_y = 334.1\,\text{cm/s} \tag{1.4}$$

Table 6.3 Elbow flexion marker results: linear velocity and acceleration
vector components

Frame	Time	Displacement		Velocity		Acceleration	
		x	y	x	y	x	y
	(s)	(cm)		(cm/s)		(cm/s)	
0	0.000	35.60	0.00	0.0			
1	0.017	35.60	0.08	− 0.2	18.7		
2	0.033	35.59	0.62	− 1.8	59.1	− 266.4	3,074.6
3	0.050	35.54	2.05	− 9.0	121.2	− 846.6	4,138.8
4	0.067	35.29	4.67	− 30.0	197.1	− 1,957.4	4,583.9
5	0.083	34.54	8.62	− 74.3	274.0	− 3,548.2	4,133.8
6	0.100	32.82	13.80	− 148.3	334.9	− 5,228.0	2,576.7
7	0.117	29.60	19.78	− 248.6	360.0	− 6,310.7	− 22.2
8	0.133	24.53	25.80	− 358.7	334.1	− 6,099.5	− 3,133.5
9	0.150	17.64	30.92	− 452.0	255.5	− 4,309.9	− 5,824.6
10	0.167	9.46	34.32	− 502.4	139.9	− 1,341.7	− 7,155.4
11	0.183	0.89	35.59	− 496.7	16.9	− 1,863.6	− 6,687.4
12	0.200	− 7.10	34.88	− 440.2	− 83.0	− 4,325.3	− 4,723.7
13	0.217	− 13.79	32.82	− 352.5	− 140.6	− 5,516.4	− 2,097.4
14	0.233	− 18.85	30.20	− 256.3	− 152.9	− 5,504.2	296.4
15	0.250	− 22.33	27.72	− 169.0	− 130.7	− 4,722.2	1,873.5
16	0.267	− 24.49	25.84	− 98.9	− 90.5	− 3,625.0	2,461.5
17	0.283	− 25.63	24.71	− 48.1	− 48.6	− 2,475.5	2,193.2
18	0.300	− 26.09	24.22	− 16.4	− 17.4		
19	0.317	− 26.18	24.13	0.0			

The application of equation (16) with marker velocity information for frames 7
and 9, calculated as shown and presented in Table 6.3, yields the linear acceleration vector components for frame 8:

$$a_x = \frac{[-452.0 - (-248.6)]\,\text{cm/s}}{2(0.01667)\,\text{s}} \qquad (1.5)$$

or

$$a_x = -6,100\,\text{cm/s}^2 \qquad (1.6)$$

and

$$a_y = \frac{(255.5 - 360.0)\,\text{cm/s}}{2(0.01667)} \qquad (1.7)$$

or

$$a_y = -3,134\,\text{cm/s}^2 \qquad (1.8)$$

Numerical differentiation is an error-magnifying process: if the position data are "noisy" to begin with, the results of applying equations (14) and (15) or (16) are poor at best. The reader is advised to investigate data smoothing techniques, such as the use of cubic splines (Zernicke et al. 1976), digital filtering (Winter et al. 1974), or Fourier series expansions (Hatze 1981). In addition, the numerical differentiation technique examined previously, the central difference relationship, is but one of several available (for example, forward and backward difference approximations or extrapolation techniques [Gerald et al. 1984]).

The calculation of body segment angular velocities and angular accelerations involves another application of the general central difference relationship given by equations (12) and (13) once the segment angular displacements are known. To this end, refer to Figure 6.13 and note that the projection of the segment vector $\mathbf{r}_{2/1}$ into the xy (or sagittal) plane; $\mathbf{r}'_{2/1}$ may be written as

$$\mathbf{r}'_{2/1} = (x_2 - x_1)\,\mathbf{i} + (y_2 - y_1)\,\mathbf{j} \tag{17}$$

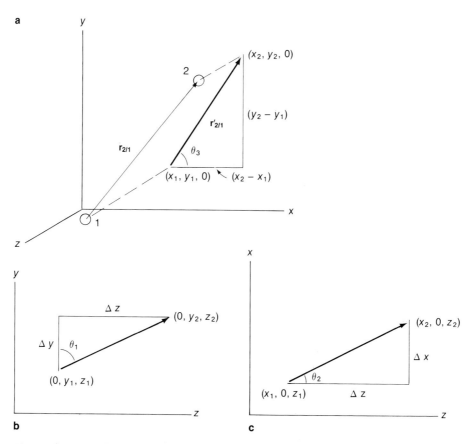

Figure 6.13 Projection of two representative body segment markers into the (a) sagittal (xy) plane, the (b) frontal (yz) plane, and the (c) transverse (xz) plane.

and the angle that this projection makes with the x axis may then be defined as

$$\Theta_3 = \tan^{-1} \left(\frac{y_2 - y_1}{x_2 - x_1} \right) \tag{18}$$

Therefore, the rate of change of Θ_x with respect to time is in fact the z component of the angular velocity vector, or

$$\omega_z = \dot{\Theta}_3 \tag{19}$$

and the z component of the angular acceleration vector is the first derivative of the z component of the angular velocity vector with respect to time, or

$$\alpha_z = \dot{\omega}_z \tag{20}$$

Following this same line of reasoning, illustrated further in Figure 6.13 in determining the complete expression of the angular velocity vector for the mth segment yields

$$\omega_\mathbf{m} = \dot{\Theta}_1 \mid_m \mathbf{i} + \dot{\Theta}_2 \mid_m \mathbf{j} + \dot{\Theta}_3 \mid_m \mathbf{k} \tag{21}$$

where

$$\Theta_1 \mid_m = \tan^{-1} \left(\frac{z_2 \mid_m - z_1 \mid_m}{y_2 \mid_m - y_1 \mid_m} \right)$$

$$\Theta_2 \mid_m = \tan^{-1} \left(\frac{x_2 \mid_m - x_1 \mid_m}{z_2 \mid_m - z_1 \mid_m} \right) \tag{22}$$

$$\Theta_3 \mid_m = \tan^{-1} \left(\frac{y_2 \mid_m - y_1 \mid_m}{x_2 \mid_m - x_1 \mid_m} \right)$$

where the subscripts 1 and 2 refer to two markers associated with the mth body segment and, similarly, an expression for the angular acceleration vector of the mth segment,

$$\alpha_\mathbf{m} = \frac{d}{dt} \dot{\omega}_x \mid_m \mathbf{i} + \dot{\omega}_y \mid_m \mathbf{j} + \omega_z \mid_m \mathbf{k} \tag{23}$$

where

$\omega_x \mid_m, \omega_y \mid_m, \omega_z \mid_m = $ components of the mth segment angular velocity in the x, y, and z component directions, respectively

Equation (12) may be applied to equations (21) and (23) as follows,

$$\omega_m = \frac{\Theta_1 \mid_m \mid_{j+1} - \Theta_1 \mid_m \mid_{j-1}}{2t} \mathbf{i} + \frac{\Theta_2 \mid_m \mid_{j+1} - \Theta_2 \mid_m \mid_{j-1}}{2t} \mathbf{j}$$

$$+ \frac{\Theta_3 \mid_m \mid_{j+1} - \Theta_3 \mid_m \mid_{j-1}}{2t} \mathbf{k} \tag{24}$$

where, for example, the notation $\Theta_1 \mid_m \mid_{j+1}$ refers to the mth body segment orientation shown in the $(j + 1)$th frame as viewed from the x axis or in the yz plane and

$$\alpha_i = \frac{\omega_x \mid_m \mid_{j+1} - \omega_x \mid_m \mid_{j-1}}{2t} \mathbf{i} + \frac{\omega_y \mid_m \mid_{j+1} - \omega_y \mid_m \mid_{j-1}}{2t} \mathbf{j}$$

$$+ \frac{\omega_z \mid_m \mid_{j+1} - \omega_z \mid_m \mid_{j-1}}{2t} \mathbf{k} \tag{25}$$

where, similarly, the notation $\omega_x \mid_m \mid_{j+1}$ represents the angular velocity of the mth segment in the $(j + 1)$th frame about the x axis.

Example 2:   Returning to the example begun earlier (the individual flexing a forearm in the sagittal plane about a fixed elbow axis such that the coordinates presented in Table 6.2 define the wrist marker displacement with time), determine the angular displacement, velocity, and acceleration associated with the forearm rotation about the elbow.

Solution: Determine angular displacement of the forearm as a function of time by returning to the marker coordinate data presented in Table 6.2 and employing one or more of the relationships defined by equation (22). With angular displacement(s) known, calculate the associated angular velocities by applying equation (24). Finally, use the angular velocity information in equation (25) to determine angular acceleration. This process may be illustrated for frame 8 by substituting the coordinate information from frame 8 (see Table 6.2) into the expression for Θ_3 in the set of equations (22), as follows:

$$\Theta_3 = \tan^{-1} \frac{(25.80 - 0.0) \, \text{cm}}{(24.53 - 0.0) \, \text{cm}} \tag{2.1}$$

or

$$\Theta_3 = 0.81 \text{ radians (rad)} \tag{2.2}$$

Note that the coordinates of the elbow marker are assumed to be (0,0), or an inertially fixed origin. Continuing, one may determine the angular velocity for time approximately equal to 0.13 s (frame 8) by substituting angular displacement data from frames 7 and 9 into equation (24), or

$$\omega_3 = \frac{(1.1 - 0.6)\,\text{rad}}{2(0.01667)\,\text{s}}$$ (2.3)

or

$$\omega_3 = 14\,\text{rad/s}$$ (2.4)

Substitution of angular velocity data (presented in Table 6.4) into equation (25) yields angular acceleration results, as follows:

$$\alpha_3 = \frac{(14.7 - 12.4)\,\text{rad/s}}{2(0.01667)\,\text{s}}$$ (2.5)

or

$$\alpha_3 = 70\,\text{rad/s}^2$$ (2.6)

Table 6.4 Elbow flexion marker motion results: angular displacement, velocity, and acceleration

Frame	Time	Coordinates		Displacement	Velocity	Acceleration
	(s)	x (cm)	y	(rad)	(rad/s)	(rad/s^2)
0	0.000	35.60	0.00	0.0		
1	0.017	35.60	0.08	0.0	0.5	
2	0.033	35.59	0.62	0.0	1.7	86.7
3	0.050	35.54	2.05	0.1	3.4	118.4
4	0.067	35.29	4.67	0.1	5.6	137.5
5	0.083	34.54	8.62	0.2	8.0	141.9
6	0.100	32.82	13.80	0.4	10.3	131.3
7	0.117	29.60	19.78	0.6	12.4	106.6
8	0.133	24.53	25.80	0.8	13.9	70.6
9	0.150	17.64	30.92	1.1	14.7	27.1
10	0.167	9.46	34.32	1.3	14.8	− 15.6
11	0.183	0.89	35.59	1.5	14.2	− 60.0
12	0.200	− 7.10	34.88	1.8	12.8	− 104.8
13	0.217	− 13.79	32.82	2.0	10.7	− 131.6
14	0.233	− 18.85	30.20	2.1	8.4	− 141.2
15	0.250	− 22.33	27.72	2.3	6.0	− 139.3
16	0.267	− 24.49	25.84	2.3	3.8	− 122.6
17	0.283	− 25.63	24.71	2.4	1.9	− 92.9
18	0.300	− 26.09	24.22	2.4	0.7	
19	0.317	− 26.18	24.13	2.4		

Table 6.4 gives complete angular displacement, velocity, and acceleration results related to this example.

At this point, the kinematics of segment motion are in a form that can be related to the motion kinetics through the application of Newton's relationships, equations (1) and (2).

Newtonian Statics and Dynamics

As indicated earlier, the basis of virtually all clinically based analysis (not assessment) of biomechanical measurements is Newtonian or classical mechanics or work/power relationships. In the discussion that follows, the fundamentals associated with these areas of analysis are briefly reviewed, in three categories: (1) determination of the force system associated with a rigid body in static equilibrium: (2) analysis of the motion of the rigid body, that is, rigid body dynamics; and (3) calculation of the mechanical work performed during rigid body motion. In this context, the term *rigid body* refers to either an anatomically complete structure, (the whole body) as a series of interconnected, interrelated linkages or to any particular segment of the entire structure (for example, a single limb, in which the "external forces" are joint reactions). The coverage given these mechanically complex concepts is brief; the reader will find more extensive discussion in mechanics texts (for example, Greenwood [1965] or Ginsberg and Genin [1984]).

Rigid body equilibrium of a spatial force system

Rigid body equilibrium is a condition in which the rate of change of linear momentum with time, or the absolute acceleration of the body, is equal to zero. This is a special case of Newton's second law (equation [1]): the time rate of change of the linear momentum of the body is linearly proportional to the force acting on it and occurs in the same direction of the force. Specifically, requirements for rigid body equilibrium are (1) that the vector sum of all externally applied forces acting on the rigid body equals zero, or

$$\Sigma \mathbf{F} = \mathbf{0} \tag{26}$$

and (2) that the vector sum of the moments (relative to any point) of the externally applied forces equals zero, or

$$\Sigma \mathbf{M} = \mathbf{0} \tag{27}$$

For general nonconcurrent, nonparallel force systems, equations (26) and (27) may be employed to calculate up to six unknown external reactions, such as forces and moments, through the simultaneous solution of six scalar relationships:

$$\Sigma F_x = 0 \tag{28}$$

$$\Sigma F_y = 0 \tag{29}$$

$$\Sigma\, F_z = 0 \tag{30}$$

$$\Sigma\, M_x = 0 \tag{31}$$

$$\Sigma\, M_y = 0 \tag{32}$$

$$\Sigma\, M_z = 0 \tag{33}$$

where the subscripts x, y, and z still refer to three orthogonal component directions associated with the force system.

Example 3:   A Russell's traction applies a tensile force to a fractured femur for immobilization. If the weight of the shank and foot shown is approximately 6.1 percent of the total weight (Winter 1979) of the 150-lb man whose leg is shown (Figure 6.14), calculate the magnitude of the weight that must be suspended from the cable at point C to maintain the position of the leg as shown. In addition, calculate the average force (tensile) applied to the thigh (femur plus musculature) under these conditions. Neglect friction and the size of all pulleys (adapted from Hibbeler 1983).

Solution: Isolating the body of interest allows the representation of the force system in the form of a free-body diagram shown in Figure 6.15. Note that the tension in the cable, T, is constant because of the frictionless pulleys.

The conditions necessary and sufficient for equilibrium are defined by

$$\Sigma\, \mathbf{F} = \mathbf{0}: \qquad \mathbf{F}_1 + \mathbf{F}_2 + \mathbf{F}_3 + \mathbf{F}_{\text{femur}} - m g \mathbf{j} = \mathbf{0} \tag{3.1}$$

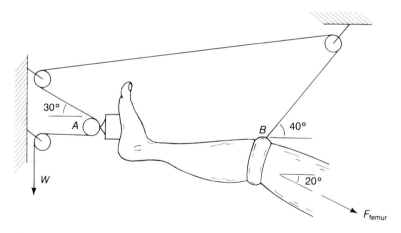

Figure 6.14   Russel's traction mechanism for clinically loading lower extremity limbs (after Hibbeler, R. C. (1983) *Engineering Mechanics—Statics,* 3d ed. Macmillan Publishing co., Inc., New York, pp. 174 and 196).

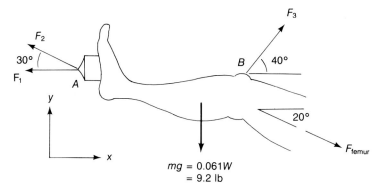

Figure 6.15   Free-body diagram of the Russel's traction mechanism.

where,

$$\mathbf{F_1} = -F_1\mathbf{i} = -T\mathbf{i} \tag{3.2}$$

$$\mathbf{F_2} = (-F_2 \cos 30°)\mathbf{i} + (F_2 \sin 30°)\mathbf{j}$$

$$= (-T \cos 30°)\mathbf{i} + (T \sin 30°)\mathbf{j} \tag{3.3}$$

$$\mathbf{F_3} = (F_3 \cos 40°)\mathbf{i} + (F_3 \sin 40°)\mathbf{j}$$

$$= (T \cos 40°)\mathbf{i} + (T \sin 40°)\mathbf{j} \tag{3.4}$$

$$\mathbf{F_{femur}} = (F_{femur} \cos 20°)\mathbf{i} - (F_{femur} \sin 20°)\mathbf{j} \tag{3.5}$$

$$mg = 0.061 \times 150 \, \text{lb} \, \mathbf{j} = 9.2 \, \text{lb} \, \mathbf{j} \tag{3.6}$$

Examining the **i** and **j** components of equation (3.1) yields

i component $-T - (T \cos 30°) + T \cos 40°$

$$+ F_{femur} \cos 20° = 0 \tag{3.7}$$

j component: $T \sin 30° + T \sin 40° - F_{femur} \sin 20°$

$$- mg = 0 \tag{3.8}$$

Equations (3.7) and (3.8) may be solved simultaneously for

$$T = 12.4 \, \text{lb} \tag{3.9}$$

$$F_{femur} = 14.5 \, \text{lb} \tag{3.10}$$

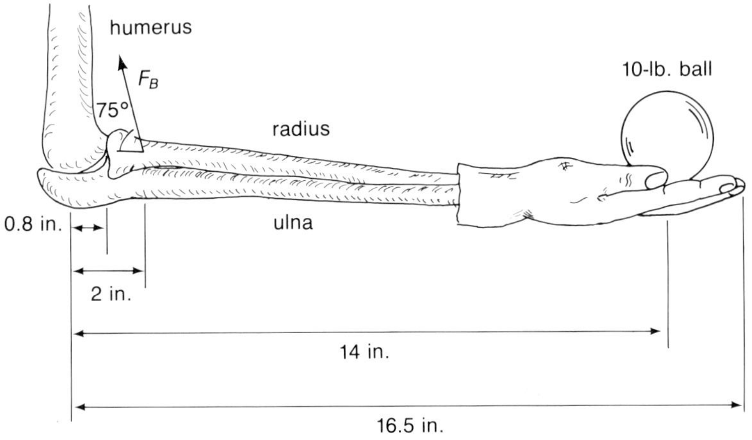

Figure 6.16 Forearm held statically fixed in a 90° flexion with a 10-lb load applied at the hand (after Hibbeler, R. C. (1983) *Engineering Mechanics—Statics,* 3d ed. Macmillan Publishing Co., Inc., New York, pp. 174 and 196).

Example 4: A 150-lb woman is holding a 10-lb ball in the palm of her hand. Anthropometrically, the forearm and hand represent approximately 2.2 percent of the total body mass, and its center of gravity is at a point located approximately 68 percent of the segment length distal to the elbow axis (Winter 1979). Assume that the system of forces is shown in static equilibrium, and that the humerus exerts a horizontal normal force $\mathbf{F_c}$ on the radius and a vertical normal force $\mathbf{F_a}$ on the ulna as shown (Figure 6.16). Determine these reactions and the force $\mathbf{F_b}$ that the biceps brachii muscle applies to the forearm. Note: this model assumes that the contribution of the brachialis muscle in forearm flexion is small by comparison to the biceps brachii and that the force in the passive triceps brachii (which serves to extend the forearm) is zero. Neglect friction (adapted from Hibbeler 1983).

Solution: Isolating the body of interest allows one to represent the force system in the form of a free-body diagram (Figure 6.17).

The equilibrium equations may be written by employing the definition of the moment of a force as the vector cross-product of a position vector and the force vector,

$$\mathbf{M_m} = \mathbf{r_{n/m}} \times \mathbf{F} \tag{34}$$

where

$\mathbf{r_{n/m}}$ = position vector from a point (*m*) of reference to the line of action of a particular force $\mathbf{F}$ applied at point *n*.

Therefore, in the problem at hand,

$$\Sigma\,\mathbf{M}_o = \mathbf{0}: \quad \mathbf{r_{e/o}} \times \mathbf{F_a} + \mathbf{r_{b/o}} \times (-10\,\text{lb})\mathbf{j}$$

$$+ \mathbf{r_{b/o}} \times (-3.5\,\text{lb})\mathbf{j} = 0 \tag{4.1}$$

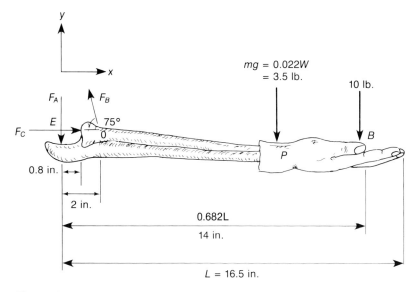

Figure 6.17   Free-body diagram of a statically loaded forearm.

where

$$\mathbf{r}_{e/o} = (-2 \text{ in})\mathbf{i} \tag{4.2}$$

$$\mathbf{F_a} = -F_a\mathbf{j} \tag{4.3}$$

$$\mathbf{r}_{b/o} = (12 \text{ in})\mathbf{i} \tag{4.4}$$

$$\mathbf{r}_{p/o} = (0.68 \times 16.5 \text{ in}) \mathbf{i} = (9.25 \text{ in})\mathbf{i} \tag{4.5}$$

Examining the **k** component of equation (4.1),

$$2F_a - 152.4 \text{ lb} = 0 \tag{4.6}$$

yields

$$F_a = 76.2 \text{ lb} \tag{4.7}$$

To solve for F_b and F_c, consider,

$$\Sigma \mathbf{F} = \mathbf{0}: \qquad -F_a\mathbf{j} + \mathbf{F_b} + F_c\mathbf{i}$$
$$-(10 \text{ lb})\mathbf{j} - (3.5 \text{ lb})\mathbf{j} = \mathbf{0} \tag{4.8}$$

where,

$$\mathbf{F_b} = \{-F_b \cos 75°\mathbf{i} + F_b \sin 75°\mathbf{j}\} \text{ lb} \tag{4.9}$$

Examining the **i** and **j** components,

i component: $F_c - F_b \cos 75° = 0$ (4.10)

j component: $-F_a - 13.5 \text{ lb} + F_b \sin 75° = 0$ (4.11)

yields

$$F_b = 92.9 \text{ lb} \tag{4.12}$$

$$F_c = 24 \text{ lb} \tag{4.13}$$

Both Examples 3 and 4 illustrate use of available anthropometric data (Dempster 1955) (describing such quantities as the location of segment center of mass, segment weight, or mass percentages of whole body weight or mass) and inertial characteristics that come into play in considering a dynamic, as opposed to a static, problem.

Motion of rigid bodies

The description of the dynamics problem begins at fundamentally the same place as the two static examples discussed, namely the construction of a free-body diagram of the segment or linkage of segments under examination. This is followed by a computation of appropriate kinematic quantities, such as linear and angular accelerations, that may be applied to equations (1) and (2). Consider an extension to the forearm problem (Example 3) given previously, stated as follows:

Example 5: A 150-lb man is flexing his elbow in the sagittal (xy) plane while holding his humerus stationary. Under these circumstances, it is convenient to locate the origin of the fixed coordinate system at the center of rotation of the elbow joint. The forearm may be represented in a "linkage" model with the following assumptions:

1 Each segment has a fixed point mass center located at the center of gravity
2 The location of the segment center of gravity (in relation to the distal/proximal ends) does not change during the movement
3 The segment inertial characteristics remain constant during the movement
4 The joint is modeled as a "pin"-jointed link

A free-body diagram incorporating these assumptions and modeling this action is shown in Figure 6.18, with

F_E = resultant joint reaction vector

M_E = resultant muscle moment generated about the joint center of rotation

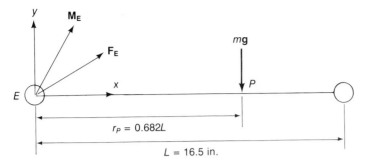

Figure 6.18   Linkage model of a forearm undergoing planar flexion about the elbow.

It is noted that the resultant muscle moment includes contributions made by the biceps brachii in active contraction as well as the triceps brachii in passive elongation. Determining the individual contribution of all of the involved muscle groups leads to an indeterminate system and, consequently, supercedes the scope of this presentation but is addressed briefly.

Solution: From a kinematic measurement system, assume that the angular velocity and angular acceleration of the forearm have been determined to be 1.6 rad/s and 1.0 rad/s², respectively. Examining Newton's second law for this planar motion yields

$$\Sigma\, F_x \;=\; ma_x \tag{5.1}$$

$$\Sigma\, F_y \;=\; ma_y \tag{5.2}$$

$$\Sigma\, F_z \;=\; 0 \tag{5.3}$$

because $a_z = 0$ for planar motion and

$$\Sigma\, M_x \;=\; \Sigma\, M_y \;=\; 0 \tag{5.4}$$

$$\Sigma\, M_z \;=\; I_p \alpha_z \tag{5.5}$$

because $\alpha_x = \alpha_y = 0$. To determine expressions for a_x and a_y, employ the relationship between $\mathbf{a_E}$ and $\mathbf{a_p}$,

$$\mathbf{a_P} \;=\; \mathbf{a_E} \;+\; \boldsymbol{\alpha} \times \mathbf{r_{P/E}} \;+\; \boldsymbol{\omega} \times (\boldsymbol{\omega} \times \mathbf{r_{P/E}}) \tag{5.6}$$

where

$$\mathbf{a_E} \;=\; \mathbf{0}$$
$$\boldsymbol{\alpha} \;=\; \alpha z \mathbf{k}$$
$$\mathbf{r_{P/E}} \;=\; r_p \mathbf{i}$$
$$\boldsymbol{\omega} \times (\boldsymbol{\omega} \times \mathbf{r_{P/E}}) \;=\; -\omega_z^2\, \mathbf{r_{P/E}} \;=\; -\omega_z^2\, r_p \mathbf{i}$$

Rewriting equation (5.6),

$$\mathbf{a_p} = r_P\alpha_z\mathbf{j} - r_P\omega_z^2\,\mathbf{i} \tag{5.7}$$

or

$$a_x = -r_P\omega_z^2 \tag{5.8}$$

and

$$a_y = r_P\alpha_z \tag{5.9}$$

Substituting the expressions for a_x into equation (5.1), a_y into equation (5.2), and a_z into equation (5.3) yields

$$F_x = ma_x: \qquad F_{Ex} = -mr_p\omega_z^2 \tag{5.10}$$

$$F_y = ma_y: \qquad F_{Ey} - mg = mr_p\alpha_z \tag{5.11}$$

$$F_z = 0: \qquad F_{Ez} = 0 \tag{5.12}$$

and substituting the appropriate values for m, r_p, ω_z, and α_z gives

$$\mathbf{F_E} = \{-0.26\mathbf{i} + 3.6\mathbf{j}\}\,\text{lb} \tag{5.13}$$

Anthropometric data again yield an approximate centroidal radius of gyration for the forearm/hand segment of $0.468L$. Therefore, the moment of inertia about point P (the center of gravity) is

$$I_P = m(0.468L)^2 \tag{5.14}$$

where L is again the length of the body segment, in this case, 16.5 in. Expanding equation (2) yields

$$\Sigma\,\mathbf{M_P} = I_P\alpha: \qquad \mathbf{M_E} + \mathbf{r_{E/P}} \times \mathbf{F_E} = I_P\alpha \tag{5.15}$$

or

$$\Sigma\,M_x\,|_P = 0: \qquad M_{Ex} = 0 \tag{5.16}$$

$$\Sigma\,M_y\,|_P = 0: \qquad M_{Ey} = 0 \tag{5.17}$$

$$\Sigma\,M_z\,|_P = I_P\alpha_z: \qquad M_{Ez} - F_{E}r_P = I_P\alpha_z \tag{5.18}$$

Again substituting values for the constants gives

$$M_{Ez} = 3.4\,\text{lb}\cdot\text{ft} = 41\,\text{lb}\cdot\text{in.} \tag{5.19}$$

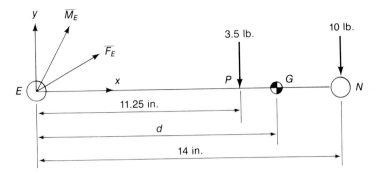

Figure 6.19   Linkage model of a forearm undergoing planar flexion about the elbow with a 10-lb vertical load applied at the hand.

Example 6:   The 150-lb individual in Example 3 is again flexing his elbow in the sagittal (xy) plane (not allowing his elbow to translate) while holding the 10 lb-ball from Example 3 in the palm of his hand. A free-body diagram of the linkage model for this case is shown in Figure 6.19, with

$\mathbf{F_E}$ = resultant joint reaction vector

$\mathbf{M_E}$ = resultant muscle moment generated about the joint center of rotation

Solution: Again, assume that the angular velocity and angular acceleration of the forearm have been determined to be 1.6 rad/s and 1.0 rad/s², respectively. As before, Newton's second law for this planar motion may be employed:

$$\Sigma \mathbf{F} = m\mathbf{a} \tag{6.1}$$

$$\Sigma \mathbf{M} = I_g \alpha \tag{6.2}$$

where a_z, α_x, and α_y are assumed to be equal to zero to yield,

$$\Sigma \mathbf{F} = m\mathbf{a}: \quad \mathbf{F_E} - m_{forearm}g\mathbf{j} - m_{ball}g\mathbf{j} = m_{total}\mathbf{a_G} \tag{6.3}$$

where

$$m_{total} = m_{forearm} + m_{ball} \tag{6.4}$$

The acceleration of the forearm and ball $\mathbf{a_G}$ may be determined as before (equation [3.6]) if the location of the composite center of gravity for the system is known. The location of point G, distance d in Figure 6.19, may be calculated by the general method for determining the center of gravity of a composite body, as follows:

$$d = \frac{\Sigma x_i W_i}{\Sigma W_i} \tag{35}$$

or, in this case

$$d = \frac{(11.25\ \text{in})(3.5\ \text{lb}) + (14\ \text{in})(10\ \text{lb})}{3.5\ \text{lb} + 10\ \text{lb}} \tag{6.5}$$

$$d = 13.3\ \text{in} = 1.1\ \text{ft} \tag{6.6}$$

Now,

$$\mathbf{a_G} = \mathbf{a_E} + \boldsymbol{\alpha} \times \mathbf{r}_{G/E} + \boldsymbol{\omega} \times (\boldsymbol{\omega} \times \mathbf{r}_{G/E}) \tag{6.7}$$

where

$$\mathbf{a_E} = \mathbf{0}$$
$$\boldsymbol{\alpha} = \alpha_z \mathbf{k}$$
$$\mathbf{r}_{G/E} = (1.1\ \text{ft})\mathbf{i}$$
$$\boldsymbol{\omega} \times (\boldsymbol{\omega} \times \mathbf{r}_{G/E}) = -\omega_z^2\ \mathbf{r}_{G/E} = -\omega_z^2\ (1.1\ \text{ft})\mathbf{i}$$

or

$$\mathbf{a_G} = \{(-2.8)\mathbf{i} + (1.1)\mathbf{j}\}\quad \text{ft/s}^2 \tag{6.8}$$

At this point, equation (6.3) may be solved for

$$\mathbf{F_E} = \{-1.2\mathbf{i} + 14\mathbf{j}\}\quad \text{lb} \tag{6.9}$$

The magnitude of the moment of inertia about the composite center of gravity, point G (required for the solution of equation [6.2]), may be determined through an application of the parallel axis theorem:

$$I_G = \{I_p + m\left(\frac{13.3\ \text{in} - 11.25\ \text{in}}{12\ \text{in/ft}}\right)^2\}_{\text{forearm}}$$
$$+ \{m\left(\frac{14\ \text{in} - 13.3\ \text{in}}{12\ \text{in/ft}}\right)^2\}_{\text{ball}} \tag{6.10}$$

where I_p (0.045 ft^4) is the moment of inertia of the forearm/hand about the physiological center of gravity, and the ball is assumed to be a "particle" (with no centroidal moment of inertia). Equation (6.2) may be expanded as follows

$$\Sigma\ \mathbf{M_G} = I_G\alpha: \quad \mathbf{M_E} + \mathbf{r}_{E/G} \times \mathbf{F_E} = I_G\alpha_z\mathbf{k} \tag{6.11}$$

and solved for the resultant moment about the elbow.

$$M_{Ez} = 15.4\ \text{lb}\cdot\text{ft} = 185\ \text{lb}\cdot\text{in.} \tag{6.12}$$

Analyses of this type are numerous; King (1984) provides a very extensive review article summarizing many biomechanical modeling techniques and applications. For additional information related specifically to joint forces and moments, the reader can consult Kairento and Hellen (1981), Mann and coworkers (1981), Nissan (1981), Vaughn and collaborators (1982b, 1982c), and Boccardi and associates (1981). Techniques are being developed and refined to address the inherent "indeterminant" nature of the bone-on-bone joint reaction problem. Representative works include Crowninshield and Brand (1981), Chao and Rim (1973), Patriarco and coworkers (1981), and Vaughn and associates (1982a, 1982c).

Mechanical work and power

Discussing the external mechanical work done during movement is relatively straightforward; for example, displacing a force along its line of action can be described as "work done on the force." The problem becomes more difficult if the work done on passive muscles or done by contracting muscles is included in the analysis, and yet this is the very objective. If through the analysis of muscle moments, the instantaneous muscle moment is combined with the instantaneous angular velocity of the segment, an indication of the instantaneous power results:

$$P = M_i\omega_i \qquad (36)$$

where

P = instantaneous power
M_i = net muscle moment in a coordinate direction
ω_i = angular velocity in a coordinate direction

This power relationship, equation (36), is integrated numerically to determine the net work done by a group of muscles over a time, for example, a cycle. Care is necessary in applying this technique because, as expected, the sign of both the net instantaneous muscle moment and instantaneous angular velocity change over a cycle of motion.

One may determine the work done on forces through the numerical integration of

$$dW = \mathbf{F}\cdot d\mathbf{s} \qquad (37)$$

where

dW = differential work on force $\mathbf{F}$ over distance $d\mathbf{s}$

or

$$W = \int \mathbf{F}\cdot d\mathbf{s} \qquad (38)$$

The total mechanical work done during a particular motion or movement (for example, gait) is growing in popularity as a prediction of pre- and posttherapy change. For additional illustrations and discussion, the following, among others, have published research results: Cooper (1981), Cavagna and associates (1977a, 1977b), Ito and Kami (1981), and Zarrugh (1981a, 1981b).

ASSESSMENT

The methods of data collection and analysis presented here ultimately provide a great deal of information for the clinician to employ in assessment. For example, Gage (1983) at the Newington Children's Hospital describes the use of lower extremity displacement/position information, correlated with selected EMG activity in the pre- and postexamination of patients with cerebral palsy. Gage also illustrates the use of "energy costs," pre- and postoperatively, as an additional assessment parameter. Although this latter application demonstrates a creative utilization of the power of the motion analysis system, recall that all the systems described can also deliver additional kinematic (for example, segment velocities and accelerations) and kinetic (ground force reactions, for instance) information. This example illustrates that at this point in the technological evolution of the hardware (and software) associated with biomechanical systems, it is generally accepted that the capability of the available technology is not being fully utilized. It should be pointed out that this is not the responsibility of the system users alone, but of the system designers and the biomechanicians in collaboration with the users. Cappozzo (1983) summarizes this dilemma, as follows,

> A workshop on clinical application of gait analysis systems was held, not a long time ago, at the University of Dundee, Scotland (30 March–1 April 1981). Participants included internationally recognized workers in the field. They were asked to identify the various techniques of gait analysis and the extent to which they can assist the clinical team in making clinical decisions. From the three-day discussion a state of the art emerged. "A rather disappointing state of the art" was the comment of many observers. It should however be emphasized that the disappointment did not apply to the hardware. It was acknowledged that instrumentation is well advanced and has reached a level of reliability and patient acceptability that permits its use in the clinical environment. Reference normal data are available, and those that are missing are reasonably easy to be acquired. What is really missing is a conceptual background. The approaches to clinical gait analysis and evaluation are not supported by general theories. The best concrete achievements have their foundation in theory, in abstraction, and gait analysis, in this sense, is no exception. We biomechanicians have been working hard, during the last decades, designing new instruments and experimental methodologies, applying old analytical techniques to our new problems. We have been gathering a great deal of numbers regarding the various aspects of human locomotion. Now, I think, more efforts should be devoted to speculation. We should try to interpret the phenomena we have observed, we should try to identify, through the generalization of single observations, the laws that govern them. In other words, we should go back to a more genuine scientific operation.

A reiteration of these concerns provides some sense of the future directions associated with the development of assessment systems. With reference to the clinical setting in particular, biomechanical measurement/description/analysis has reached a point at which fundamental questions related to the interpretation of data, such as the following, must be readdressed:

1   What is fundamental to the patterns of gait for an individual? How might these fundamental characteristics be best described and presented for assessment purposes?

2   Is it realistic to think in terms of "normal" for amputee gait, cerebral palsy gait, and so on? Should these types of gait disorders be examined and evaluated with more regard to efficiency than to normalcy?

3   What is the most effective method for correlating kinematic, kinetic, and EMG data? How might these data be presented for improved assessment application—through sophisticated computer graphics techniques?

4   Are the techniques described in this discussion clinically efficient and cost-effective in the diagnosis/prognosis of physical disabilities? Or are they most appropriate as research tools?

5   How might the clinical motions measurement systems employed today be adapted for broader application, such as sports biomechanics, thus, conceivably, reducing the initial costs of these systems?

The "assessment" phase of biomechanical evaluations is and will continue to be the most ambiguous and least readily definable area. At this point, measurement system designers and users are asking and must ask difficult questions related to the utilization of the available measurement data and descriptive information to push assessment techniques forward in an effective, cost-efficient manner.

REFERENCES

Astrand, P., and Rodahl, K. 1977. *Textbook of work physiology.* New York: McGraw-Hill.

Boccardi, S., Pedotti, A., Rodano, R., and Santambrogio, G. C. 1981. Evaluation of muscular moments at the lower limb joints by an on-line processing of kinematic data and ground reaction. *Biomech* 14(1):33–45.

Cappozzo. 1983. Considerations on clinical gait evaluation. *Biomech* 16(4):302.

Carollo, J. J. 1981. Clinical gait analysis. *Med Electron* April 1981, pp. 95–99.

Cavagna, G. A., Heglund, N. C., and Taylor, C. R. 1977a. Mechanical work in terrestrial locomotion: Two basic mechanisms for minimizing energy expenditure. *Am J Physiol* 233(5):243–261.

Cavagna, G. A., and Kaneko, M. 1977b. Mechanical work and efficiency in level walking and running. *J Physiol* 268(2):647–681.

Cavanaugh, P. R., and Lafortune, M. A. 1980. Ground reaction forces in distance running. *J Biomech* 13(5):397–406.

Chao, E. Y., and Rim, K. 1973. Application of optimization principles in determining the applied moments in human leg joints during gait. *J Biomech* 6(5):497–510.

Chao, E. Y., Laughman, R. K., and Stauffer, R. N. 1980. Biomechanical gait evaluation of pre- and post-operative total knee replacement patients. *Arch Orthop Trauma Surg* 97(4):309–317.

Clark, T. E., Lafortune, M. A., Williams, K. R., and Cavanaugh, P. R. 1980. The relationship between center of pressure location and rear foot movement in distance running. *Med Sci Sports Exerc* 12(2):92.

Cohen, A., Orin, D. E., and Marsolais, E. B. 1980. The gait laboratory force plate at the Cleveland VA Medical Center. *Bull Prosthet Res* 10-33:90–97.

Cooper, L. 1981. Calculating external work in walking from force plate data. *Bull Prosthet Res* BPR 10-35, 18(1):318–320.

Coutts, K. D. 1980. Ground reaction forces and angles during volleyball spike jump. *Med Sci Sports Exerc* 12(2):96.

Crowninshield, R. D., and Brand, R. A. 1981. A physiologically based criterion of muscle force prediction in locomotion. *J Biomech* 14(11):793–801.

Davis, R. B., and Burger, A. S. 1985. The Scandinavian flexible prosthetic limb socket: Interface pressure distributions during stance. Proceedings of the 11th Northeast Bioengineering Conference, Worchester, Massachusetts.

Dempster, W. T. 1955. Space requirements of the seated operator. WADC Technical Report 55-159, University of Michigan.

Draganich, L. F., Andriocci, T. P., and Strongwater, A. M. 1980. Electronic measurement of instantaneous foot-floor contact patterns during gait. *J Biomech* 13:875–880.

Gage, J. R. 1983. Gait analysis for decision-making in cerebral palsy. *Bull Hosp Joint Dis Orthop Inst* XLIII(2):147–163.

Gage, J. R. 1984. Clinical assessment of gait through motion analysis. *IEEE Frontiers of Engineering and Computing in Health Care—1984.* Proceedings of the Sixth Annual Conference of the IEEE Engineering in Medicine and Biology Society, pp. 648–650.

Gerald, C. F., and Wheatley, P. O. 1984. *Applied numerical analysis.* Reading Mass.: Addison-Wesley.

Ginsberg, J. H., and Genin, J. 1984. *Statics and dynamics.* New York: John Wiley.

Golbranson, F. L., and Wirta, R. W. 1981. The use of gait analysis to study gait patterns of the lower-limb amputee. *Bull Prosthet Res* BPR 10–35, 18(1):153–155.

Grahammer J., and Gregor, J. R. 1979. Force plate evaluations of weightlifting and vertical jumping. *Med Sci Sports Exerc* 11:106.

Greenwood, D. T. 1965. *Principles of dynamics.* Englewood Cliffs, N.J.: Prentice-Hall.

Groh, H., and Baumann, W. 1976. Joint muscle forces acting in the leg during gait. *T Biomechanics V-A,* Baltimore: University Park Press, 328–333.

Hagy, J. 1981. Serial frame (Vanguard) motion analysis. *Bull Prosthet Res* BPR 10–35, 18(1):288.

Hatze, H. 1981. The use of optimally regularized fourier series for estimating higher order derivatives of noisy biomechanical data, *J Biomech* 14:13–18.

Hibbeler, R. C. 1983. *Engineering Mechanics—Statics,* (3rd ed.) New York: Macmillan, pp. 174 and 196.

Ito, A., and Komi, P. V. 1981. Estimation of positive mechanical work efficiency in running at slow and fast speeds. *VIIIth International Congress of Biomechanics,* Nagoya, Japan.

Jarrett, M. O., Moore, P. R., and Swanson, A. J. G. 1980. Assessment of gait using components of the ground force vector, *Med Biol Eng Comput* 16:685–688.

Judge, G. 1975. Measurement of knee torque during the swing phase of gait. *Eng Med* 4(3):13–17.

Kairento, A. L., and Hellen, G. 1981. Biomechanical analysis of walking. *Biomech* 14(10):671–678.

King, A. I. 1984. A review of biomechanical models. *J Biomech Eng* 106:97–103.

Kunz, H., and Kaufmann, D. A. 1981. Biomechanical analysis of sprinting: Decathletes versus champions. *Br J Sports Med* 15(3):171–181.

Lamoreux, L. 1981. Exoskeletal goniometry. *Bull Prosthet Res* BPR 10–35, 18(1):288–290.

Lord, M. 1981. Foot pressure measurements: A review of methodology. *J Biomech Eng* 3(4):91–99.

Mann, R. W., Rowell, D., Conati, F., Tetewsky, A. T., and Antonsson, E. 1981. Precise, rapid, automatic, 3-d position and orientation information from multiple moving bodies. *VIIIth International Congress of Biomechanics,* Nagoya, Japan. p. 233.

Marsolais, E. B. 1981. Engineering applications in orthotic and prosthetic treatment of musculoskeletal defects. *Bull Prosthet Res* BPR 10–35, 18(1):129–130.

Mason, B. R., Bates, B. T., James, S. L., and Ostering, L. R. 1979. Ground reaction forces during running. *Med Sci Sports Exerc* 11:86.

Morris, J. R. 1972. Accelerometry in gait analysis. *Br J Surg* 59(11):899.

Morris, J. R. 1973. Accelerometry—A technique for the measurement of human body movements. *J Biomech* 6(6):729–736.

Murray, M. P., Sepic, S. B., Gardner, G. M., and Mollinger, L. A. 1981. Gait patterns of above-knee amputees using constant-friction knee components. *Bull Prosthet Res* 17(2):35–45.

Nissan, M. 1981. The use of a permutation approach in the solution of joint biomechanics: The knee. *Eng Med* 10(1):39–43.

Patriarco, A. G., Mann, R. W., Simon, S. R., and Mansour, J. M. 1981. An evaluation of the approaches of optimization models in the prediction of muscle forces during human gait. *J Biomech* 14(8):513–525.

Perry, J., and Antonelli, D. 1981. Evaluation of CARS-UBC triaxial gonoimeter. *Bull Prosthet Res* BPR 10–35, 18(1):225–226.

Plaja, J., Maldonado, F., and Goig, J. R. 1976. Accelerometric and goniometric patterns of normal and pathologic gait. *Biomechanics V-A*. Baltimore: University Park Press. pp. 347–351.

Rae, J. W.,and Cockrell, J. L. 1971. Interface pressure and stress distribution in prosthetic fitting. Bull Prosthet Res 8:64–111.

Smidt, G. L., Deusinger, R. H., Arora, J., and Albright, J. P. 1977. An automated accelerometry system for gait analysis. *J Biomech* 10(5–6):367–375.

Stokes, I. A. F., Hutton, W. C., and Evans, M. J. 1974. Force distribution under the foot—A dynamic measuring system. *Biomed Eng* 9:140–143.

Taylor, K. D. 1984. An automated clinical gait analysis laboratory. *IEEE Frontiers of Engineering and Computing in Health Care—1984,* Proceedings of the Sixth Annual Conference of the IEEE Engineering in Medicine and Biology Society. pp. 651–656.

Taylor, K. D., Mottier, F. M., Cohen, W., Simmons, D. W., Pavlak, R., Cornell, D. P., and Hankins, G. B. 1982. An automated motion measurement system for clinical gait analysis. *J Biomech* 15:505–516.

Vaughan, C. L., Andrews, J. G., and Hay, J. G. 1982a. Selection of body segment parameters by optimization methods. *J Biomech Eng* 104:38–44.

Vaughan, C. G., Hay, J. G., and Andrew, J. G. 1982b. Closed loop problems in biomechanics. Part I: A classification system. *J Biomech* 15(3):197–200.

Vaughan, C. L., Hay, J. G., and Andrew, J. G. 1982c. Closed loop problems in biomechanics. Part II: An optimization approach. *J Biomech* 15(3):201–210.

Williams, K. R., and Cavanaugh, P. R. 1980. Kinetics and kinematics of the foot-ground interface during the golf swing. *Med Sci Sports Exerc* 12(2):96.

Winter, D. A. 1979. *Biomechanics of human movement.* New York: Wiley.

Winter, D. A., Sidwall, H. G., and Hobson, D. A. 1974. Measurement and reduction of noise in kinematics of locomotion. *J Biomech* 7:157–159.

Woltring, H. J. 1980. Planar control in multi-camera calibration for 3-d gait studies. *J Biomech* 13(1):39–48.

Wyss, U. P., and Pollack, V. A. 1980. Locomotion analysis in two or three dimensions using a newly developed data acquisition system. *Human locomotion. I: Proceedings of Canadian Society for Biomechanics.* p. 90–91.

Zarrugh, M. Y. 1981a. Power requirements and mechanical efficiency of treadmill walking. *J Biomech* 14(3):157–165.

Zarrugh, M. Y. 1981b. Kinematic prediction of intersegment loads and power at the joints of the leg in walking. *J Biomech* 14(10):713–725.

Zernicke, R. F. Caldwell, G., and Roberts, E. M. 1976. Fitting biomechanical data with cubic spline functions. *Res Q* 47:9–19.

Part Four

Computer Technology: Medical Applications

CHAPTER 7

Computers and Medical Instrumentation*

Joseph D. Bronzino, Ph.D., P.E.

The Vernon Roosa Professor of Applied Science Trinity
 College
Director of the joint Trinity College/Hartford Graduate
 Center
Biomedical Engineering Program
Hartford, Connecticut

INTRODUCTION

Of the technological innovations of the twentieth century, the electronic computer looms a true giant. During the past two decades, the expansion of computer technology has been explosive, involving almost every facet of human activity. Today computers are nearly everywhere, especially in the field of medical instrumentation. The infusion of microcomputer-based computerized systems in the medical arena has greatly accelerated, with every indication that this trend will continue. Throughout the remaining portion of the 1980s, it is anticipated that computer-based systems will be extensively utilized in the automation of clinical chemistry laboratories, the monitoring of critically ill patients, and the development of various diagnostic support systems, such as electrocardiographic (ECG) interpretation and pulmonary function analysis. As a result, computers will have a significant impact upon the very nature of the health care process.

*The material in this chapter has been condensed from Bronzino, J. D., "Computer Applications for Patient Care," published by Addison-Wesley, 1982. Reproduced with permission.

Because of the awesome potential of this remarkable technological innovation, all members of the health care delivery team—physicians, nurses, administrators, and biomedical engineers—must become familiar with the basic concepts of computing and the effective utilization of computer systems within the health care environment. With this in mind, this chapter provides an overview of some basic concepts of computer technology, highlighting applications in the field of medical instrumentation. These applications emphasize primarily the computer-based systems developed for the automation of the clinical laboratories and intensive care units.

BASIC COMPUTER CONCEPTS

Initially the computer was designed as a tool to manipulate numbers and thus solve arithmetic problems. However, during its development, researchers recognized that any machine that can manipulate numbers can also manipulate any "symbol" that can be represented in numeric form. This feature is extremely important, for humans create, use, and manipulate many symbols that represent events and facts in the world about us. These symbols and the concepts they represent are essentially termed *information*.

A computer then can be viewed as an information processing machine. It is a device capable of performing computations and making logical decisions, at speeds much faster than are possible for their human counterparts. If we comprehend the generality of this definition we can readily understand why a computer can be applied in virtually every human endeavor. Its only limitation is that the computer requires instruction about what to do in terms of its own internal basic operations.

Modern computers range in size from the miniaturized microcomputers in hand-held calculators to the large multiunit systems in national computer centers. However, regardless of their physical characteristics or application, most computers have a common organizational structure. That is, a computer must accept information (in the form of instructions and data), store this information so that it can be retrieved as desired, perform calculations (and other manipulations) on the data, and provide the results of the computation process, all in a controllable fashion. Thus, to process "information" a machine must contain the following five logical elements (Figure 7.1):

1 The *input,* or receiving unit, of a computer accepts information entered by humans from various input devices for processing by other units in the machine.

2 The *memory,* or storage unit, retains the information entered by the input device so that it is available to the processing units as needed. In addition, information that has already been processed is also stored here until it is placed into the appropriate output devices.

3 The *arithmetic and logic unit* (ALU) performs all the arithmetic calculations such as addition, subtraction, multiplication, and division. These four oper-

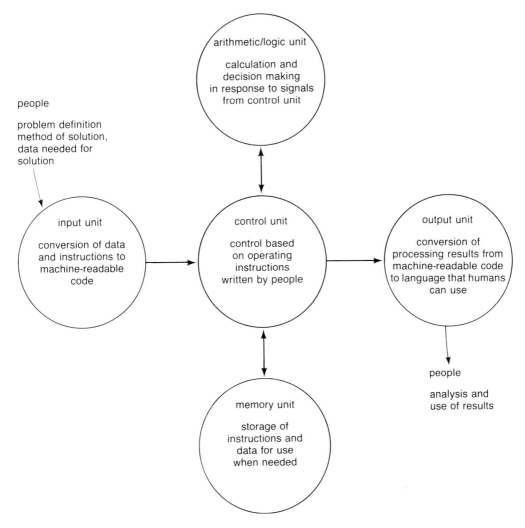

Figure 7.1   Diagram of the basic logic elements of a digital computer.

ations are also used in a variety of ways to perform other calculations. In addition, the ALU can perform logical operations, such as comparing information entered from the input unit to information already stored in memory.

4 The *control unit* directs the overall functioning of all other units and controls the flow of information among them during the processing procedures. In turn, the instructions written into the machine in the form of a computer program control this unit.

5 The *output* unit takes the information processed by the machine and displays it in various formats (tables, graphs, and so on) for review by humans.

Modern computing systems employ the latest advances in solid-state electronics to provide an extremely accurate, reliable, versatile, and high-speed tool. But how does this information handling process actually take place? The answer to this question is extremely important; however, we can understand what a computer does only by understanding its basic operation. It is therefore necessary to provide some explanation of the internal operation of digital machines, from the machine language that enables the computer to enter and handle information to the interaction of the various components to process this information in a manner prescribed by the operator. To start, let us define the term *digital computer*.

The Digital Computer

The term *digital computer* identifies an electronic device capable of manipulating bits of information under the control of sequenced instructions stored within its memory. Electronic devices, of course, respond to electrical signals. Therefore, to enable these signals to represent information, recognizable codes easily and reliably deciphered within the device are necessary. In a digital computer these codes are based on the binary system, which uses two binary digits (1 and 0) so that one number (1) represents the presence of an electrical pulse at a given time, and the other (0) denotes its absence. Binary signals then can represent both instructions and data. Consequently, binary number system provides the basic language of the digital computer.

Binary Number System

The system of numbers commonly employed within modern digital computers is termed *binary* (having a base of 2), compared to the *octal* system, which has a base of 8, and decimal system, which has a base of 10. Table 7.1 presents the symbols of the binary, octal, and decimal systems. The base of a number system indicates two important features: (1) the number of symbols available in the system and (2) the positional value of the digits used in that system. That is, the digits have different values because of their different positions.

We live in a decimal world (probably because we have ten fingers). The selection of the base (in this case 10) of this very familiar number system is quite arbitrary. It could easily have been 8, or 5, or 2. Its chief feature, however, is the posi-

Table 7.1   Selected number system

Base	Name	Symbols
2	Binary	0, 1
8	Octal	0, 1, 2, 3, 4, 5, 6, 7
10	Decimal	0, 1, 2, 3, 4, 5, 6, 7, 8, 9

tional value of the digits in any decimal number. The expression 4102, for example, is simply a convenient way of expressing the following sum:

$$
\begin{aligned}
4 \times 1{,}000 &= 4{,}000 \\
+1 \times 100 &= +100 \\
+0 \times 10 &= +0 \\
+2 \times 1 &= \underline{+2} \\
& \quad\; 4102
\end{aligned}
$$

As can be seen, in the decimal system, the positional values are increasing powers of the base 10, beginning with 10 raised to the zero power (10^0) $= 1$. As another example, consider the decimal number 374; this means three hundreds, seven tens, and four ones: $374 = (3 \times 10^2) + (7 \times 10^1) + (4 \times 10^0)$.

Using the binary system the process is the same, except that the base power is 2, not 10. Counting in the binary system then is identical to counting in any other system except for the obvious inconvenience of running out of symbols more quickly. For example, consider the binary number 10110 represented in the following way:

$$
\begin{aligned}
1 \times 2^4 &= 16 \\
+0 \times 2^3 &= +0 \\
+1 \times 2^2 &= +4 \\
+1 \times 2^1 &= +2 \\
+0 \times 2^0 &= \underline{0} \\
& \quad\; 22
\end{aligned}
$$

Thus, the binary number 10110 represents the decimal number 22. In a similar manner the binary number 111 represents $1 \times 2^2 + 1 \times 2^1 + 1 \times 2^0$, or the decimal number 7. By computing each element as shown, any binary number can be converted into its more familiar decimal counterpart.

The most elementary piece of information in the binary system is one binary digit, or _bit_. It will be noted that the word _bit_ is derived from binary digit. A group of 8 bits is known as a _byte_. These two terms are quite commonly used and form an important part of the computer jargon. The number of bits used in defining a particular number or symbol is important for another reason: it defines or limits the number of different arrangements of 1's and 0's that are possible. For example, in using just 2 bits it is possible to obtain only four different arrangements of 1's and 0's: 00, 01, 10, and 11, while 16 different meanings can be communicated by using 4 bits. In general, if n bits are used, then 2^n meanings can be established. One of the most common computer codes involves the use of 8 bits, thereby providing 2^8, or 256, possible meanings.

The octal system, having the base number of 8, operates in similar manner to that of both the decimal and binary systems. In this case, however, we can use eight symbols, 0 to 7, and determine the potential value by using powers of 8. For example, the octal number $(201)_8$ can be converted to the equivalent decimal number as follows:

$$2 \times 8^2 = 128$$
$$0 \times 8^1 = 0$$
$$1 \times 8^0 = 8$$
$$\overline{136}$$

Therefore $(201)_8 = (136)_{10}$.

Some examples of binary octal and decimal equivalent values are illustrated in Table 7.2.

Any *number* can be represented in decimal, octal, or binary notation, even a very large one. For example, the number eleven thousand, six hundred and eighty three is represented by $(11683)_{10}$, $(26643)_8$, or $(010110110100011)_2$. In binary notation, however, large numbers require such a long string of symbols that they are often difficult to read. As a result, the bits used to represent the numbers are often assembled in succeeding groups of threes. For example, let the string 010110110100011 be grouped in the following subsets: 010 = 2, 110 = 6, 100 = 4, and 011 = 3. By putting these subsets in consecutive order we have $(26643)_8$; that is, we have generated a number in the octal system. In this way, the length of the number is shortened threefold, and the monotonous succession of 0's and 1's is relieved. Thus, an octal number is a short equivalent of a rather lengthy binary number. This feature is quite important since conversion between octal and binary is far easier than conversion between decimal and binary.

Coding in Binary

As the preceding discussion indicates, any decimal number can be converted to binary notation. This information can then be entered into the computer and appro-

Table 7.2 Different number systems

Binary	Octal	Decimal	Number
0000	00	00	Zero
0001	01	01	One
0010	02	02	Two
0011	03	03	Three
0100	04	04	Four
0101	05	05	Five
0110	06	06	Six
0111	07	07	Seven
1000	10	08	Eight
1001	11	09	Nine
1010	12	10	Ten
—	13	11	Eleven
—	14	12	Twelve
—	15	13	Thirteen
—	16	14	Fourteen
—	17	15	Fifteen

(Fill in the blanks in the binary column.)

Table 7.3   BCD code for letters of the alphabet

A	110001	J	100001	S	010010
B	110010	K	100010	T	010011
C	110011	L	100000	U	010100
D	110100	M	100101	V	010101
E	110101	N	100101	W	010110
F	110110	O	100110	X	011111
G	110111	P	100111	Y	011000
H	1101000	Q	10000	Z	011001
I	1101001	R	101001		

priate arithmetic operations performed within the machine, again by using binary notation. However, we do not deal solely with numbers; we also handle alphabetic information. So that letters or certain characters are properly interpreted and communicated to a machine that deals soley with long strings of 0's and 1's, it is necessary to develop the notion of *coding*: the code relates data to a fixed array of binary digits or bits so that the specific arrangement has only one meaning. The system of expressing decimal digits in a equivalent representation is known as *binary coded decimal* (BCD). An early BCD system developed by IBM, for example, represented letters of the alphabet as in Table 7.3.

Using this code, if you typed in *JOE,* the computer would interpret it as *J* = 100001, *O* = 100110, *E* = 110101, which in turn can be used as a code that would permit the computer to recognize (at least in binary notation) the operator at the terminal.

Binary Logic: Hardware

Working with long strings of 1's and 0's would be cumbersome for humans, but it is simple for a digital computer. Composed mostly of parts that are essentially on-off switches, the machines are perfectly suited for binary computation. When a switch is open, it corresponds to the binary digit 0; closed, it stands for the digit 1. Figure 7.2 illustrates a number of commonly employed devices that exhibit this binary mode of operation.

But how does the computer make sense of the binary numbers represented by its open and closed switches? At the heart of the answer is the work of the gifted 19th-century mathematician George Boole, who devised a system of algebra, or mathematical logic, that can reliably determine whether a statement is true or false. Since a Boolean proposition is either true or false, by using Boolean algebra only three logical functions are needed to process these true and false statements or, in computer terms, 1's and 0's. The functions are called *NOT, AND,* and *OR,* and their operation can be readily duplicated today by inexpensive integrated circuits containing numerous electronic switches-transistors. These devices and the functions they represent are called *logic gates* (because they pass on information only according to the rules built into them). Incredible as it may seem, such gates can, in the proper combinations, perform all the computer's high-speed prestidigitations.

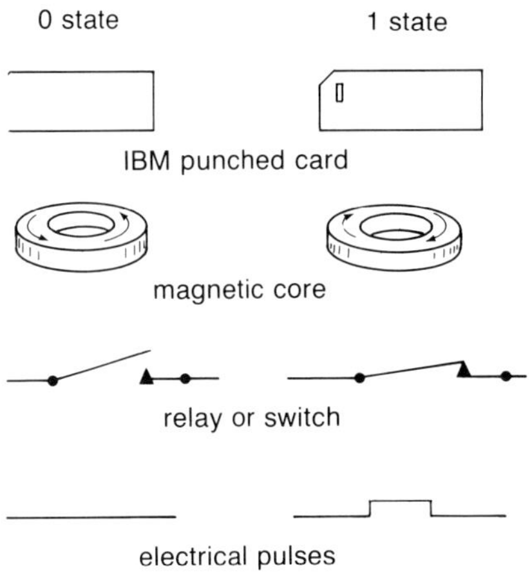

0 state   1 state

IBM punched card

magnetic core

relay or switch

electrical pulses

Figure 7.2   Schematic diagrams of commonly employed devices that are capable of provide and "O" and "l" states.

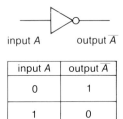

input A output $\overline{A}$

input A	output $\overline{A}$
0	1
1	0

Figure 7.3   Definition and symbol for the NOT operation.

The *NOT* function represents an algebraic means to represent the logical complement of any other state. The *NOT* circuit is a very simple one since its response is the inverse of any input such as A. The result of such an operation is represented by the symbol $\overline{A}$, which means "not A." The electronic device, or "gate," that performs the *NOT* operation is called an *inverter* (see Figure 7.3).

Now let us see the way the AND and OR gates are obtained. If two switches A and B are connected into a circuit, they can be arranged in two different ways, either in parallel or in series (see Figure 7.4). In the series circuit both *A AND B* must be closed (TRUE) for a circuit to be conductive. In Boolean terms this would be expressed as $A \wedge B \equiv C$, where the symbol $\wedge$ is the logic symbol for AND, and the column of three dashes mean "identical to." Therefore, the AND operation of the two variables A and B is 0 if either A or B is 0, and 1 if they are both 1. Figure 7.5 shows the functional relationship between the input and output variables. This logical "truth table," as it is called, represents the switch closed, conductive, or true state by 1 and the switch open, nonconductive, or false state by 0. In binary arithmetic $1 \times 1 = 1$; therefore, the *AND* statement is the logical equivalent of multiplication and can be written $A \cdot B \equiv C$.

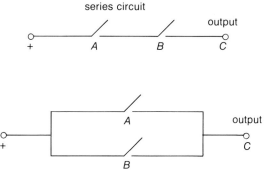

Figure 7.4 Circuit diagrams illustrating the arrangment of switches A and B for series and parllel operation.

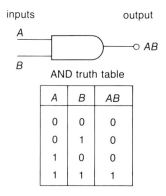

Figure 7.5 Definition and symbol for the AND operation.

In the case of the parallel circuit, on the other hand, *A OR B* must be closed (true) to enable the circuit to conduct. In Boolean terms, this would generally be written $A \vee B = C$. The *OR* operation of the variables A and B is 1 if both are 0 and 1 if either A or B is 1. Figures 7.6 shows the symbol for an OR gate and provides the truth table describing the relationship between its input and output variable. As can be seen, the normal or INCLUSIVE-OR gate gives 1 when either A or B is 1 and also when A and B are both 1. However, it will be recalled that in binary arithmetic $0 + 0 = 0$, $0 + 1 = 1$, and $1 + 1 = 0$ with carry $= 1$. To implement the carry operation the normal OR gate is not used. Rather the EXCLUSIVE-OR gate, presented in Figure 7.7, is employed and is the equivalent of binary addition. This function may be represented by $A + B = C$ with the $\oplus$ sign indicating the EXCLUSIVE-OR gate can be easily realized or constructed by using NOT, AND, and OR gates as Figure 7.8 illustrates. It is suggested that the reader verify the logic statement $A \cdot \bar{B} + \bar{A} \cdot B = A \oplus B$ illustrated in this figure. (Hint: use truth tables.)

inputs
outputs
A
B
A + B

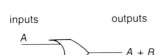

OR truth table

A	B	A + B
0	0	0
0	1	1
1	0	1
1	1	1

Figure 7.6 Definition and symbol for the OR operation.

inputs
output
A
B
$A \oplus B$

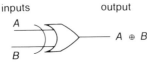

EXCLUSIVE-OR truth table

A	B	$A \oplus B$
0	0	0
0	1	1
1	0	1
1	1	0

Figure 7.7 Definition and symbol for the EXCLUSIVE - OR operation.

A
B
A
$\overline{B}$
$A\overline{B}$
A
$\overline{A}$
B
$\overline{A}B$
$A\overline{B} + \overline{A}B = A \oplus B$

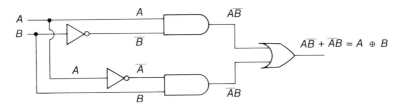

Figure 7.8 Circuit diagram illustrating the arrangement of logic elements to realize the EXCLUSIVE - OR operation.

Although electrical circuits composed of switches are a convenient way to represent the AND, OR, and NOT operations, in computers the actual electronic components implementing these actions are not ordinary switches. Instead of "off" and "on," the actual imputs are voltage or current pulses, and the output from the arrangement of transistors is either a corresponding pulse or the lack of one. A "clock" generates input pulses at a steady (and very high) frequency; this stream of voltage pulses flowing through the wiring of the computer determines its behavior. The technical problems of design and production are not of conern to us here but must be solved by the engineers involved in the manufacture and development of computers.

The principle application of Boolean algebra, however, is in the design and analysis of digital computer circuits. These electronic circuits within the digital computer consist of switching circuits that are binary in nature. Figure 7.9 illustrates the electronic symbols for those circuits that perform the *AND, OR,* and *NOT* functions. These circuits are interconnected within the machine to yield a desired result such as addition of two binary numbers. In this way combinations of *AND, OR,* and *NOT* functions enable the computer to handle arithmetic and logic functions.

The design of the electronic hardware to treat electrical signals as if they represent numbers constitutes the *hardware* aspect of the computer. The design begins with a statement of the function (such as arithmetic operations: addition, multiplication, and so on) to be performed and the constraints on them. From this beginning, following principles based upon digital logic circuits, the implementation follows naturally. A computer therefore comprises a very large number of electronic components arranged to handle information (such as numbers) in binary format and to follow a sequence of instructions dealing with the processes to which this information will be subjected.

The discussion to this point has dealt with the hardware characteristics of the digital computer, with no mention of the way the computer knows what to do with the information it receives or the order in which these calculations are to be accomplished. And yet, the computer, that is, its hardware component, can do nothing

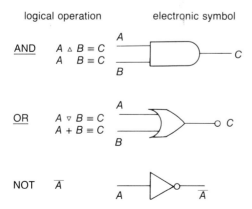

Figure 7.9 Summary of the logic statements and symbols for AND, OR and NOT operations.

without a set of instructions, or *program,* to execute. Thus, the *software* aspect of the computer, the development of computer languages and programs, is also essential for computer function. The capability so often referred to as a computer is neither the hardware nor the invisible software: it is the two together. The software concept, programming the computer, is discussed next.

The Process of Computer Programming: The Software

The term *digital computer* as defined at the beginning of this chapter describes a machine capable of manipulating bits of information under control of sequenced instructions called *computer programs* stored within the memory of the machine. These programs guide the computer through an orderly series of steps to assure that the information is processed according to a desired procedure specified by computer programmers. Since the computer requires instructions in order to solve specific problems, computer programming is the process of telling the computer when and how to utilize its various components to solve these problems. Thus, the process of generating programs, or software packages, consists of a number of distinct steps: (1) defining the problem, (2) determining the operations that the computer must perform in a sequential manner to solve a particular problem, (3) selecting a "language" (or code) that is most appropriate or available for preparation of the program, (4) coding the operations to be performed in accordance with the rules of that language, and (5) entering the program into the computer's memory. Once it is in the memory of the machine, this stored program is processed to achieve the desired results whenever it is called into action.

A key word in the preceding definition is *sequenced.* Sequencing is not a new concept; any set of ordered instructions involves a sequence. For example, to obtain the "average" of ten numbers, a definite sequence of operations must be followed. First, the ten numbers must be entered into the machine, and each is added to the previous one as it is entered so that when all ten numbers have been placed into the machine the sum of all ten numbers is obtained. Then this total is divided by the number of data points entered, in this case ten, and the average value is computed. The series of steps is sequential. Although one may program the computation process differently, once the program is established the steps specified by it are followed in order. Thus, if there are but four steps or instructions (*A, B, C,* and *D*) in a given program, then instruction *C* cannot be executed until steps *A* and *B* have been completed, and instruction *D* cannot be undertaken until step *C* is accomplished. Such a process would be extremely slow for human beings, but the computer can perform these instructions at speeds thousands and even millions of times faster than humans can. As a result, these computations, although followed one after the other, are completed in a relatively short period of time.

It was recognized, however, that the power of a digital computer would be enhanced if it had the ability to make logical decisions. Therefore, all modern computers provide this capability. This decision making ability means that when the computer has two possible actions, it can be programmed to select one or the other, depending on the outcome of a previous event. For example, consider the use of the computer to keep in order a single file of records, which may be patient records, such as those individuals admitted to a particular service in a hospital such as the radiology department. All of the records are to be in the file in ascending sequence by account number. Therefore, as records are entered, one at a time, one must decide where to store the incoming record (identified by its account number). Therefore, the account number of the incoming record should always be higher than that of the preceding record. Any incoming record lower than the previous record is recognized as an out-of-sequence condition, and the program transfers to another routine (or set of instructions), which is initiated to take corrective action. After each high comparison, the record is placed into storage, where it is compared with the next record until it reaches its proper location in the file.

Another example of the utility of the decision making capacity incorporated within the digital computer is its use to monitor the heart rate of a patient in an intensive care unit. In this case, one supplies the monitored heart beat, and the computer calculates the heart rate. If the calculated value of the heart rate is above or below a preselected value, the computer activates an alarm to alert the attending staff that a problem exists. If the value is within preselected values (often called a *window*), the computer continues to calculate the heart rate over the next time period. The computer, however, *must be programmed* to decide whether to activate the alarm circuitry or simply to proceed with the monitoring process: it does not make this decision itself. However, to accomplish this task successfully, the medical staff of the intensive care unit must interact with computer programmers to ensure that the specific tasks required are incorporated into the program developed to direct the activity of the computer.

Computer Languages

Computer programs are a sequence of instructions written for the computer in a language that the machine understands. Some programming languages are directly understandable by the computer, but others require additional translational steps. Although hundreds of computer languages are in use today, they all basically fall into one of three categories.

1 Machine languages
2 Assembly languages
3 High-level languages

Machine language is the natural language of a particular computer. It is closely related to the actual construction of the digital logic circuits (discussed previously) within the machine. Consequently, a machine language instruction generally consists of a code in binary notation (long strings of 1's and 0's) that directs the computer via the logic gates to perform some specific operation such as add, subtract, store, read, write, or move. For example, the string of bits 0110 can indicate a "move" operation. As a result, any computer can directly understand the machine language developed for it. However, machine languages are extremely machine dependent: each computer has its own machine language, which may be different from those of other models or types of computers. Consequently, programmers must be familiar with the basic set of instructions inherent in each machine before they can begin to communicate with it.

Each machine language instruction consists of an operation code and one or more operands. The *operation code* specifies the operation to be performed, and the *operand* identifies the quantities to be operated on, for example, the numbers to be added or the locations where data are stored. Consider the following machine language instruction with two operands.

Operation Code	Operand 1	Operand 2
0110	1101	1111

As stated, the operation code refers to the part of the instruction that specifies the operation to be performed; in this case, let us assume that 0110 is the binary representation for "MOV." The operands, on the other hand, provide information regarding the place within the computer where the data to be processed are located. In this case, the contents of memory location 1111 are to be MOVED to memory location 1101.

Obviously, coding a program in machine language is difficult. It requires the programmer to remember not only the specific machine language representation for each operation code, but also the addresses of the operands in each instruction. Therefore, although machine languages provide a means to communicate directly with the machine, they are usually inconvenient for the majority of human operators, who do not have a thorough knowledge of the computer.

Unfortunately, until the 1950s machine languages were the only ones available. Therefore, anyone who wanted to work with a particular computer had to learn the special language of that machine. As a result even a simple problem in arithmetic represented a major problem in programming. Consequently, other approaches became necessary. The first simplification was the development of symbolic languages, or mnemonics. Nearly everyone uses mnemonic symbols as a quick, easy-to-remember shorthand for longer expressions. For baseball fans *K* for "strikeout" and *BB* for "base on balls" are familiar examples. Equally common are such symbols as *RN* for registered nurse, *NIH* for National Institute of Health, and *DOD* for Department of Defense. Using this concept, computer programmers developed their own shorthand codes that enabled them to write instructions in alphabetic symbols. These symbols were easier to remember than their binary equivalents in machine language and consequently significantly reduced the time necessary to program a problem.

Languages consisting of these English-like abbreviations are called *assembly languages*. In this type of language, all operation codes have a mnemonic designation, and all machine addresses and other operands in the instruction are written with symbolic notation. As an example, the letters *LA,* instead of a long string of ones and zeros, can represent the program instruction to load the address (location of data or instruction) into the computer's memory, and *ADD* can tell the computer to add two operands specified in the other portion of the instruction.

Table 7.4 Assembler language coding form

Location	Operation	Operand 1	Operand 2	Comments
BEGIN	MOVE	*D*	*A*	Move *A* to *D*
	ADD	*D*	*B*	Add *B* to *D*
	STOP			End of Program
A:	(value of *A*)			
B:	(value of *B*)			
D:	(result of *A* + *B*)			

Using symbolic labels and instruction mnemonics, one can create the simple program in Table 7.4 to calculate the sum of two numbers, $D = A + B$.

However, before the computer can use this program, it must translate these symbolic instructions into machine language form. As a result, computer programs called *assemblers* were developed to read and translate assembler language programs to object programs in machine code. It will be noted that in the program in Table 7.4 symbolic names designate the address or location used to store data (such as the values of *A* and *B*) or the results. Somehow address values must be assigned for them. The advantage of the assembler is that it can do this automatically for the programmer. As the assembler encounters each of these symbolic locations it assigns it to a particular location. Therefore, this type of language helps the programmer to specify exact memory locations for the data and for the operations to be conducted. However, although this type of program does relieve the programmer of many intricate coding details, it still requires an intimated knowledge of the computer.

Macroinstructions were another big step forward. With a macroinstruction, the programmer, in one statement, can cause the computer to go through a long sequence of previously written steps. They were and are used for functions that keep recurring in any computer program. For example, with one macroinstruction to read a record stored in memory, the computer automatically goes through the many individual steps required, and the programmer does not have to write out each step.

As technology improved and computer speed increased, internal processing of an instruction took only millionths of a second instead of the thousandths of a second required in the 1940s and early 1950s, and computers were designed to compute, record input, and generate output simultaneously. If a computer could be programmed to translate *LA* to machine language, it could be programmed to translate words like *COMPUTE, MULTIPLY, SQUARE ROOT,* too. Higher-level languages, along with appropriate language translation programs called *compilers* or interpreters, were developed to do just that, speeding up the process of programming computers significantly.

Higher-level languages contain single statements that accomplish tasks that often required many machine language or assembly language statements. They permit instructions to be written in a manner closely resembling English and con-

Table 7.5   Common higher-level computer languages

FORTRAN   (Acronym for Formula Translation): Developed in 1956 to solve mathematical problems in the sciences and most widely used higher-level programming language. Has had a series of revisions known as *FORTRAN II, FORTRAN III,* and *FORTRAN IV.*

BASIC TM   (Beginners All-purpose Symbolic Instruction Code): Ideal for instruction in computer concepts and programming. Used frequently by occasional programmers.

COBOL   (Common Business Oriented Language): Most widely used by professional programmers and used in hospital accounting systems.

ALGOL   (ALGOrithmic Language): Mostly outside the United States, the most popular language for engineers, natural scientists, and mathematicians.

MUMPS   (Massachusetts General Hospital Utility Multi-Programming System): Applicable to many areas of health care delivery in which storage and manipulation of large textual data bases are of primary concern.

tain commonly used mathematical notations. High-level languages are much more desirable from a programming standpoint than other types of computer languages. They are easy to learn and easy to use. Although they sacrifice speed, computer time, and computer memory, they do allow ease of operation and provide extremely valuable diagnostic services (such as being able to debug the program as it is being written) that more than offset these disadvantages. A number of languages that permit the operator to generate rather useful and complex programs without understanding the internal operations of the computer have been developed. Table 7.5 provides a brief description of the four most frequently used programming languages.

As a result of the advances in these higher-level languages computer users now have a wide variety of programming aids that they can tailor to their individual needs. Although these tools are better and faster than ever, still the individual with the flow diagram and coding sheet must solve the problem. Today's powerful programming aids can provide assistance only after a correct method for solving the problem has been worked out. Once it is, converting the solution to the detailed instructions a computer needs to perform the operations required to provide the information or answers requested of it is not difficult.

The Microcomputer

In recent years the size and shape of the digital computer have changed as a result of the advances in solid-state electronics that preceded the development of *microprocessors,* which are essentially integrated circuits (ICs) impressed on small silicon chips possessing enormous computing capacity. These microprocessors, hooked to input/output devices and additional memory, constitute the *microcomputer.* Figure 7.10 illustrates the typical functional organization or architecture of a microcomputer. Referring to the initial definition, we see that a microcomputer system is a digital computer containing all five basic sections of a computer: (1) the input unit, (2) the control and (3) arithmetic units contained within the microprocessor, (4) the memory unit, and (5) the output unit. It is classed as a micro-

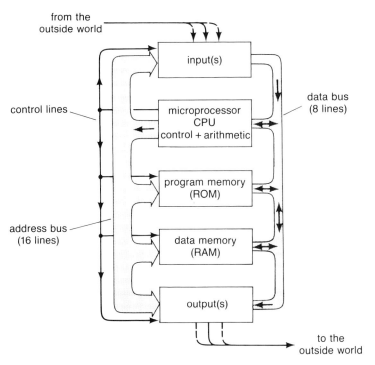

from the
outside world

input(s)

control lines

data bus
(8 lines)

microprocessor
CPU
control + arithmetic

program memory
(ROM)

address bus
(16 lines)

data memory
(RAM)

output(s)

to the
outside world

Figure 7.10 Schematic diagram illustrating internal
organization of a typical microcomputer.

computer only because of its small size and low cost. The microprocessor generally
forms the central processing unit (CPU) section of a microcomputer system and
regulates all the units of the system by control lines. Besides the control lines, the
address bus (16 parallel conductors) selects a certain memory location, input port,
or output port. The *data bus* (eight parallel conductors) on the right is a two-way
path for transferring data in and out of the microprocessor unit. It is important to
note that the microprocessor unit (MPU) can send data to or receive data from the
memory using the data bus.

If a program that is stored permanently is usually placed in a memory device
called a *read-only memory* (ROM), which is usually a permanently programmed
memory chip (IC). Temporary data memory is usually stored in an IC device called
a *read/write memory* (RWM). In common practice, the read/write memory is referred to as a *random-access memory* (RAM). Temporary microcomputer user
programs are also stored in the RAM section of memory, along with data. The
RAM and ROM sections of memory are usually shown as separate units because
they are usually separate ICs.

It is to be pointed out that this system represents the general organization of a
microcomputer. Since more than 20 companies produce a wide variety of general-
purpose microprocessors, and even more companies assemble microprocessors,
memories, and other components into microcomputer systems, it is not possible to
cover the many computer products that are presently available. Most microcomputers would have the minimum features mentioned plus several more. For clarity,

however, it is customary to omit the necessary power supply, clock, and some feedback lines to the microprocessor unit, with the understanding that any MPU requires connections to power supply and clock.

When learning about a new microprocessor, any user or programmer must study the following (Tokheim 1983):

1 Microprocessor architecture handles the arrangement of registers in the CPU, the number of bits in the address and data buses, and so on.

2 The instruction set is a listing of the operations the microprocessor can perform. This includes transferring data and performing arithmetic and logical operations, data testing, branching instructions, and input/output operations and involves a variety of addressing modes.

3 A minimal system using the microprocessor may contain a microprocessor, a clock, a RAM, a ROM, input/output ports, an address decoder, and a power supply. Sometimes separate ICs or components perform these functions; however, some microprocessor units contain most of these capabilities.

4 Control signals include outputs that direct other ICs (such as RAMs, ROMs, and I/O ports) when to operate. Some typical control signals might govern memory reading and writing or input/output reading and writing.

5 Pin functions perform special inputs and outputs of the microprocessor. Other pins might be power supply, clock, serial data I/O, interrupt inputs, and bus control.

Although these details are beyond the scope of this presentation, it is important to emphasize that the design of microcomputer systems for any application requires in-depth understanding of these components. The final point, however, is that microcomputer-based systems are ideal for *dedicated* use: for computations that are standard and are frequently utilized. Consequently, the microcomputer is an ideal tool in the development of modern medical instrumentation systems.

Computer Operations: Hardware and Software Interaction

To explain the way a computer operates, let us re-examine the essential elements of the comptuer introduced earlier in this chapter in terms of the various hardware components that make up a digital computer system (Figure 7.11). In the simplest terms, information that may be data or the program itself goes into the machine via various input devices such as a terminal or card reader. This information is stored within the memory unit of the machine and directed to the central processing unit as needed.

Since the memory unit is such an important element of the computer, it is necessary to discuss it in some detail. In the context of electronics, *memory* usually refers to a device for storing digital information. The most widely used digital memories are *read/write memories* that perform read and write operations at an identical or similar rate. Important characteristics include storage capacity, cost per bit, reliability, speed of operation (defined in terms of access time), cycle time, and data-transfer rate. Access time is simply the time required to read or write at

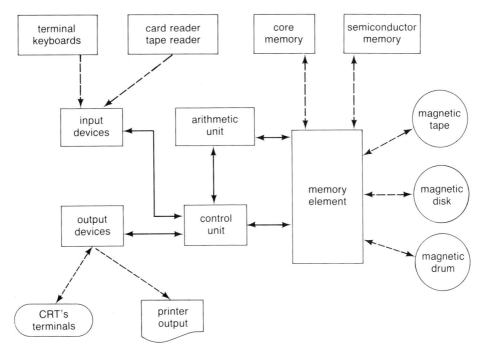

Figure 7.11   Block diagram illustrating the hardware aspects
of a digital computer system.

any storage location. Some memories, such as RAMs, have the same access time to *any* storage location, whereas serial access and block access memories have access times that depend on the storage location selected. *Cycle time,* on the other hand, is the specified minimum period of time random-access memories can complete a read or write operation, and *data-transfer rate* is the speed at which information is transferred to or from sequential storage locations.

Digital memories can be conveniently classified as either entirely electronic devices or moving-surface devices. Each has distinct advantages and therefore an appropriate place in today's computer systems. Several kinds of electronic memory devices exist, but most high-speed machines designed in the 1960s and presently in service use magnetic cores. These are tiny "doughnuts" the size of pinheads that are made of a special material. Each core can at any time be magnetized in either of two directions. One direction stands for a binary 0, the other direction for a binary 1. By arranging these cores in a column, we can therefore store any binary number. Thousands of cores are strung together on criss-crossed wires inside a frame that looks something like a square tennis racket. Thus, in two dimensions, there are essentially a number of rows (in the horizontal direction) and columns (in the vertical direction) of these basic memory elements. By extending this visualization to include a third dimension that gives the appearance of a wire cage, and then stacking these units on top of each other, it is possible to build up a basic magnetic card memory unit. Typical core memories have a storage capacity of 10^6 to 10^7 bits and an average access time of 1 microsecond (μs) and cost approximtely 1 cent per bit.

These ferrite-core memories, however, are being largely succeeded in new designs by semiconductor memories that provide faster data access, smaller power consumption, and significantly lower cost. These new electronic memory systems have been made possible by the development of large-scale integrations (LSI) techniques that permit the mass fabrication of microscopically scaled arrays of electronic elements and all their interconnections on a tiny chip of silicon. In general, a LSI memory chip carrying N bits is organized so that it has one read/write channel and N addresses. Usually N is a power of 2 such as 1,024, 4,096, or 16,384, in which cases the chip is referred to as *1K, 4K,* or *16K*. Internally, the N storage cells are physically arranged in an array and are selected by the two array lines on which they lie. The chip usually carries two decoders that select these two lines from a binary code. Hence the number of address lines to the chip is relatively small (10 for 1K, 12 for 4K, and 14 for 16K). These chips are mounted directly on a printed board or packaged in separate cans, which typically have 16 pins, mounted on printed boards. To complete the memory system, of course, power supplies and coupling circuits are necessary. It is interesting to note that the resulting system cost per bit is in general almost ten times greater than that for the chip alone.

New memory devices are continually appearing on the scene as a result of the emerging new electronic technologies. Some of these innovations include electron-beam addressable memories (EBAM), charge-coupled device (CCD) memories, and magnetic-bubble memories (MBM). These new memory devices are essentially serial access devices in which the stored bits circulate as if they were in a closed pipeline. Each stored bit is transferred sequentially through 64 or more storage locations between the time it is written into memory and the first time it becomes available for reading. The rate at which bits are shifted from one storage site to the next in a CCD memory is about the same as the cycle time for a random-access memory. Thus the largest access time for a serial memory with 64 storage locations is 64 times the cycle time for a random-access memory. They are, therefore, somewhat slower than semiconductor memories. However, in many applications serial access is entirely satisfactory. For example, for a computer to refresh the information presented in a conventional video display, which is scanned point by point in a repeated linear pattern, a serial access memory is quite appropriate.

Moving surface memory devices, on the other hand, are quite different. These devices provide information storage in localized areas of a thin magnetic film coated onto a nonmagnetic supporting surface, which may be flexible, in the form of a tape or disk made out of plastic, or rigid, in the form of a disk or drum. In these devices, the magnetic film and the read/write head, which consists of a simple electromagnet, move in relation to one another to bring a storage site into position for the writing or reading of information.

The simplest digital magnetic-type memories are adapted from audio-cassette type recorders. One such cassette is capable of storing 10^7 bits and has an access time from 10 to 100 s. Stacks of disks that look like phonograph records are also used. These play back information in much the same way that a phonograph record plays back music. Large magnetic disk memories can store 10^9 to 10^{10} bits on one or more disk surfaces mounted on a single spindle rotated by a single motor and usually have an average access time of 20 ms.

These moving surface memory devices essentially act as external memory units for the computer and are used when data do not change frequently. Magnetic disks and magnetic drums are *block-accessed devices;* that is, data are transferred at a rate determined by the surface velocity and the density of the data storage on the surface. Typical transfer rates range from 10^6 to 10^7 bits per second. Consequently, these devices allow data transfer back and forth to the core memory at a very fast rate. Magnetic tape, on the other hand, provides a slow, but inexpensive and almost infinite auxiliary memory for computer systems. It can hold huge quantities of data: a single $10\frac{1}{2}$ in. reel of tape can hold the contents of 250,000 punched cards. In a magnetic tape system consisting of a tape drive and a replaceable reel of half-inch magnetic tape, magnetic changes can be introduced on the surface of the tape and then be sensed as the tape passed across the read/write heads. It records and reads serially (in a progressive order) so that it may require a considerable amount of time (a minute or two, which is a long time compared to the time the computer takes to perform a set of arithmetic instructions). As a result, magnetic tapes are not used for random searches but rather for access to bulk data.

Various input/output devices essentially permit users to communicate directly with the computer and to view the results of the calculations it performs. The input devices transfer the information from its original form, usually a handwritten, typed, or printed document, into machine-readable form. For this purpose, punched cards and punched paper tape are generated to act as inputs for data or the program. In analyzing information obtained from monitoring or laboratory equipment, analog electrical signals are converted into the appropriate digital format by analog-to-digital converters (ADCs). Printers and teletypewriters are the most commonly used output devices, but once again it is possible to convert a sequence of digital numbers into an analog signal by means of a digitial-to-analog converter (DAC) and to have the electrical signal control external devices (such as humidifiers or air conditioners to control the room environment). Thus, computers can communicate directly with other machines to achieve a specific objective (such as regulating the air temperature and humidity of incubators to ensure that premature infants have an appropriate environment).

These input/output (I/O) devices allow rapid processing of data and are not suited to the slower rate at which a person can type (150 words per minute, maximum). However, in many situations it is appropriate for an individual to communicate directly with the computer. For example, during medical history taking at a screening clinic, the patient responds directly to questions displayed at a console terminal. After the patient responds, the computer files the response and goes on to the next question. On the other hand, in a modern eye clinic, the intraocular pressure obtained during tonometry may be automated and displayed for the clinician in a graphical format easier to interpret than a column of numbers. In this situation, while the data are being taken, specific calculations to assist in the decision making process can be requested and provided to the physician before the patient leaves the laboratory.

The principal mechanism in the display console is the *cathode-ray tube* (CRT); output is displayed in the form of letters, numbers, curves, and lines. With an interactive display console available, one can combine the rapid calculation and information processing capability of the computer with the integrative ability of the human operator. In this way the operator can explore the results obtained and perhaps be more creative since the machine's power can facilitate this creative effort.

The computer with all its hardware, software, and information processing capabilities must still be applied to specific tasks to achieve any useful purpose. Many of these applications have changed the organizations that use them, sometimes dramatically, more often subtly. In the health care field these applications are increasing at an incredible rate and will change the very nature of health care delivery in the future. Health service professionals must adapt themselves to this change. Just as the computer has afforded changes in so many other fields, its implementation will enable the medical profession to keep abreast of the increasing demands brought upon it and distribute better care among a far greater number of people. It is impossible here to review all the possible computer applications in medicine; consequently we will focus our attention on those applications that automate the clinical chemistry laboratories and monitor critically ill patients.

COMPUTERS IN THE CLINICAL LABORATORY

The primary information required for any clinical decision is usually the medical data collected during the care of patients. These data are often processed in clinical laboratories, which have historically provided the chemical, hematological, microbiological, and blood banking services for hospitalized patients and outpatients (Williams 1969). The traditional organization of these clinical laboratories usually includes the disciplines of hematology, chemistry, and microbiology with the breakdown of activities within these disciplines as follows (Martinek 1972):

1 Hematology primarily involves monitoring the activity of a single physiological process, the formation and development of erythrocytes (red blood cells).

2 Clinical chemistry is based on the technical science of chemistry and is oriented primarily to the application of clinical methods without regard for any specific physiological system or anatomical group of organs or diseases. According to the International Federation of Clinical Chemistry, the discipline encompasses the study of the chemical aspects of human life in health and illness and the application of chemical laboratory methods to diagnosis, control treatment, and prevent disease.

3 Clinical microbiology, which includes bacteriology, serology, immunology, virology, and other related disciplines, primarily focuses on the detection of a large number of extraneous biological agents (the microbes). In addition, it involves blood bank operations limited to the collection and preservation of blood and its characterization for compatibility and therapeutic use.

The activities within these clinical laboratories chiefly entail providing information about the presence of any "pathological" condition. If *physiology* is defined as the study of the normal function of cells, tissues, and organs, then pathology is the study of disease-induced alterations in the human body. The various laboratory procedures, including chemical tests, microscopic examinations, tissue cultures, and the like, conducted within the clinical laboratory are vital if the appropriate health professionals are to diagnose and monitor the course of a particular disease properly. To be of clinical value this information must be accurate, easily accessible, and as rapidly processed as possible.

A clinical laboratory today has the primary function of obtaining appropriate medical data about a particular patient for review by the attending physician. To accomplish this task, the staff must collect samples, process tests, report the results, and somehow store all the relevant data collected on each patient. In essence all of the steps required to develop modern microcomputer-based instrumentation equipment are found here.

Over the years, the performance of these steps by manual methods has become increasingly difficult as the number and type of determinations have grown in complexity as well as volume. In 1960, for example, clinical laboratories had equipment and methods limited to 12 or so different biochemical determinations (Dickson 1969); today more than 400 different tests are available within the confines of this facility. These tests range from a rather simple physical measurement of specific gravity to such sophisticated techniques as atomic absorption spectrophotometry. The volume of these tests conducted each year has also grown at an ever-increasing rate, reaching the 10 billion mark by the mid-1980s. These are staggering numbers and illustrate, in part, the importance of this scientifically based information in the treatment of patients.

Over the past 20 years a number of extremely successful systems have evolved, some of which are available from commercial vendors. Microcomputers have been directly interfaced with a wide variety of laboratory instruments for on-line analysis of data, and automation of rather complex computations has become indispensable in many laboratories (Whitcomb et al. 1978). Presently, computer systems are being designed for use in clinical laboratories to store, retrieve, route, sort, and verify the flow of laboratory information and thereby provide an efficient and cost-effective means of handling patient data. As computer technology has become less expensive and more flexible, it has become apparent that the computerization of a clinical laboratory requires that laboratory personnel as well as engineers assist in the conceptual planning of the computerized system being designed for a particular laboratory (Lincoln 1978). Therefore, a discussion of the computerization of the clinical laboratory requires an understanding of the nature of the tests, procedures, and equipment employed in the hematology and clinical chemistry laboratories.

Hematology

Hematology is the study of the structure and gross anatomy of the blood and blood-forming tissue. The proper functioning of this important process is essential to good health. The circulatory system, for example, is the most important mode of transport within the body, bringing nutrients to the numerous cells within the body and removing a variety of their waste products. In the process, a great number of raw materials remain in suspension in the blood to be used on demand by tissues and cells. Thus, the contents of the general chemical milieu of the body may be estimated from the analytic tests of the many constituents that normally circulate within the vascular system (Ray 1974). These tests are conducted within the hematology laboratory and include sedimentation rates, hematocrit, and counts of blood cells and other particulate matter in blood.

The blood consists mainly of a fluid or plasma in which are suspended the formed elements, principally erythrocytes (red cells), leukocytes (white cells), and platelets. To perform most tests, blood must be anticoagulated upon removal from the body to prevent clotting. When such blood stands quietly, the erythrocytes gradually fall to the bottom. The rate at which they settle, the *sedimentation rate,* usually is measured in millimeters per hour. The sedimentation rate, a nonspecific test, is a general indicator of physiology and metabolism. Normally, the sedimentation process occurs slowly, but in many diseases, the rate is rapid and, in some cases, proportional to the severity of the disease. The sedimentation rate can therefore be used, not only as a diagnostic aid, but as an indicator of the progress of a particular disease.

Permitting the prolonged settling of a blood sample in a tube or by centrifuge allows the percentage of red blood cells in the whole blood column to be measured. This parameter, the *hematocrit,* is essentially a measure of the volume occupied by erythrocytes in a given volume of blood and is usually expressed as a percentage. If the red cells are then chemically fractured so that all of the hemoglobin (which makes up almost 35 percent of the red blood cell) is released from them, the total amount of hemoglobin can be determined by colorimetry. *Hemoglobin* (Hb), therefore, is simply a measure of the amount of hemoglobin in a given volume of blood and is expressed in units of gram-percentage.

In addition, by smearing a drop of blood onto the surface of a glass slide and then using appropriate staining techniques, the clinician can detect *various cells* by direct microscopic indentification. This type of *differential counting* of the various constituents in the blood provides evidence of particular infections or disease states (such as leukemias) that may involve one cell type in particular. The *reticulocyte count,* for example, provides a measure of the capability of bone marrow to respond to therapy and the effectiveness of such therapy. It may also alert the physician of excessive drug treatment as in the case of chemotherapy leukemia.

In the hematology laboratory, a group of tests called a *complete blood count* (CBC) is one of the most commonly performed blood assays. These tests include hematocrit, hemoglobin, red blood cell count (RBC), white blood cell count (WBC), and a differential count. Other indices or measures are derived from these basic data. For example, mean corpuscular volume (MCV), mean corpuscular hemoglobin (MCH), and mean corpuscular hemoglobin concentration (MCHC) can be estimated by the following equation:

$$MVC = (\text{hematocrit} \times 10)/RBC$$

MVC represents the mean volume of the red blood cells in blood and cubic micrometers ($cm^3 \times 10^{-6}$). On the other hand, MCH provides a measure of the average content of hemoglobin per erythrocyte in micromicrograms ($g \times 10^{-12}$), calculated by the following equation:

$$MCH = [Hb(g/100\,mL) \times 10]/RBC\,(10^6/mm^3)$$

Whereas MCH represents the mean weight of hemoglobin per erythrocyte, MCHC expresses the mean *concentration* of hemoglobin in each erythrocyte and is calculated according to the following formula:

$$MCHC = Hb\,(g/100\,mL) \times 100/\text{hematocrit}$$

The tests and procedures of the hematology laboratory are performed on specimens of bone marrow, whole blood, and cells or other material in blood. Collection of these specimens varies from surgical procedures required to collect bone marrow to drawing of blood samples. Usually the collection occurs at the bedside of inpatients, and ambulatory patients go the the laboratory for blood collection.

Once the specimen arrives at the hematology laboratory, it undergoes one (or all) of five general types of tests: (1) microscopic examination of smeared or sectional tissues, (2) counting of the many kinds of cells and cell fragments, (3) determination of color after treatment with various reagents, (4) electrophoresis, and (5) mechanical fragility and sedimentation procedures (Garrett 1976).

Usually, the hematology laboratory possesses at least one high-volume analyzer, a Coulter counter (see Figure 7.12). This device performs all the preceding determinations except differential counts on individual blood samples introduced by the operating technician.

In this device a small specimen of blood is diluted and placed into a chamber where a vacuum forces the cells through an aperture passageway, whose diameter is only slightly greater than the average cell size (8 μm), into another (receiving) chamber on the other side of the narrow aperture. Since electrodes are immersed in both chambers, the electrical potential changes between the two electrodes as each cell passes through the aperture. This change of electrical potential generates an impulse that is automatically counted and totaled. It is important to note that one may adjust the counting circuit in this device quite accurately to accept or reject particles within a certain size range (1 to 20 mm). Therefore, in addition to simple counts, the clinician can obtain from the Coulter counter data related to the particle size distribution and mean particle size. Attachments to these instruments include a hematocrit calculator and a mean cell volume calculator, with which by the number of pulses multiplied by the mean cell volume determines the hematocrit, and the total pulse voltage divided by the number of pulses determines the mean cell volume.

In general, the Coulter technique permits the counting of particles regardless of their size, shape, form, or orientation as long as they can pass through the aperture. Table 7.6 summarizes the types of tests performed within a typical hematology

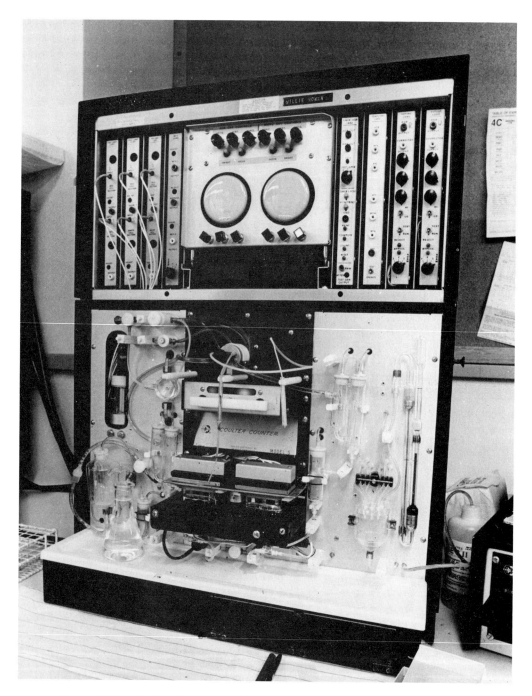

Figure 7.12   Coulter Counter used in the counting of blood components-all numbers, sizes and hemoglobin content (courtesy of the Saint Francis Hospital and Medical Center, Hartford, Connecticut).

Table 7.6 Types of tests performed in typical hematology laboratory

Test Type	Device	Units	Normal Range	Average Number/Day*
CBC (complete blood count)	Coulter	—	—	150–275
WBC	Coulter	Number $\times$ 10^3	4.5–10.0	
RBC	Coulter	Number $\times$ 10^6	M 4.4–6.0 F 4.2–5.5	
MCV	Coulter	3	82–96	
MCH	Coulter	g	27–44	
MCHC	Coulter	%	31–35	
Hgb†	Coulter	g%	M 14–18 F 12–16	50–75
Hematocrit†	Coulter	%	M 40–54 F 37–47	50–75
Platelet	Microscope and counter	$10^3/mm^3$	150–400	15–30
Reticulocyte	Microscope and counter	%RBC	0.5–1.5	10–20
Sedimentation rate	Graduated cylinders	mm/h	M 0–15 F 0–20	30–50
Differential count	Microscope and counter	%WBC		275–300

*Typical values for a 900- to 1,000-bed hospital.

†Tests performed as part of the CBC that are also requested separately.

laboratory, their units, the normal range of values, and the device that performs each type of test. It should be quite clear that the Coulter counter is by far the most widely used analyzer in the hematology laboratory; consequently, the initial concern in automating any hematology laboratory involves primarily the Coulter counter.

Clinical Chemistry

The cure and prevention of disease requires knowledge of the structure and function of the body in both health and disease. Over the years, clinical chemistry has contributed significantly to the early detection of disease processes as well as to the nature of responses of organs and body systems to therapy. Therefore, it has become extremely important for the clinical chemistry laboratory to provide rapid and reliable analysis of a wide range of body constituents.

As an example, let us consider the mineral content of the body. Seven minerals occur in sufficient content in the body to be considered of prime importance:

1 Calcium (Ca)
2 Phosphorus (P)
3 Sodium (Na)
4 Magnesium (Mg)
5 Potassium (K)
6 Chlorine (Cl)
7 Iron (Fe)

Six additional minerals, although occurring only in small quantities, are nevertheless important for healthy function; these are sulfur, iodine, copper, maganese, cobalt, and zinc. In addition to these 13 essential elements are, of course, the major constituents of all tissue cells—carbon, hydrogen, nitrogen, and oxygen—which are all metabolically derived from protein (amino acids), fats (fatty acids), and carbohydrates. The necessary amounts of all these elements are usually available in one's average dietary intake (Ray 1974). However, inadequate amounts may occur in the presence of certain deficiencies or disease states. Furthermore, many of these disorders are functional (metabolic) and appear to produce no definite change in tissue structure except for certain target organs such as the liver or kidney. Monitoring for disturbances in the normal levels of each of these elements is, therefore, essential.

Abnormal variations in the body or blood content of these minerals lead to a number of pathological conditions sometimes having lethal consequences. For example, abnormally low iron content results in inadequate quantity of the iron-compounded red cell pigment, hemoglobin. Since hemoglobin in turn is necessary for the transfer of oxygen through the blood, this anemia leads to tissue oxygen deprivation. Consequently, a deficiency in one of these essential minerals may have a "rippling effect" upon various physiological systems. Thus, testing the mineral content in various body fluids, within the clinical chemistry laboratory, provides vital information regarding the "health" status of a patient.

Unlike the "clean" chemistry ordinarily found in analytic techniques, the great "soup mix" of the body fluids contains numerous combination possibilities of many substances, several of which interfere with one another during analysis. Therefore, sophisticated means of separating or isolating the particular substance being measured are necessary.

Fortunately, a very small number of these substances constitute the majority of procedures in the clinical chemistry laboratory. In fact, probably 75 percent of the expected test load consists of one or more of the 20 tests listed in Table 7.7. Commercially available biochemical assay apparatus has been designed for these tests. In general, these devices employ a particular physical principle in order to obtain a measure of the substances present in a particular sample of body fluid. They include such devices as colorimeters, spectrophotometers, fluorometers, and chromatographs.

Table 7.7   Standard clinical chemistry laboratory tests

Blood serum glucose	Uric acid
Blood urea nitrogen (BUN)	Lactic dehydrogenose (LDH) (enzyme)
Creatinine	Cholesterol
Bilirubin	Potassium
Total protein	Calcium
Sodium	Serum glutamic-pyruvate transaminase (SGPT) (enzyme)
Albumiin (Alb)	Carbon dioxide (CO_2)
Alkaline phosphatase	Amylase (enzyme)
Serum glutamic-oxalacetic transaminase (SGOT) (enzyme)	Thyroxine
	Creatine-phosphokinase (CPK)
	Chloride

The majority of tests to be automated are basically quite simple. A sample is mixed with a reagent; the resulting reaction effects a change in the mixture proportional to the amount of chemical (being tested) in the sample. Most of these tests involve a change in light's transmission through a substance absorbed by the mixture. This is equivalent to saying that the mixture can change color or change the way it reacts to dyes over a period of time. Looking at the absorbance and transmission of light through mixture forms the basis of spectroscopy.

In 1957, Skeggs described a single-channel automatic chemical analyzer that became a working prototype of the continuous flow system widely adopted for use in clinical chemistry laboratories, the Auto Analyzer (Technicion Instruments Corporation, Tarrytown, New York). The Auto Analyzer is essentially a train of interconnected modules that automate the time-consuming step-by-step procedures of manual analysis. Sampling may be performed on a wide variety of biologic materials: whole blood, plasma, serum, urine, cerebrospinal fluid, and so on. The operation of the instrument is based upon a continuous flow concept that allows a great deal of versatility and flexibility.

In *autoanalysis,* chemical reactions take place in continuously flowing air segmented streams. Air bubbles continuously separate the flowing streams of samples and reagents, thereby maintaining sample integrity and eliminating cross-mixing of samples. The flow of the stream (or streams) is directed through plastic tubing from module to module, each of which automatically carries out a different analytical function. Briefly, its operation follows a rather logical sequence of steps. The analytical train starts with a sampler. After loading of properly identified samples into the cups on the sampler, a multichannel proportioning pump operating continuously moves the samples, one following another, and a number of streams of reagents into the system. Sample and reagents are brought together under controlled conditions (time, temperature, concentrations), causing a chemical reaction and the appearance of a specific color. Color intensity of the analytical stream is measured in a colorimeter, with the results, a series of peaks, displayed on a strip chart recorder. This type of display provides the operator with a means of visually monitoring the performance of the equipment; assuming that the performance ap-

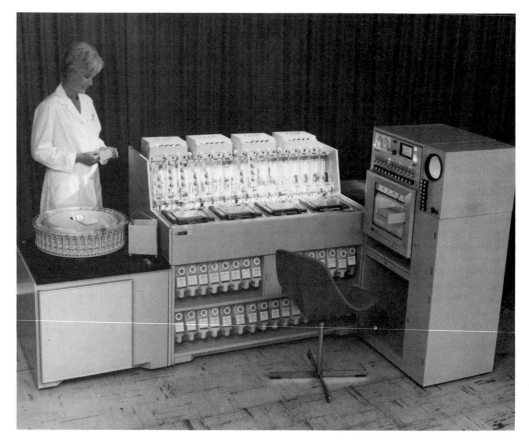

Figure 7.13 A 12-Channel continous type analyzer SMA 12/60 (from Bronzino, JD: *Computer Applications for Patient Care,* Reading, Mass.: Addison-Wesley, 1982).

pears to be satisfactory, the individual peak heights are simply read off and converted into the corresponding concentrations for the substance being measured.

Fundamental to Auto Analyzer techniques is the exposure of known standards to exactly the same reaction steps used for the unknown samples. The concentrations of the unknowns are continuously plotted against the known concentrations. For this reason, reactions need not be carried to completion as in conventional chemistry procedures. The detection techniques utilized with this device include colorimetry, spectrophotometry, flame photometry, fluorometry, and atomic absorption spectrometry.

In this type of analysis, changeover from one chemical determination to another is a relatively simple procedure requiring minutes. In short, one Auto Analyzer can perform the majority of wet-chemical tests commonly requested in the clinical chemistry laboratory.

With the development of the sequential multiple analyzer (SMA) system (Skeggs and Hochstrasser 1964), laboratory output further increased, and perfor-

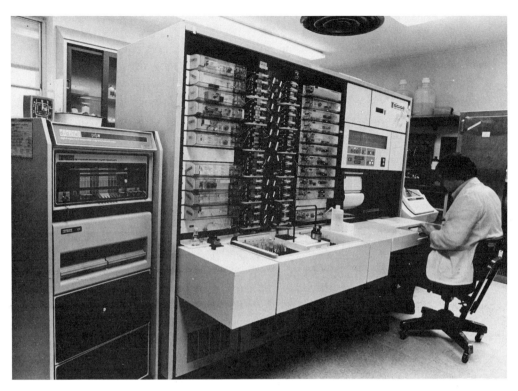

Figure 7.14 The sequential multiple analysis computer (SMAC) system (from Bronzino, JD: *Computer Applications for Patient Care,* Reading, Mass.: Addison-Wesley, 1982).

mance time decreased. By adding channels, it became possible to perform some determinations simultaneously. For example, glucose/BUN and Cl/CO_2 were among the tests combined. In many cases, this was accomplished merely by adding streams and another colorimeter and recording system. The SMA 6 (6 channels), SMA 12/60 (12 channels) (see Figure 7.13), and 22-channel SMAC were all refinements of this type of approach (Figure 7.14). The SMA 12/60 analyzes unmeasured individual serum samples for 12 selected biochemical parameters at the rate of 60 samples per hour. The results (concentration levels) obtained from this device are usually presented in a graphic format form, the *serum chemistry graph,* and the availability of this comprehensive chemical profile for each patient is a major factor for this device's wide acceptance.

One significant shortcoming of sampling as it is carried out today is that the sample, once collected, represents only one measurement point in time. Consequently, any values obtained reflect only that one point. In many cases, continuous or repeated on-line sampling covering a longer period or several periods is more desirable and can be expected to be incorporated into clinical testing techniques in the future.

Several of the presently available automatic analyzers include small built-in microprocessors that allow computations and improved data presentation. As mentioned previously, early analytical instruments used analog meter displays for data presentation so that the labortory technician had to record the results. The next step was analog recording on calibrated paper. Digital read-out and print-out, however, now available in modern analyzers, are frequently used to simplifying data presentation.

In recent years, a number of automated laboratory instruments using techniques that differ from the established ones have been developed. The continuous flow technique, because of its ability to provide only one measurement, an end-point determination, per sample, is partially, being upstaged by discrete systems that take a specimen, proportion it into separate discrete analysis chambers, and process each test independently.

A new concept in discrete sample analysis, for example, that uses a centrifuge with several compartments to fill, mix, hold, read, and flush the various specimens to be analyzed has been developed (Anderson 1970). In this microanalytical system, centrifugal force adds aliquots of a reagent to several discrete samples and propels these reaction mixtures radially into separate, equally spaced cuvettes on the outer edge of an analytical rotor. The total centrifugal reagent-sample addition and mixing steps require less than 5 s, with the initial absorbance measurements obtained in approximately 5 s from the start of the reaction. This type of instrument, therefore, can provide dynamic or reaction rate information (Tiffany 1974). Particularly useful in this regard are certain enzyme measurements. Such kinetjc determinations are not performed on many of the continuous flow automatic analyzers, which primarily determine reaction end points.

This fast centrifugal analyzer generates data at such a rapid rate that computerization is almost required. It, therefore, represents a new trend in chemical analysis and a significant advance in the continual development of flexible instrumentation that is sophisticated in principle, but simple in operation and function. It demonstrates that appropriate instrumentation can be produced at lower cost than the large automated clinical analyzers presently available entail.

Eastman Kodak's recent entry into the field of clinical chemistry has provided a unique and innovative approach to the measurement of various analytes in biological fluids. Through transfer of some aspects of a large body of knowledge, gained over the years in film technology, Kodak has developed techniques for incorporating in dry form, on single-use slides, all the chemicals required for quantitating various constituents in serum or other body fluids. In conjunction with these thin-film slides, instrumentation allows the rapid, accurate, and precise measurement of these constituents.

At present two types of analysis use the Kodak technology (referred to as *Ektachem*). In the first, based upon colorimetry, a small volume (10 microliters [μL]) of sample is applied to the upper surface of the slide. The substance to be measured diffuses in a controlled manner through this upper "spreading layer" to the layer or layers below, wherein are contained the chemicals required to develop a characteristic colored complex. The density of the color is then measured by reflectance densitometry and related to the concentration of the analyte in the sample (Figure 7.15).

A second type of thin-film technology employed by the Ektachem system is based upon potentiometric measurement by ion-selective electrodes contained on

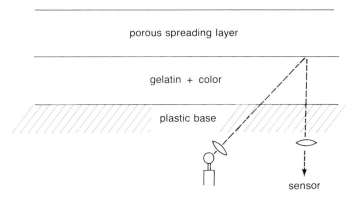

Figure 7.15   The Kodak Ektachem clinical chemistry slide for colorimetry (from Bronzino, JD: *Computer Applications for Patient Care,* Reading, Mass.: Addison-Wesley, 1982).

multilayered films. Each slide consists of two half-cells to which are applied 10 μL of sample and reference fluid, respectively. Connecting the two half-cells is a paper bridge. When moistened by sample and reference fluid this bridge provides a liquid junction between the half-cells. A potentiometer measures the voltage difference generated by the ion species for which the electrodes are selective, and the ion's concentration is then calculated (see Figure 7.16).

All of the modules required for slide and sample disposition, measurement, and read-out are integrated into a compact system, the Ektachem 400, which contains nine microprocessors that form four separate computers. The computer effects master control of all analyzer functions of the control unit. This unit receives operator input, monitors and directs the other computers, and handles output of data.

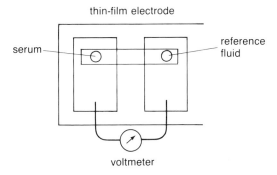

Figure 7.16   The Kodak Ektachem clinical chemistry slide for potentiometry (from Bronzino, JD: *Computer Applications for Patient Care,* Reading, Mass.: Addison-Wesley, 1982).

The Ektachem 400 recently received an extensive field evaluation at St. Francis Hospital and Medical Center, Hartford, Connecticut. During this trial program, this system's enormous potential for becoming a mainstay of the clinical chemistry laboratories of the future was quite apparent. Aside from the unique nature of the thin-film/slide technology, the system has several other distinct advantages. For example, it frees the laboratory from storing a large number of separate reagents and accessories, has very low space requirements for slide storage, and requires only the availability of 110 volts of alternating current (Vac) for its operation.

Throughout these tests, the Ektachem proved to be a rapid and reliable system for performing those clinical chemistry tests evaluated (glucose, BUN, sodium, potassium, chloride, CO_2, amylase, total protein, albumin, total). One can only speculate as to its future capabilities: fluorescence assays, kinetic enzyme measurements, and a host of others are probable. Observing the future directions this newest clinical chemistry analytic approach will take should prove interesting.

Computerization Concepts in the Clinical Laboratory

Traditionally, attempts to computerize the clinical laboratory have tended to separate the data acquisition functions of the laboratory from essentially clerical tasks (including cumulative, patient, ward, and physician-oriented reports, status reports of particular tests, and worksheet and label generation). The managerial aspect of potential computerization, however, is by far the more complex and more difficult to implement of the two tasks (Lipkin and Lipkin 1975; Wist et al. 1982).

A somewhat similar, but perhaps more productive, view of the laboratory is to consider the following two levels of potential computerization: (1) the instrumental/process control level (IPC) and (2) the central laboratory computer (CLC). This division reflects a distinction between decentralized autonomy, which increases processing efficiency within a unit, and central regulation, which promotes patient-oriented integration of data from a variety of sources. To achieve a successful system, a balance between these two levels in the laboratory is necessary. These two levels will be considered individually.

The instrument level

The first level, the IPC concept, consists of a set of computers or simple processors, each characterized by inputs that are specimens and associated identification data and digital outputs that represent results, analytical conditions, and associated identification data. Typically, Coulter counters and sequential multiple analyzers both fall into this category and because of their high-volume activity make computerization quite attractive.

The reliability of the analytical results and the capture of all data as they emerge from these devices are still important concerns as one employs computer techniques to automate these devices. However, more importantly, the IPC concept emphasizes (1) modularity and pseudoindependence of individual IPC units, which in turn permits uniformity in data protocols; (2) local control of analytical conditions in which the computation process is sufficiently understood and methods sufficiently accurate to ensure confidence in results; and (3) addition or modification of laboratory instrumentation without major interruption of overall system operation.

At the individual instrument level, computerization can be made cost-effective. For example, the program to run a Coulter counter is essentially the same in any facility. The differences among such instrumental programs are at input (specimen identification data) and output (communications protocol peculiar to the local installation) levels. Thus, each device may be designed, constructed, and programmed independently to perform its particular function.

In addition, if the data obtained from the clinical laboratory can be combined with information pertaining to each patient, it can generate "patient records." With this in mind, several of the presently available automatic analyzers now include small built-in computers that allow computations and improved data presentation. Once such device is the sequential multiple analysis plus computer (SMAC) system.

The SMAC system resulted directly from further development of the continuous flow systems, such as the SMA 8 and SMA 12/60 systems previously discussed. The basic principles of operation remain the same: samples, separated by air bubbles, are operated by means of a pump, distributed to different channels, dialyzed and heated (where needed), measured, and recorded. However, in this system, the SMAC computer is involved in virtually every phase of system operation. The computer calibrates each channel at preselected intervals, monitors all channels and modules, aids in troubleshooting, identifies samples, calculates data, and reports results. It is an excellent example of a computerized laboratory instrument.

The SMAC system is capable of measuring 20 parameters of a patient's specimen, at the rate of 150 patients per hour as compared to 12 per hour for the SMA 12/60. It contains its own microcomputer, with a CRT or video terminal and teletype writer as the primary input/output devices. Its operation is dependent not only on the apparent hardware components, but on sophisticated software routines that permit "computer-naive" individuals to operate the system.

Briefly, it operates as follows. Test requests and pertinent patient data are entered at the keyboard of the SMAC video terminal. This informtion may include the patient's name, hospital number and location, physician's name, and so on. To assist the operator, the SMAC video screen presents a step-by-step format to ensure correct order of data entry. Test requests may be entered by either total profile, organ profile, single test, or any combination of tests, which are displayed on the video screen for the convenience of the operator. The SMAC system stores all the input information and automatically matches the test requests with the sample, significantly reducing data collection and clerical errors. The computer associated with the SMAC system also performs function checks on basic system performance during start-up. These include reagent absorbance referenced to water, proper standardization factors, proper dwell time for each individual test, and checks for shift and noise. After completing this check procedure, the computer produces a detailed report listing values for all of the preceding parameters. This document then becomes part of the daily laboratory quality control procedures.

As the sample enters the flow cell, the computer begins a series of control and monitor routines that check the overall shape and characteristics of the "peak curves," comparing them to an experimentally derived ideal curve for the particular chemical element being evaluated. If the curve is within certain preset limits, absorbance is converted to concentration and "outputted" when all other parameters for that patient have been determined. If these limits are exceeded, on the other hand, the computer brings the malfunction to the attention of the operator by means of an audible alarm and indicates which module is malfunctioning, the test(s) affected, and the nature of the problem. The operator can then decide whether to correct the problem immediately or to shut down the affected channel and attend to the problem later. It, therefore, provides valuable information regarding continuous overall performance.

These systems run quickly and efficiently, a virtual assembly line for chemical reactions. The use of such systems has aroused some concerns, however. The older analytical instruments used for their standards a pure substance in an aqueous base; for example, glucose dissolved in water gives a known glucose concentration. Running this through the older analytical system provides a good calibration and check on the accuracy of the devices. However, with the complexities of the SMAC systems, establishing a complete standard of comparison for all samples is not possible. That is, it is difficult to know whether the standards used to calibrate the system are in fact accurate in all the compound concentrations contained in the standard. Though the differences found so far are small, they are of concern to those interested in the degree of accuracy of the data provided to the physician, who must make a clinical decision based upon them.

Another example of the IPC concept is the incorporation of on-board computers into various instruments and systems of instruments. For example, the FINNIGAN 4000 system joins three sophisticated pieces of chemical analysis equipment together: the gas chromatograph, the mass spectrometer, and the minicomputer (Figure 7.17). In this system the gas chromatograph serves to separate the sample's components (for example, a mixture of different drugs in a toxicological specimen). The components, thus separated, are introduced by way of an interface into the mass spectrometer portion of the system. Here the characteristic mass spectra of the individual compounds are generated, the mass spectrometer functioning, therefore, as a very sensitive and sophisticated form of "detector" for the gas chromatograph.

The FINNIGAN system uses the on-board minicomputer for several reasons. First of all, it controls the operation of the mass spectrometer and handles the volumus amount of data coming from it. Second, the 16K of core, 16-bit CPU, and 24-million-bit disk memory are used for another unique feature: the library look-up. With an extensive memory capacity the computer can store several thousand mass spectra on its disk. It can then take the mass spectrum of the sample and try to match it with those it has, thereby identifying the compound. This feature is particularly useful in toxicology, where the time required for identification is critical to the delivery of health care.

In this device, computational power is needed primarily during the data acquisition stage and the library searches. However, when the chemical identification features are not being used, the on-board general purpose-computer can be

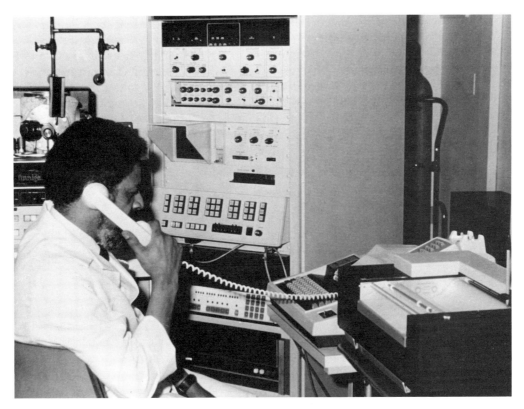

Figure 7.17 Computerized gas chramatograph mass spectrometer system containing a computer terminal, and telecommunication link (courtesy of the Saint Francis Hospital and Medical Center, Hartford, Connecticut).

programmed by BASIC and can even be used to play computer games using the graphics system associated with this device. The FINNIGAN system is a good example of on-board computerization; however, because it is a dedicated machine, it cannot help with the running of the laboratory.

The introduction of more and more microprocessors into the clinical laboratories (Westlake 1975; Titus 1977; Williams 1975; Preston 1984) offers other possibilities: the interfacing of these devices to a central computer for data processing and integration of medical data with other pertinent patient information. Such an approach would also help the laboratory to perform its managerial functions.

The management level

The incorporation of a computerized management system or central clinical laboratory computer (CLC) is possible at two different levels. The first concerns primarily the control and integration of various laboratory instruments to transfer data processed directly from the various analytical devices into a computerized patient record. The second deals with the many clerical functions of the laboratory, such as recording, verifying, and reporting medical data.

In the first case, a controlling laboratory computer (Figure 7.18) can "call" an instrument by presenting it with an appropriately identified specimen or reference standard. The anlytical device performs its tests, computes the results, and outputs a string of data in an appropriate digital format. In this type of modular general system, a specific instrument that presents its own digital face to the world performs each determination. Each instrument then is specifically adapted to its particular task and contains a digital interface, buffer, and controller. These are, vis-à-vis the analysis, specifically adapted to the procedure, its calibration, and the anticipated vagaries of analytical conditions. The output, on the other hand, consists of a small series of standard-length digital words that represent the result, identification, and any other parameterization data for each determination. Such output is delivered to the central laboratory computer for final processing and storage.

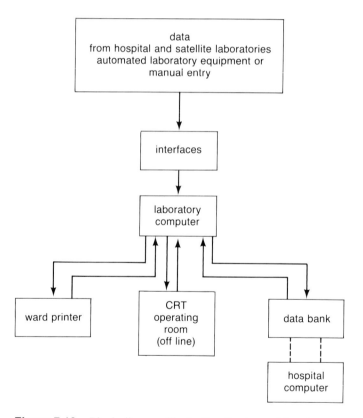

Figure 7.18   Block diagram illustrating the type of input obtained from data - acquisition stations and subsequent "output" routes that are available once the information is assembled and processed (from Bronzino, JD: *Computer Applications for Patient Care,* Reading, Mass.: Addison-Wesley, 1982).

For this type of situation, the computerization of the clinical laboratory's instruments involves not only the hardware aspects, but software complexities required to integrate each instrument properly. Each device must give its data to the main computer before new data replace them. Some instruments may have more data items per second than others. In the middle of the information exchange process is the computer, which is continually integrating these instruments. Standardized digital circuits and connector "buses" make the task of getting the correct signals to flow easier.

Interfacing the instrumentation in the clinical laboratory therefore results in the creation of one overall computerized system. There are many problems in timing, data transmission, etc., but it has been done before.

For example, at the Hopkins Medical Laboratory in Providence, Rhode Island, a Digital Equipment Corporation PDL computer system with specialized software generates laboratory reports and provides medical billing, record keeping, and business management functions. This represents a considerable task for a clinical laboratory that, with its main facility and four branch collection stations, serves approximately 750 patients a week for hundreds of physicians and 18 nursing homes throughout the entire state.

In this facility, a sample, or walk-in patient, arrives at the main laboratory; the patient's name, address, physician required tests and assigned identification number are entered into the system through the keyboard of a video display terminal. This patient-related information and the final laboratory test results are obtained in a printed format on a DEC writer. The computer automatically indicates any abnormal laboratory results by placing an asterisk beside the value. In this way, the physician is quickly alerted to any abnormalities. The speed of this system is such that for all tests completed in the morning a report is generated and in the mail by the end of the lunch hour. Afternoon tests are generally completed by 4:30 so that reports are also generated and mailed at the end of the work day. For nursing home patients, reports are sent to both the nursing home and the physician's office.

Since federal regulations require maintenance of hard-copy patient records for a 5-yr period, the computer has met this requirement in a more organized fashion, reducing the storage space for such records. In addition, the system generates bills for the laboratory when no one is in it. This computerized system and others like it have enhanced the overall operation of the clinical laboratory.

Clinical laboratories offer services to the hospital, the private physician, the clinic, and comprehensive health testing organizations. The basic job of the laboratory is providing reliable data on biological specimens to support a physician's preliminary diagnosis. It can monitor the course of therapy and, presumably in the future, identify a disease while there is still time to prevent its further development. These data are obtained through chemical, microbiological, and morphological analyses on blood, urine, spinal and synovial fluids, and tissues. In view of the every-increasing demands and requirements on these laboratories, they can be successful in performing high-quality specimen analysis only by using fully automated equipment. The term *automated* is obviously broad, including modules such as automatic pipettes, specific systems such as automatic cell counters, and general systems that include computers. True automation initiates work and guarantees its correct accomplishment. Therefore, by this definition, a majority of clinical laboratories are not presently automated, since none of the anlyzing apparatus used today is self-correcting. However, the automation of clinical laboratories is essential if laboratory scientists are to shoulder their expanded responsibilities with success. To achieve the goal of complete automation requires extensive use of electronic data processing and cooperation of laboratory scientists and engineers.

Available systems, however, represent only the beginning. Automation as it exists today has made few if any inroads into other clinical laboratory sciences such as microbiology. It is generally agreed that before real progress in the automation of clinical laboratories is possible, the entire field of laboratory science must be intensely reviewed and its approaches revised. In general, however, major progress can only result from the development of new instruments capable of detecting minute amounts of biological compounds and the incorporation of data processing equipment and techniques designed to provide automated analysis. Most laboratories have no need for a large computer. Mini- and microcomputer systems that can easily assemble and accumulate 1 day's laboratory data at a cost considerably lower than with large machines have been developed. The "microcomputer," the smallest processor available yet, will become integral to many future systems.

This process is underway. As we move toward the end of the 20th century computers and microcomputers will continue to change many instruments and methodologies employed in the clinical laboratory, with continued emphasis on (1) upgrading of the data handling processes within these laboratories; (2) increasing automatic collation of test results on the same patient from all over the laboratory; (3) developing more instrument self-monitoring, fault-finding, and operator alerts; (4) providing greater availability of ongoing automatic quality control data; and (5) broadening use of effective patient and sample identification systems (Alpert 1979).

As one continues to gaze into the future, it is quite reasonable to predict that these laboratories at the turn of the century will be designed around the computer. Indeed, all analytical instruments will be essentially computer accessories, interconnected with a central computer that collates results for a patient from several instruments and calls for the tests to be performed in logical order. Cheaper, faster, smaller, and more powerful computing facilities that can be expected from the postsilicon era of the late 1980s and early 1990s (Kulikowsi and Weiss 1979) will perform these processes and others not even conceived in today's laboratory.

The benefits to be derived by this continuing evolution of automated clinical laboratory systems are quite appealing. For example, automation enables the laboratory to provide more rapid service with a reduction in the time elapsed from the receipt of a biological sample to the delivery of information to the physician from days or hours to minutes. It also enables the physician to arrive at a proper diagnosis more quickly through a computer presentation of all tests performed on each patient on a single printout sheet or the screen of an interactive display terminal. Because of the scarcity and cost of skilled labor, the exploitation of automation in this setting provides for optimal utilization of professional and technical labor. Finally, the repetitive nature of most laboratory tests makes them ideal for automation; for example, only 10 to 20 tests account for almost 14 percent of the workload in the average clinical laboratory. With an automated chemistry system two technicians can run more than 40 times the number of tests than a more highly qualified worker using the same manual chemistry techniques can run.

Throughout the United States, approximately 7,000 clinical laboratories (including those within hospitals) are supervised by clinical chemists or clinical pathologists, microbiologists, and so on. However, surprisingly, these laboratories account for only 25 percent of the total clinical laboratory work performed in this country each year. Small laboratories in general practitioners' and internists' offices and the small commercial laboratories scattered throughout the country perform the other 75 percent. Thus, the magnitude of the economic impact of clinical laboratory services has been significant and will only increase as the activities of even these smaller laboratories are tied into regional systems.

In recent years, to a large extent the automation of many clinical laboratories has not only been successful in technical terms but also has received wide acceptance within the medical community. It is generally agreed that these automated hospital facilities represent a cornerstone of a patient management system that can be expanded to include automated multiphasic health testing and computerized patient records.

COMPUTERIZED PATIENT MONITORING

Computerized patient monitoring systems may be viewed as consisting of three distinct processes: (1) the detection phase, in which the measuring instruments provide data regarding a specific physiological variable (such as heart rate, ECG, and temperature); (2) the interpretive phase, in which this information is ranked (prioritized) and assembled to provide an overview of the patient's status; and (3) the analysis and computation phase, in which a digital computer evaluates the "nature" of the input information using programmed instructions, displays pertinent data, stores specific aspects of the data for further use, and even directly controls various devices such as infusion pumps. Each component part is important.

In the critical care environment, where sudden changes are more ominous, success or failure of the system depends on the precision of the monitoring devices and the manner and speed with which the information is conveyed to the medical staff. Consider, for example, the importance of the clinical decisions necessary for addressing exactly which information is to be collected and the way it is to be presented to the clinician. Without a plan or set of guidelines outlining the use of this information (that is, its assimilation, interpretation, and display), such a tool will only confuse those it is supposed to serve. Only those computerized systems that effectively incorporate all three of these elements can be effective tools in monitoring the critically ill.

The next section highlights the physiological measures of interest to the clinician: the way they are monitored and some of the basic concepts to be incorporated in the development of automated systems for intensive care units. It also explores operation of computerized patient monitoring systems and ways they can assist health professionals in meeting their responsibilities in this type of environment, discusses the goals that future systems must meet, and provides several examples of computerized patient monitoring systems currently used in a variety of clinical settings.

Physiological Monitoring

The goal of physiological monitoring is to measure and display physiological signals that characterize the functioning of a biological system (Terdiman 1974). Certain types of physiological signals, such as bioelectric activity, can be directly sensed and recorded. Others, such as arterial blood pressure, are usually transduced to an electrical form for ease of communication, analysis, and display. Still other variables, such as cardiac output, must be derived from indirect measurements. Actually, the number of parameters that are monitored *continuously* at this time is quite limited. Heart rate, various systematic and cavity pressures, respiration rate, and temperature are available in basic systems; with more sophisticated monitors, waveform analysis, transcutaneous blood gases, and respiratory gas concentrations are possible. A substantial portion of the monitoring systems commercially available essentially monitors the same three or four parameters.

It is obvious that any monitoring in the clinical situation should be conducted so that what is being measured has value; however, in each medical institution situations occur that may cause the collection of specific physiological data to be of little clinical use (Friedman and Gustafson 1977; De Asla and Bryan-Brown 1979). Consider, for example, some of the common pitfalls one may experience in a clinical setting:

1 The physiological parameter being monitored is redundant or only marginally relevant.

2 Measurements are made for which staff members do not have sufficient experience or expertise to interpret the results.

3 Such large volumes of information are produced that "data overload" occurs, preventing staff members from evaluating the data in a clinically useful way.

4 Staff members are unaware of factors affecting the accuracy of a measurement. Certainly, inaccurate data have no value whatsoever and may even be detrimental to patient care.

5 Equipment is overdesigned and too sophisticated for the task at hand or is just too difficult to use.

To avoid these dilemmas, health professionals must interact continuously with biomedical instrumentation industry to ensure that the appropriate type of patient monitoring equipment is designed and utilized for each specific application.

Among physiological parameters, such variables as heart rate, temperature, blood pressure, and respiration clearly necessitate monitoring. It should be noted, however, that changes in several biochemical aspects of the body (pH, P_{O_2}, P_{CO_2}) and electrolytes occur much earlier than changes on the electrocardiogram and may even be more important than the more obvious measures. However, use of

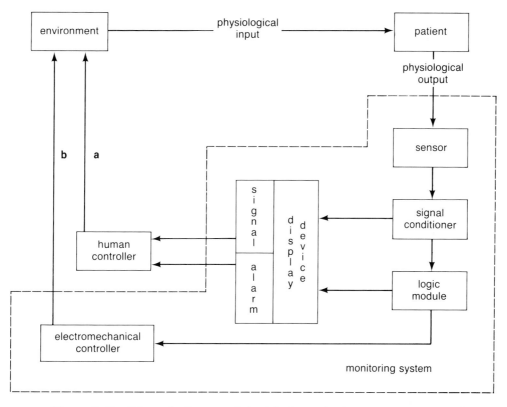

Figure 7.19 Schematic diagram of physiologic monitoring system showing basic components and signal flow pathways. Pathway (a) contains a human interaction in the feedback loop, while (b) contains an electromechanical controller in the feedback loop (from Bronzino, JD: *Computer Applications for Patient Care,* Reading, Mass.: Addison-Wesley, 1982).

these more "subtle" parameters requires additional clinical research studies before it will be widely accepted in the medical community.

Any patient monitoring system has a number of essential components. These components may be divided into the following five categories (Terdiman 1974): sensor, signal conditioner, display device, logic module, and controller (see Figure 7.19).

Sensor

The properties of various electrodes and transducers used to detect physiological signals are well known (Geddes and Baker 1968). Those most commonly used in physiological monitoring systems include surface area contact electrodes for electrocardiography and electroencephalography, intravascular and respiratory pressure transducers, ultrasonic and electromagnetic flow rate detectors, and chemical and pH electrodes. The output of each of these sensors is an electrical signal that is directly related to the measured physiological paramenter. (See chapter 2).

Signal conditioner

The electrical signals available at each sensor must often be amplified and shaped before they can be transmitted for review by the clinician. The signal conditioner extracts the information of interest from the input signal and conditions it for display, recording, or analysis. To accomplish this, it usually consists of a number of electrical devices such as detectors, amplifiers, filters, and other signal transformation devices.

Display device

The display unit receives an electrical signal from the signal conditioning module and converts it into an appropriate display. Various types of displays include dial indicators, digital displays, cathode-ray tubes, signal lights, audible alarms, and hard-copy displays. The latter category may be further expanded to include strip chart and XY recorders, photographs, microfilm, and even computer printouts.

Logic module (computer)

The logic module compares a signal to a reference level, as in the case of a limit check, or performs more complex analyses. A common example of the former is a cardiac monitor that compares heart rate to preset upper and lower limits; this process uses specialized digital electronic circuits. However, if it is desired to include computation of specific desired parameters such as cardiac output to determine the Fourier transform of specific signals, or to analyze specific components of each electrocardiogram, then a digital computer is used. The extent of the hardware and software required by a particular analysis depends on its nature and complexity.

Controller

The type of control used, if any, also depends on the application. A passive control system, for example, provides for human interaction in the maintenance of a clinical state. It usually provides visual or auditory alarms triggered whenever a physiological signal falls outside a present range. When an alarm occurs, the intended response requires that a human observer attempt to bring the physiological signal back within its normal range by exerting some direct or indirect controlling action on the physiological system through, for example, drugs or other therapeutic measures (Figure 7.19[a]).

Active control usually entails a direct feedback path between the logic module and a controller of the physiological input. In the infusion pump example cited earlier, it is possible to employ a digital computer to convert the measured urine output and central venous pressure to a signal that activates the motor of an infusion pump and to maintain a specified fluid balance (Figure 7.19[b]).

Clearly any monitoring system receives one or more inputs through its sensors and may produce a variety of outputs for display. A minimal monitoring system must contain a sensor, signal conditioner, and display device. The exact uses of patient monitoring systems within the hospital depend upon the nature of the illness and the "hospital unit" handling that particular condition. In general, patient monitoring equipment is utilized on one of the following areas:

1 *Diagnostic areas:* Clinical areas in which unstable patient status or initiation of procedures that may affect patient status requires monitoring. Examples are the emergency room, special procedures in the radiology department, and the cardiac catheterization lab.

2 *Treatment areas:* Clinical areas such as the operating room or delivery room where specific invasive or noninvasive procedures designed to improve patient status are performed but may result in status deterioration.

3 *Surveillance areas:* Clinical areas in which patients are monitored during stabilization and recuperative periods, such as surgical, medical, coronary, and neonatal intensive care units. Intermediate care or "step-down" units also fall into this category since patients have progressed through critical stages and are not necessarily bedridden but still require monitoring of heart rate on an ambulatory telemetric basis.

The patient monitoring equipment presently being utilized in these critical care areas involves primarily bedside monitoring stations and some sort of centralized facility usually termed the *nurse* (or central) *station* (Figure 7.20). The standard bedside monitoring station is essentially a compact and simple-structured unit that provides a quick and comprehensive picture of monitored patient parameters, such as heart rate and ECG. The bedside monitors usually contain fairly small oscilloscope (CRT) screens that display parameter values and waveforms of each patient. In the nurse or central station, the primary goal is to achieve multiple-bed supervision. As a result, a number of bedside monitors are usually grouped together in an array to enable the nurse at a central station to monitor ECGs from several patients simultaneously.

In recent years, the "modular concept" has been widely accepted and employed in patient monitoring equipment, permitting clinicians to select a variety of physiological monitoring units for each patient. In the process it has been possible for them to observe the dynamic characteristics of specific parameters for each patient in their care. Many modern units are compact, have responsive display capabilities, and permit printouts of each parameter. In some units, alarm systems alert the nurse or other observers by audible or visible signals in the event of a critical condition (for example, whenever the heart rate falls below 60 or exceeds 150 beats per minute). In others, electrical circuits indicate that an electrode has become disconnected or that a mechanical failure has occurred somewhere else in the monitoring system. Although these systems are not without problems (noise and movement artifacts, false triggering of alarm circuits), they have been successful in detecting the presence of life-threatening events. The information made available by these systems can provide better care to critically ill patients. With this in mind, let us examine the operation of automated patient monitoring systems and the design criteria they must meet now and in the future.

Successful application of computer technology to the monitoring of critically ill patients requires definitive, quantitative descriptions of waveforms that must be

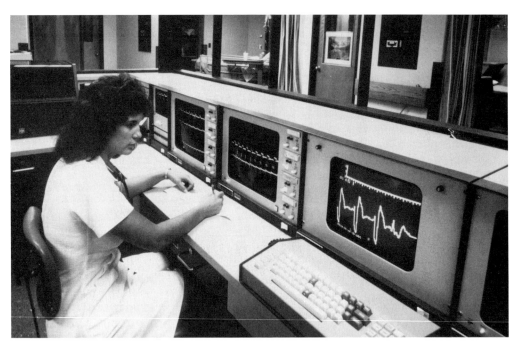

Figure 7.20   A patient monitoring system permit the nursing staff at central station to keep track of patient's chemical status (courtesy of Hewlett-Packard, Waltham, Mass.).

identified and the specific conditions that must be detected. It is the explicit nature of programming the computer that imposes such demanding specifications. Therefore, the development of computer programs with sufficient sophistication to recognize specific life-threatening patterns reliably has proved extremely difficult. The ability of the human observer to correlate an observed pattern with previous experience or training and to identify the event is not understood well enough to allow precise description and quantitation of the pattern-recognition procedure that must precede the design of appropriate computer programs. Detection of P waves, for example, has been especially unreliable. Most arrhythmia-detection programs have therefore been designed to classify ventricular arrhythmias in terms of R–R intervals and the shape of the QRS complex (Sheppard and Kouchoukos 1978).

Various computerized systems have been developed for automatic rhythm analysis (Cox et al. 1968; Haywood et al. 1970; Geddes and Warner 1971; Feldman et al. 1971; Oliver et al. 1971; Sweene et al. 1973; Yanowitz et al. 1974;). For almost all of these arrhythmia detection systems, an essential step in the analysis of the ECG is the detection of the QRS complex. Most systems accomplish this by taking the first derivative or slope of the ECG signal. When the absolute value of the first derivative exceeds the empirically determined threshold, the presence of a QRS complex is suspected. This tentative QRS is then usually subjected to a "reasonableness" criterion to exclude artifact. Systems that attempt to identify P and T waves do so by using the QRS as a starting point in the search for these waves.

Most arrhythmia detecting systems use measurements of QRS width, offset, amplitude, and area to classify complexes into a set of morphological families. The morphology of a given QRS complex is then compared to some stored representation of the "normal" QRS for that patient (Prody 1977). This stored normal is usually acquired by the system as part of a stand-up procedure, often with the patient's own normal QRS as a template. If the comparison is within certain limits, the QRS recorded is deemed normal. If it is not, then it is considered abnormal and indicative of the occurrence of a premature ventricular contraction (PVC). Early results with this approach were encouraging. During this past decade, the accuracy of detecting ventricular ectopic beats improved from approximately 70 to 90 percent. Unfortuantely, many of these early approaches were plagued by relatively high error rates, especially in the percentage of false negative results.

The ARGUS (Noll et al. 1974) arrhythmia monitoring system deserves special mention since its widely accepted AZTEC (Cox et al. 1968) preprocessing algorithm has been employed in many systems. Incorporating Digital Equipment Corporation minicomputer (PDP-11) and microcomputer (LSI-11) computer technology, a modern version of this system, ARGUS/PLUS, offered by Mennen Medical, is an on-line computerized patient monitoring system based on the modular philosophy. The system is capable of examining each patient's cardiac activity continuously, classifying every heart beat as to type, and alerting medical personnel to events that may lead to life-threatening conditions.

Figure 7.21 depicts the flow of information to and within the ARGUS/PLUS system. An A/D converter residing in a microprocessor (in this case, an LSI-11 Arrhythmial Pre-Processor) samples ECG signals directly. Following analysis and morphological determination of each incoming QRS complex, this microprocessor provides a serial stream of arrhythmia-related parameters to the central computer (another LSI-11) for further processing and presentation on the video screen. This central computer has complete control of the interactions with I/O periphrals, such as the video displays, chart recorder, and system keyboard. The operator can simply request any of the system functions via the keyboard with the central computer directing all the outputs to the appropriate video display. Acquired data from the Arrhythmia Pre-Processor are stored within the central computer as well as on storage disks to facilitate long-term parameter trending.

ARGUS has been extensively evaluated and found to detect QRSs consistently with an accuracy of 99 percent and to identify 90 percent of the premature ventricular beats correctly (Fozzard and Kinias 1974). Despite these good results, clinical acceptance of commercially available systems has been slow. It has been speculated that the lack of enthusiasm for most of these systems results from the emphasis placed on premature ventricular contractions, with virtually no attention to detection of other premonitory arrhythmias or atrial activity. If only PVCs can be detected by these systems, many clinicians believe that the impact of automated arrhythmia detection on patient care may not be sufficient to justify the cost of such a system (Sheppard and Kouchoukos 1978).

Another example of an arrhythmia monitoring system commercially available for the early detection and warning of ventricular premature beats and most other premonitoring or life-threatening cardiac arrhythmias was developed jointly by the Medical Products Group of Hewlett-Packard and the Cardiology Division

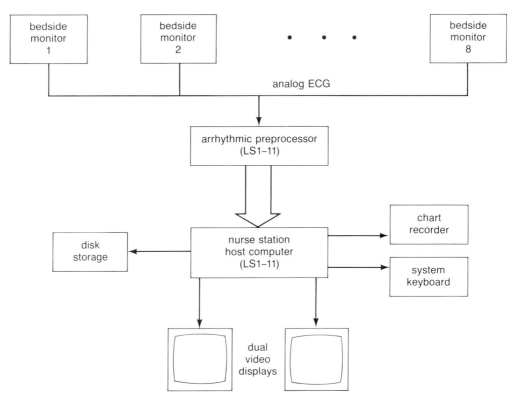

Figure 7.21   Schematic representation of information flow in ARGUS/PLUS system.

of the Stanford University School of Medicine. This system provides a continuous display of the current status of up to 24 patients, enabling the staff to verify the condition of each immediately. The system status condition for each patient includes alarm status, rhythm status, extopic beat status, and monitoring status on a continuous basis. Whenever an alarm sounds, a nurse need only look quickly at the screen to determine the patient and condition causing the alarm. Although the system does not recognize all cardiac arrhythmias, it does provide highly efficient, round-the-clock surveillance of coronary care patients.

In regard to the accuracy of this system in detecting PVCs, evaluation tests conducted at Stanford University show that this system was capable of detecting about 84 percent of all PVCs, while incorrectly identifying approximately 0.16 percent (or about 1/1000) of all beats as PVCs. In arrhythmic monitoring no single set of programmable criteria yet produced is comparable to the performance of a trained cardiologist (and one must bear in mind that even cardiologists may disagree on specific criteria). Alert, constant observation of ECG waveforms by trained, dedicated, intelligent personnel, on duty 100 percent of the time, would equal or better the performance of any computerized system, but such an approach is economically impractical. Although no available computer system can accurately distinguish among all of the dozens of different arrhythmias, no human observer could be expected to monitor and analyze, in real time, the ECG signals of eight (much less 16) patients around-the-clock.

When one attempts to evaluate computerized monitoring systems the question to ask is not whether these measurement systems can save lives, but rather how effective they are in making the nursing staff aware of specific events, logging their occurrence, and reducing clerical function.

There has been some concern in medical quarters that the presence of this electronic instrumentation has had a negative effect on the personal involvement of patients and the hospital staff responsible for their care. Thus, even with the available instrumentation, the nurses on duty and the physician must observe the patient and not simply the display monitor. This is a valid concern but should be kept in perspective; no device will ever replace the nurse or physician. It can only assist them to perform their tasks more efficiently and effectively. The computer therefore is simply a tool that health professionals can add to their arsenal of weapons that will enable them to provide better care for their patients.

REFERENCES

Alpert, N. C. 1979. Laboratory instruments in the year 2000: Streamlined—but much like today's. *Med Lab Obs* 11:120–127.

Anderson, N. G. 1970. Basic principles of fast analyzers. *Am J Clin Pathol* 52:778.

Bronzino, J. D. 1982. *Computer applications for patient care.* Waltham, Mass.: Addison-Wesley.

Cox, J. R., Nolle, F. M., and Fozzard, H. A. 1968. AZTEC, a preprocessing program for real-time ECG rhythm analysis. *IEEE Trans Biomed Eng* 15:128–129.

De Asla, R. A., and Boyan-Brown, C. W. 1979. The clinically valuable variable. *Med Instrum* 13:325–326.

Dickson, J. F. 1969. Automation of clinical laboratories. *Proc IEEE* 57:1974–1985.

Feldman, C. C, Amazeen, P. G., and Klein, M. D. 1971. Computer detection of ventricular ectopic beats. *Comput Biomed Res* 3:666–674.

Fozzard, H., and Kinias, P. 1974. ECG Monitoring: A review of developmental systems. In *Computer Cardiology.* Long Beach, Calif.: IEEE Computer Society.

Freidman, R. B., and Gustafson, D. H. 1977. Computers in clinical medicine, a critical review, (guest editorial). *Comput Biomed Res* 10:199–204.

Garrett, R. D. 1976. *Hospital Computer Systems and Procedures,* Vol. II. New York: Medical Systems Mason/Charter.

Geddes, L. A., and Baker, L. E. 1968. *Principles of applied biomedical instrumentation.* New York: Wiley.

Geddes, L. A., and Warner, H. R. 1971. A PUC detection program. *Comput Biomed Res* 4:493–508.

Haywood, C. J., Murtony, U. K., and Harvey, G. A. 1970. On-line real time computer algorithm for monitoring the ECG waveform. *Comput Biomed Res* 3:15–25.

Kulikowski, C. A., and Weiss, S. M. 1979. Laboratory computers in the year 2000: Call them intelligence amplifying systems. *Med Lab Obs* 11:150–163.

Lincoln, T. L. 1978. Computers in the clinical laboratory: What we have learned. *Med Instrum* 12:223–236.

Lipkin, L. E., and Lipkin, B. S. 1975. Computers in the clinical pathologic laboratory: Chemistry and image processing. *Ann Rev Biophys Bioeng* 4:529–577.

Martinek, R. 1972. Automated analytical systems. *Med Electron Data* 3:33–39.

Noll, F. M., Cox, J. R., Jr., and Oliver, G. C. 1974. The Argus arrhythmia guard system. In *Computer Cardiology.* Long Beach, Calif.: IEEE Computer Society. pp. 201–204.

Oliver, G. E., Nocc, F. M., and Wolff, G. A. 1971. Detection of premature ventricular contractions with a clinical system for monitoring electrocardiographic rhythms. *Comput Biomed Res* 4:523–541.

Prody, L. 1977. Computer arrhythmia detection. In Oliver, J. (ed.) *Computer electrocardiography: Present status and criteria.* Mt. Kisco, N.Y.: Futura. pp. 322–323.

Preston, K., Fagen, C. M., Huang, H. K., and Pryor, T. A. 1984. Computing in medicine. *Computer* 17:294–313.

Ray, C. D. 1974. Clinical pathology and clinical chemistry. In Ray, C. D. (ed.) *Mutual Engineering.* Chicago: Year Book. pp. 743–776.

Sheppard, L. C., and Kouchoukos, N. T. 1978. Computers as monitors. *Anesthesiology* 45:250–259.

Skeggs, C. T., Jr., and Hochstrasser, H. 1957. Multiple automatic sequential analysis. *Clin Chem* 10:918.

Sweeve, C. A., Van Bemmel, J. H., and Hergeueld, S. J. 1973. Pattern recognition for ECG monitoring. An interactive method for classification of ventricular complexes. *Comput Biomed Res* 6:150–160.

Terdiman, J. 1974. Physiological monitoring systems. In Collen, M. F. (ed.) *Hospital computer systems.* New York: Wiley. pp. 241–273.

Tiffany, T. O. 1974. Centrifugal fast analyzers in clinical laboratory analysis. In King, J. W., and Faulkner, W. R. (eds.) *Critical reviews in clinical laboratory sciences,* vol. 5. Cleveland: CRC Press. pp. 129–191.

Titus, J. A. 1977. The impact of microcomputers on automated instrumentation in medicine. Proceedings of the 5th annual symposium on computer applications in medicine. New York: IEEE Press. pp. 99–103.

Tokheim, R. L. 1983. *Microprocessor Fundamentals.* New York: McGraw-Hill.

Westlake, G. 1975. Microprocessors, programmable calculators and minicomputers in the clinical laboratory. *Assoc Adv Med Instrum Clin Eng News* 3:1–3.

Whitcomb, C. C., Vogt, C. P., and Wilbur, N. M. 1978. Clinical laboratory data processing with a central hospital computer *Comput Biol Med* 8:197–206.

Williams, C. Z. 1969. Automation in clinical laboratories. In Dickson, J. F. and Brown, J. H. V., (eds.) *Future goals of engineering in biology and medicine.* New York: Academic Press.

Williams, C. Z. 1975. Why Automation? In Kinney, T. D., and Melville, R. S. (eds.) *Conference: Evaluation of uses of automation in the clinical laboratory.* Sponsored by the National Institute of General Medical Sciences, DHEW. pp. 5–15.

Wist, A. O., Horowitz, R. E., and Megargle, R. 1982. Computers in the clinical laboratory in applications of computers in medicine. In Schwartz, M. D. (ed.) Catalog no. TH0095-0. IEEE Press.

Yanowitz, F., Kinias P., and Rawling, D. 1974. Accuracy of a continuous real-time ECG dyrythmic monitoring system. *Circulation.* 50:65–72, 86.

Part Five

Diagnostic Support Systems

CHAPTER 8

Basic Science and Practice of Nuclear Medicine

Richard P. Spencer, M.D., Ph.D. and Fazle Hosain, D. Phil.

Department of Nuclear Medicine
University of Connecticut Health Center
  Farmington, Connecticut

INTRODUCTION

One of the major problems still facing physicians today is making a proper diagnosis, that is, determining exactly what is wrong with a patient. This step is absolutely essential to insure appropriate medical treatment, monitoring, and follow-up. But exactly how is such a diagnosis made? Even today beginning of this process starts with the taking of the patient's medical history and a thorough physical examination. The medical history compiled after a detailed discussion with the patient about the illness provides clues regarding origin (when it began), frequency (whether it occurred before), duration (the length of time it has occurred), and possible causes (whether anyone in the family has anything like it). Thus, depending upon answers to these questions the clinician can focus on appropriate points and steer away from others. From the discussion of the patient's history, attention moves to the physical examination, which indicates to the clinician the probable site(s) of concern. Unfortunately the patient's medical history and physical examination are often not sufficient to establish the nature or extent of the patient's disorder. To progress any further in establishing a proper diagnosis the clinician must employ "diagnostic aids," specialized technological tools. Diagnostic aids presently available are quite varied. For example, one may involve the sampling of body fluids or excreta to gather data on the content of various components (for example, blood can be assayed for the content of electrolytes, enzymes, red blood cells, white blood cells, and a variety of complex molecules [see Chapter 7]. Since the content of any material in the blood is the net result of the processes of production and disappearance or destruction, the change in quantity with time (dQ/dt) may be expressable as

$$dQ/dt = \text{influx} - \text{efflux}$$

Although the measurement of the blood content of a substance can be useful, the parameter of interest is the result of two events (influx and efflux) that may have to be measured. Serial sampling is often necessary to determine the way in which a substance is changing. Another type of diagnostic aid may involve studying the spatial distribution of events. For example, a chest x-ray provides a means to view the spatial distribution of lung tissue (filled with air), blood vessels, and soft tissue and bone. Consequently, it provides a road map of these physiological systems in a noninvasive fashion. Some forms of noninvasive imaging such as ultrasonography and nuclear magnetic resonance imaging are discussed in Chapters 10 and 11; this chapter focuses on procedures employing ionizing radiation (radiation capable of producing ion pairs), which essentially may be classified into two general types:

1 Radiation is produced externally and passes through the patient, being detected by one or more radiation-sensitive units "behind" the subject. This is the usual form of x-ray procedure and is also applied in the technique of computerized tomography.

2 The patient receives a material that emits a detectable gamma ray. In other words, the patient is the "source" of the emissions. This technique is referred to as *emission imaging* or *emission scanning*. Tomography can also be performed by use of these emissions. This particular form, using the rays emitted by the radioactive material in the patient, is termed *emission computed tomography* (ECT).

Over 90 percent of the diagnostic procedures in nuclear medicine use emitted rays (gamma rays, or the radiation from positron annihilation). However, two other procedures are sometimes employed:

1 Fluorescence scan, in which an external source of gamma rays strikes a target and the characteristic or fluorescence x-ray is emitted. In this procedure, usually employed on the thyroid, the patient receives no radioactive material, and radiation exposure is limited to the region receiving the fluorescence activating beam.

2 Use of radioactive sources to provide monoenergetic or monochromatic photons to measure bone density.

Thus, Nuclear Medicine, that branch of medicine that employs radioactive pharmaceuticals for the purpose of assisting physicians arrive at a proper diagnosis, is the focus of this chapter. During the past four decades, this medical specialty has grown from a scientific dream to a burgeoning enterprise. Rarely in the course of medical history has a medical discipline experienced such spectacular growth and acceptance. An outgrowth of the atomic age, ushered in by the advances made in nuclear physics and technology during World War II, nuclear medicine has emerged as a powerful and effective approach in detecting and treating specific physiological abnormalities.

The field of nuclear medicine is a classic example of a medical discipline that has embraced and utilized the concepts developed in the physical sciences. Conceived as a "joint venture" of the clinician and the physical scientist, it has evolved into a science in itself with its own body of knowledge, techniques, and skills that can be systematically studied and improved. In the process, the domain of nuclear medicine has grown to include studies pertaining to (1) the creation and proper utilization of radioactive tracers (or radiopharmaceuticals), (2) the design and application of appropriate nuclear instrumentation to detect and display the activity of these radioactive elements, and (3) the determination of the relationship between the activity of the radioactive tracer and specific physiological processes (Wagner 1975).

To appreciate the present status of nuclear technology in clinical medicine, let us explore radioactivity, its detection, and the instruments available to monitor or image the activity of radioactive materials. In this way, the clinical applications presented will have more meaning and demonstrate the use of these basic concepts to provide valuable diagnostic information.

BASIC CONCEPTS OF NUCLEAR MEDICINE

The "seeds of life" for nuclear medicine were planted in 1895 when Wilhelm Conrad Roentgen announced the discovery of a new type of penetrating radiation emitted from a gas discharge tube with which he had been working (Myers and Wagner 1974). He called this radiation *x-rays* because the precise nature of the components was unknown. Even so, the achievement caused Roentgen to become the world's first Nobel prize winner. It is interesting to note that although the subsequent utilization of x-ray technology in medical and surgical diagnosis is well known, one of the most important consequences of the discovery of x-rays was the work leading to the discovery of radioactivity.

Shortly after Roentgen's discovery, the French physicist Henri Becquerel began to investigate the possibility that known fluorescent or phosphorescent substances produced a type of radiation similar to the x-rays discovered by Roentgen (Goodwin et al. 1970). As a result of these studies, in 1896 he announced that certain uranium salts also radiated, that is, emitted penetrating radiations. The rays were emitted spontaneously and continuously from all uranium compounds whether or not they were fluorescent. These results were startling, presenting the world with a new and entirely unexpected property of matter.

Urged on by scientific curiosity, Becquerel convinced Marie Curie, one of the most promising young scientists at the Ecole Polytechnique, to investigate exactly what it was in the uranium that caused the radiation he had observed (Wagner 1975). Madame Curie, who subsequently was to coin the term *radioactivity* to describe the emitting property of radioactive materials, and her husband Pierre, an established physicist by virtue of his studies of piezoelectricity, became engrossed in their search for the mysterious substance. In the course of their studies, the Curies discovered a substance far more radioactive than uranium. They called this substance *radium* and announced the discovery in 1898.

While the Curies were investigating radioactive substances, there was a tremendous flurry of activity among English scientists, who were beginning to identify the constituent components of atoms. Since the turn of the nineteenth century, Dalton's chemical theory of atoms, in which he postulated that all matter is composed of atoms that are *indivisible,* reigned supreme as the accepted view of the internal composition of matter. However, in 1897, when Thompson identified the electron as a negatively charged particle having a much smaller mass than the lightest atom, a new concept of the basic elements comprising matter had to be formulated. Our present image of atoms was developed in 1911 by Ernest Rutherford, who demonstrated that the principal mass of an atom was concentrated in a dense positively charged nucleus surrounded by a cloud of negatively charged electrons. This idea became incorporated into the planetary concept of the atom, a nucleus surrounded by very light orbiting electrons, conceived by Niels Bohr in 1913.

With this insight into the elementary structure of atoms, Rutherford was the first to recognize that radioactive emissions involve the spontaneous disintegration of atoms. After the general acceptance of this basic concept, Rutherford was awarded a Nobel prize in chemistry in 1908, and the "mystery" began to unfold. By observing the behavior of these radioactive emissions in a magnetic field, the Curies discovered that there are three distinct types of active radiation emitted from radioactive material. The three, arbitrarily called *alpha, beta,* and *gamma* by Rutherford, are now known to be (1) alpha (α) particles, which are positively charged and identical to the nucleus of the helium atom; (2) beta (β) particles, which are negatively charged electrons; and (3) gamma (γ) rays, which are pure electromagnetic radiation with zero mass and charge.

Once these foundations had been laid, the measurement of these radioactive emissions improved, and artificial radionuclides were developed and applied clinically in the years that followed. These basic discoveries by Roentgen, the Curies, and Rutherford opened up new fields in medicine and the natural sciences, and the excitement they created in their time has rarely been exceeded in the history of science (Goodwin et al. 1970).

Elementary Particles

By the 1930s, the research in this field clearly identified three elementary particles: the electron, the proton, and the neutron, usually considered the building blocks of atoms. Consider the arrangement of these particles as shown in Figure 8.1, a common view of the atom. The atom includes a number of particles: (1) one or more electrons, each having a mass of about 9.1×10^{-31} kg and a negative electrical charge of 1.6×10^{-19} C; (2) at least one proton with a mass of 1.6×10^{-27} kg, which is approximately 1,800 times that of the electron; and (3) perhaps neutrons, which have the same mass a protons but possess no charge.

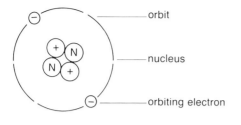

orbit

nucleus

orbiting electron

$\ominus$ = electron: mass = 9.1×10^{-31} kg
charge = -1.6×10^{-19} C

$\oplus$ = proton: mass = 1.6×10^{-27} kg
charge = $+1.6 \times 10^{-19}$ C

$\left(N\right)$ = neutron: mass = 1.6×10^{-27} kg
charge = 0

Figure 8.1 Planetary view of structure of atom. Primary mass is in nucleus, which contains protons and neutrons. Nucleus, which has a net positive charge, is surrounded by smaller orbiting electrons. In stable atoms the net charge of electrons in orbit is equal and opposite to that of the nucleus. The atom illustrated is helium.

The electrical charge carried by the electron is a fundamental property of matter, as is the mass of a particle. Since this is the smallest amount of electricity that can exist, it is usually expressed as a *negative unit charge* (-1). When expressing a unit charge in the metric system of units (meters, kilograms, and seconds), one obtains the value 1.6×10^{-19} C. The charges carried by all other atomic particles are therefore some integral multiple of this value. Consequently, it is impossible for a particle to have, for example, a charge equal to two and one-half times that of the electron.

Neutrons and protons exist together in the nucleus and have been given the collective name of *nucleons*. The total number of nucleons in the nucleus of an element is called the *atomic mass,* or *mass number,* and is represented by the symbol (A), whereas the number of protons alone is referred to as the atomic number (Z).

The various combinations of the neutron and proton that may exist in nature is illustrated by examining the makeup or composition of the nuclei of the three types of hydrogen atom (hydrogen, deuterium, and tritium). Although hydrogen has a nucleus consisting of a single proton, the combination of one proton and one neutron exists as a single particle called a *deutron* and is the nucleus of the atom called *heavy hydrogen,* or deuterium. Extending this concept further, the combination of two protons and two neutrons forms a stable particle—the alpha particle, which in nature exists as the nucleus of the helium atom. Alpha radiation emitted from radioactive substances consists essentially of a stream of such particles. Tritium, the third atom of hydrogen, on the other hand, has a nucleus consisting of only one proton and two neutrons.

These three types of hydrogen are examples of atoms whose nuclei have the same number of protons and therefore the same atomic number (Z) and at the same time may have a different number of neutrons and thereby a different atomic mass (A). Atoms exhibiting this characteristic were given the name *isotope* (from the Greek, meaning "same place"). The term isotope has been widely used to refer to any atom, particularly a radioactive one. However, current usage favors the word *nuclide* to refer to a particular combination of neutrons and protons. Thus isotopes are nuclides that have the same atomic number. All elements with an atomic number (Z) greater than 83, and/or atomic mass (A) greater than 209 are radioactive, that is, they decay spontaneously into other elements, and this decay causes the emission of active particles.

In order to specifically designate each individual atom, certain symbols have been developed. In the process of reading the literature in this field, it is therefore necessary to become somewhat familiar with them. Until recently, in the United States, it was the practice to place the atomic number as a subscript before and the atomic mass as a superscript after the chemical symbol of the atom ($_{53}I^{131}$). Since the chemical symbol itself also specifies the atomic number, one often omits it and simply writes I^{131}. In Europe, on the other hand, it was customarily written as a superscript prior to the chemical symbol (^{131}I). In an effort to achieve international standards, it was agreed in 1964 that the atomic mass should be placed as a superscript preceding the chemical symbol (^{131}I). When superscripts are not used, a more literal form of designation, such as cobalt 60, is commonly used. Referring to the helium atom illustrated in Figure 8.1, then, one simply writes $_2^4He$ or ^4He, where 4 is equal to the atomic weight (because of the aggregation of protons and neutrons in the nucleus) and 2 denotes the atomic number of the element.

Atomic structure and emissions

As already mentioned, Bohr's model suggested the existence of an atomic structure analogous to the planetary system. In this system electrons rotated in discrete orbits or shells around the nucleus, and the orbital diameters were determined by a quantum number (n) having integer values. These orbits were then represented by K, L, M, and N, corresponding to increasing number of n, a nomenclature still in use today. This model was further refined in 1925 by Wolfgang Pauli in terms of quantum mechanical principles; Pauli's work on atomic structure explained various observed phenomena, including the estimates for binding energy of the electrons at various orbits of an atom. The highlights of those observations involve the following: An atom is defined by four quantum numbers: (1) n is the principal quantum number, which is an integer and scalar quantity; (2) l is the angular momentum quantum number, a vector quantity which has integral values ranging from 0 to $n - 1$; (3) m_1 is the magnetic quantum number with integral values ranging from -1 through 0 to $+1$; (4) m_s is the spin magnetic quantum number, which has the values of $+\frac{1}{2}$ and $-\frac{1}{2}$. According to the *Pauli exclusion principle,* no two electrons in an atom can have the same set of quantum numbers.

In an electrically neutral atom, the number of orbital electrons exactly balances the number of positive charges in the nucleus which contains protons (positively charged masses about 1,800 times heavier than electrons) and neutrons. In 1932 Chadwick identified the neutron, which is slightly heavier than proton but without any electrical charge. The chemical properties of an atom are determined by the orbital electrons since they are predominantly responsible for molecular bonding, light spectra, fluorescence, and phosphorescence. Electrons in the inner shells, on the other hand, are more tightly bound, and may be removed from their orbits only by considerable energy such as by radiation interaction.

The amount of energy required to eject an electron from an orbit is equivalent to the binding energy for that shell, which is highest for the electrons at the innermost shell. The energy required to move an electron from an inner shell to an outer shell is equal to the difference in binding energies between the two shells. This energy requirement represents one of the natural characteristic of an element. When this characteristic energy is released as a photon, in the case of transition of an electron from an outer shell to an inner shell, it is known as a *characteristic x-ray.* However, if instead of the emission of a photon, the energy is transferred to another orbital electron, called an *Auger electron* it will be ejected from orbit. The probability for the yield of characteristic x-ray in such a transition is known as *fluorescent yield.*

Nuclear structure and stability

Protons and neutrons (also known as *nucleons*) are packed together to form the atomic *nucleus.* The *nucleus* is then defined by the number of protons, or *atomic number* (Z), and an *atomic mass number* (A), which is equivalent to the number of nucleons. Each element has a specific atomic number. Atoms with the same Z but different A are called isotopes of the same element. Different atoms having same A are called *isobars,* while those with same number of neutrons are called *isotones.*

Nucleons at the core experience a short-range nuclear force that is far greater than the electromagnetic force of repulsion between the protons. The movement of nucleons is often described by a shell model, analogous to orbital electrons. However, only a limited number of motions are allowed, and they are defined by a set of nuclear quantum numbers. The most stable arrangement is known as the *ground state.* The other two broad arrangements are (1) the *metastable state,* when the nucleus is unstable but has a relatively long lifetime before transforming into another state; and (2) the *excited state,* when the nucleus is so unstable that it has only a transient existence before transforming into another state. Thus, an atomic nucleus may have separate existence at two energy levels (one at a metastable state), known as *isomers* (both have same Z as well as same A). An unstable nucleus transforms itself to a more stable condition, either by absorbing or releasing energy (photons or particles), ultimately to a nucleus at ground state. This process is known as *radioactive transformation* or *decay.* Naturally occuring heavier elements, having Z greater than 83, are unstable.

Assessment of nuclear binding energy is important in determining the relative stability of a nuclide. This binding energy represents the minimum amount of energy required to overcome the nuclear force so as to separate the individual nucleons. This can be assessed on the basis of mass-energy equivalence as represented by $E = mc^2$, where E, m, and c represent energy, mass, and speed of light, respectively. This has led to the common practice of referring to masses in terms of electron-volts (eV). The mass of an atom is always found to be less than the sum of the masses of the individual components (neutrons, protons, and electrons). This apparent loss of mass (Δm), often called *mass defect* or *deficiency,* is responsible for the binding energy of the nucleus and is equivalent to Δmc^2. The mass of a neutral carbon 12 atom has been accepted as 12.0 atomic mass units (amu). In this scale, the sum of the masses of the components of ^{12}C would be 12.10223 amu. The difference in masses (0.10223 amu) is equivalent to 95.23 megaelectronvolts (MeV) of binding energy for this nucleus, or 7.936 MeV/nucleon for carbon 12. For nuclei with atomic mass number greater than 11, the binding energy per nucleon ranges between 7.4 and 8.8 MeV. One atomic mass unit (^{1}amu) is equal to $1.6605655 \times 10^{-24}$ g, or, using the mass-energy relation, is equivalent to 931.502 MeV. The rest-mass of an electron on the other hand is 0.511 MeV, and its kinetic energy is equivalent to the increase in relativistic mass; $(1 - 1)/(1 - v^2/c^2)^{1/2}$ (where v and c are the speeds of the electron and light, respectively).

An unstable nuclide, commonly known as a *radionuclide,* would eventually come to a stable condition with the emission of ionizing radiation after a specific probability of life expectancy. In general, there are two classifications of radionuclides: natural and artificial. Naturally occurring radionuclides are those nuclides which emit radiation spontaneously and therefore require no additional energy from external sources. Artificial radionuclides, on the other hand, are essentially man-made, produced by bombarding so-called stable nuclides with high-energy particles. Both types of radionuclides play an important role in nuclear medicine. The average life or half-life, the mode of transformation or decay, and the nature of emission (type and energy of the ionizing radiation) constitute the basic characteristics of a radionuclide. All radioactive materials, whether they occur in nature or are artificially produced, decay by the same types of processes. They emit alpha, beta, and/or gamma radiations. As just discussed, the emission of alpha and beta particles involves the disintegration of one element into another. The rate of this decay process is spoken of in terms of disintegrations per unit time or its half-life ($T\frac{1}{2}$, time for half the original number of atoms in a given radioactive element to disintegrate). Half-lives of radioactive elements range in value from thousandths of a second to millions of years. For example, ^{131}I has a half-life of 8.05 days, whereas ^{60}Co has a half-life of 5.24 years.

Sometimes, a radionuclide attains the final stable state in successive stages of transition. A radionuclide is often called *parent,* and the decay product the *daughter.* Broadly speaking, then, the modes or phases of transformation in the process of a radionuclide passage from an unstable to stable condition may be divided into six categories: (1) α (alpha), (2) β^- (negatron), (3) β^+ (positron), (4) electron capture (EC), (5) isomeric transition (IT), and (6) fission. Types (2), (3), and (4) are essentially similar, constituting a beta decay or isobaric transition.

Alpha (α) decay

Alpha particles are ionized helium atoms moving at a high velocity. The emission of an alpha particle from the nucleus would produce a different element by reducing Z by 2, and A by 4. A number of naturally occurring heavy elements undergo α decay. For example, radium (^{226}Ra) transforms to radioactive radon (^{222}Rn) by α decay. Alpha emitters are hardly used in nuclear medicine, although some of them have been considered for therapy. The emitted alpha particles are monoenergetic, with the energy approximately related to the logarithm of decay constant of the radionuclide.

Negatron (β^-) or (β^-, γ) decay

A negatron, or beta (β^-) particle, is an electron coming out of the nucleus with a certain amount of kinetic energy. The β^- decay process produces a different element by increasing Z by 1, with A remaining constant. Phosphorus 32 is a typical example of a pure β^- emitter (^{32}P is transformed to ^{32}S), which has been used for therapy. Beta particles are emitted with all energies between zero and some maximum for each discrete transition. Since this behavior seems to violate the conservation of energy, Pauli hypothesized that another unobserved particle (the neutreno) was emitted along with the beta particle. The maximum possible energy for the beta particle (β_{max}) is considered a characteristic of the radionuclide. The average energy of the beta particles is approximately equal to one-third of β_{max}. However, most of the radionuclides undergoing β^- decay also emit γ rays, almost simultaneously. There are also different probabilities of sharing the transition energy between β^- and γ ray emissions. For example, iodine 131 emits several β^- and γ rays in this process.

Positron (β^+) or (β^+, γ) decay

Positrons (β^+ or e^+) are created in the nucleus, as if a proton was converted to a neutron and a positron. The positron decay would produce a different element by decreasing Z by 1, with A being the same. For example, carbon 11 decays to the predominant stable isotope of boron (^{11}C transforms to ^{11}B). Positrons (like negatrons) share their energy with neutrinos. Positron decay is usually associated with γ-ray-emission. Moreover, the positron, once emitted, is annihilated as a result of a collision with an electron within about 10^{-9} sec. producing a pair of photons of 0.511 MeV each moving in opposite directions. A minimum transition energy of 1.022 MeV is required for any positron decay.

Electron capture (EC), or K capture

An orbital electron, usually from the inner shell (K shell), is captured by the nucleus (as if a proton captured an electron and converted itself to a neutron). An electron capture process would produce a different element by decreasing Z by 1, with A being the same (similar to B$^+$ decay). Indeed, some radionuclides have definite probabilities of undergoing either positron decay or electron capture (such as iron 52, which decays with about 42 percent EC and 58 percent β^+ emission). Further, there could be an associated gamma emission with electron capture. For example, ^{51}Cr transforms to ^{51}V (vanadium 51) with about 90 percent going directly to the ground state, but the remaining 10 percent goes to an excited state of ^{51}V, followed by transition to ground state with the emission of photons. An electron capture would also cause a vacancy in the inner shell, which would lead to the emission of a characteristic x-ray or Auger electron. Absence of high-energy electrons (beta particles) in EC would cause low radiation absorbed dose to the tissue.

Isomeric transition (IT) and internal conversion (IC)

Radionuclides at a metastable state emit only γ rays. The element remains the same with no change in A (isomeric transition). The atomic mass number of the isomer is, therefore, denoted by Am. For example, ^{99m}Tc (technetium 99m) decays to ^{99}Tc. However, there is a definite probability that instead of a photon coming out, the energy may be transferred to an inner orbital electron. This is known as *internal conversion,* and the internally converted electrons are close to monoenergetic beta particles. For example, barium 135m (decaying by IT) emits about 84 percent IC electrons. They also create a vacancy in the shell, consequently leading to the emission of characteristic x-rays and Auger electrons.

Nuclear fission

Usually a heavy nuclide may break up into two nuclides (more or less equal fragments). This may happen spontaneously, but is more likely with the capture of a neutron. The uranium fission products mostly range between atomic numbers 42 and 56. A number of medically useful radionuclides are produced as fission products, such as Xenon 133, which may be extracted by appropriate radiochemical procedures.

Transformation constant

The reduction of the number of atoms through disintegration of their nuclei is known as radioactive decay and is characteristic of all radioactive materials. Unaffected by changes in temperature, pressure, or chemical combination, the rate of the decay process remains constant, with the same number of disintegrations occurring during each interval of time. Furthermore, this decay process is a random event; consequently every atom in a radioactive element has the same probability of disintegrating.

As the decay process continues, it is clear that fewer atoms will be available to disintegrate. This fraction of the remaining number of atoms that decay per unit of time is called the *decay constant* (λ). The half-life and decay constant are obviously related, since the larger the value of the decay constant (λ), the faster the process of decay and consequently the shorter the half-life. In any event, the decay constant is an unchanging value throughout the decay process. The point of this discussion is to emphasize that each radionuclide exhibits a distinctive disintegration process because of its inherent properties, that is, its decay constant (λ) and half-life ($T_{1/2}$). All nuclides decay in the same manner, but one should not draw the conclusion that all decay at the same rate, since this is a parameter determined by the unique nature of the particular radioactive element in question.

Considering a number of atoms (N) of a specific type of radionuclide present at a time $t,$ the transformation rate can be defined by $-dN/dt$ (the minus sign denotes the decay/decrease), which would be proportional to the number of atoms, or

$$dN/dt = \lambda N$$

where λ is the transformation constant.

Taking the initial number of atoms as N_o ($N = N_o$ when $t = t_o$), we get by integration

$$N = N_o e^{-\lambda t} \tag{2}$$

The half-life, or $T_{1/2}$ (the time corresponding to transformation of 50 percent of the nuclides, when $N = No/2$), therefore may be obtained by solving for $\lambda T_{1/2}$ in equation 2.

$$T_{1/2} = \ln 2/\lambda = 0.693/\lambda$$

and the average life (T_a) can be deduced as

$$T_a = 1/\lambda = 1.443\, T_{1/2}$$

Mixture and parent-daughter

A sample of radioactive material that contains a mixture of two different unrelated species of radionuclides can be represented by a simple additive equation. Considering N_{10} and N_{20} as the number of nuclides for the two species at $t = 0$, taking λ_1 and λ_2 as corresponding transformation constants, we get

$$N = N_{10}\, e^{-\lambda_1 t} + N_{20} e^{-\lambda_2 t}$$

There are also radionuclides that produce another radionuclide in the process of transformation. The parent radionuclide is no doubt decaying, but the daughter radionuclide initially grows in number. The growth and decay patterns of the daughter radionuclide can be described by the relative values of the transformation constants of the parent and the daughter. For example, denoting parent by 1 and daughter by 2, we get

$$dN_1/dt = -\lambda_1 N_1 \quad \text{(parent)}$$

$$dN_2/dt = +\lambda_1 N_1 - \lambda_2 N_2 \quad \text{(daughter)}$$

Starting with a pure parent $N_{20} = 0$ at $t = 0$), we would get for the daughter

$$N_2 = N_{10}(e^{-\lambda_1 t} - e^{-\lambda_2 t}).\, \lambda_1/(\lambda_2 - \lambda_1)$$

Further, when $\lambda_2 >> \lambda_1$ ($e^{-\lambda_2 t} = 0$ and $\lambda_2 - \lambda_1 = \lambda_2$), we have

$$N_2 = N_1\lambda_1/\lambda_2 \quad \text{(secular equilibrium)}$$

and, when $\lambda_2 > \lambda_1$ ($e^{-\lambda_2 t} = 0$ for large values of t), we get

$$N_2 = N_1\lambda_1/(\lambda_2 - \lambda_1) \quad \text{(transient equilibrium)}$$

In the case of $\lambda_2 = \lambda_1$, with special mathematical treatment (Spencer and Hosain 1976), we get

$$N_2 = N_1\lambda t \qquad (\text{taking } \lambda_2 = \lambda_1 = \lambda)$$

But when $\lambda_2 < \lambda_1$ ($e^{-\lambda_1 t} = 0$ for large values of t), we get

$$N_2 = N_{10}e^{-\lambda_2 t}\lambda_2/(\lambda_1 - \lambda_2) \qquad (\text{no equilibrium})$$

One of the most important situations is transient equilibrium, in which one could construct a parent-daughter generator system to obtain a short-lived radionuclide from a relatively long-lived parent. Several such generator systems have been evaluated for nuclear medicine (Lebowitz and Richards 1974).

Technetium 99m ($T_{1/2} = 6$ h), which is used extensively in nuclear medicine, is obtained from molybdenum 99 ($T_{1/2} = 66$ h) generator. radioactive ^{99}Mo as molybdate is adsorbed on an alumina column, and ^{99m}Tc is eluted from time to time with isotonic saline as sodium pertechnetate.

Radionuclides and Radiopharmacy

Progress in nuclear medicine has been related to the availability of radionuclides that could be used in human subjects in appropriate chemical forms. The choice of a radionuclide depends on its physical characteristics in relation to diagnostic and therapeutic applications, and the possibility of incorporating it into an appropriate chemical compound suitable for biomedical investigation (Hosain and Hosain 1978). Since the major role of nuclear medicine today is related to diagnostic approaches based primarily on radionuclide imaging procedures it is important to understand what constitutes a radionuclide and how it is utilized. Radionuclides are initially obtained in simple chemical forms and then used to derive the intended radiochemicals. Within radiopharmacy, pharmaceutical principles are applied to the labeled compound to make it suitable for clinical use and to dispense the compound in radiopharmaceutical doses for clinical procedures under the guidelines of the Nuclear Regulatory Commission (NRC).

Nuclear reactions

The production of artifical radionuclides is based on nuclear reactions. They are obtained mostly by means of interaction of high-energy charged particles (usually protons, deuterons, or alpha particles) from cyclotrons and linear accelerators, or neutrons from nuclear reactors. Further the generator-produced radionuclides are radioactive decay products, and the parent radionuclides are obtained by nuclear reactions. It is important to note that the probability of nuclear reactions depends on the nature and energy of the incoming particle and on the relative binding energies of the target and the product nuclei. This probability can be represented by an apparent target size or cross section. When a beam of particles of flux ϕ (number of particles per second per square centimeter) impinges on a target material (exposing M moles of specific target nuclei), only a very small percentage of target nuclei is transformed. Therefore, the loss of target nuclei due to any nuclear reaction would be negligible. The rate of transformation or production of a radionuclide (taking N as Avogadro's number) is given by

$$dR/dt = \sigma \phi MN$$

where σ is a constant (having the dimension similar to area) and known as cross-section for nuclear reaction. This is expressed in units of barns (b) (10 to 24 cm^2). The radionuclide so produced would decay according to its characteristic transformation constant (λ). The yield, or the product obtained after bombarding for a time t, is then given by

$$Ac = \sigma \phi MN(1 - e^{-\lambda t})$$

where the radioactivity Ac is equal to $R\lambda$, which represents the number of transformations per second or becquerel.

The energy at which a reaction occurs with detectable yield is known as *threshold energy.* A plot of the cross section against the energy of bombarding particles is known as the *excitation function.* For larger values of t (greater than 3 times the half-life of the radionuclide produced), the activity reaches close to saturation.

It is customary to represent the nuclear reactions symbolically, in the following general form:

$$^nA(a, b)^mB + Q$$

where the target element A with atomic mass number n reacts with impinging particle a, which causes the emission of b (a nucleon, group of neuclons, or photon) and production of a nuclide B with atomic mass number m, and the release or absorption of an energy Q. Same radionuclide may be produced by different types of nuclear reactions. For example, fluorine 18 can be obtained in many different ways, and certain reactions are preferable for specific precursor compounds (Palmer et al. 1977). The reaction $^{16}O(^3He, p)^{18}F$ using a water target is good for obtaining fluoride ion, whereas $^{20}Ne(d, \alpha)^{18}F$ is favorable for obtaining anhydrous fluorine. The low-energy (thermal) neutrons are extensively used for inducing (n, γ) reactions in a nuclear reactor to produce radioisotopes of the target nuclide. The radioctivity is expressed in terms of specific activity, such as megabecquerels per milligram (MBq/mg) of carrier element. An enriched stable isotope of the target element is preferred, if available, for obtaining radionuclides with high specific activity. However, it is possible to have (n, p), (n, d), and (n, α) reactions in nuclear reactors, and they would produce carrier-free radionuclides. A radionuclide so produced may generate another radionuclide; the parent or the daughter may be recovered from the target, depending on the half-life of the parent. The fission products are obtained as a (n, f) reaction on enriched uranium in the reactor.

Chemical processing

The chemical processing to derive a medically useful compound requires several steps. First, the desired radionuclide must be recovered from the target. The recovery of radionuclides, especially in a pure form, requires considerable radiochemical processing. The radiochemical steps may be similar to ordinary chemical procedures, but they require remote handling facilities. Since a number of alternative nuclear reactions could produce the same radionuclide, the merits and demerits of different reactions are judged according to the yield and purity. A desirable radionuclide recovered from fission product may contain more radionuclide impurities. Many radionuclides have been evaluated for medical use, but the number of radionuclides used in clinical nuclear medicine has been rather limited.

Labeled compounds

A radiopharmaceutical contains a specific chemical compound labeled with a radionuclide. This may be a simple inorganic salt or a complex organic molecule. It is well recognized that the chemical properties of an element reflect some of the possible biological behaviors, and the behavior of several elements within the same group of the periodic table appears similar. For example, strontium 85 has been used to represent calcium metabolism in bone. Radionuclides are usually obtained in simple chemical forms after target processing. Many of them with minor modifications have been found valuable in nuclear medicine, such as sodium iodide 131, thallous 201 chloride, and xenon 133 gas. However, the next step in deriving biologically important radioactive chemical compounds is to incorporate the radionuclide into the desired chemical compound by chemical, biochemical, or radiation-catalyzed synthesis. The most important factor is the time involved in the synthesis in relation to the half-life of the radionuclide. Often this is a limiting factor in the use of radiopharmaceuticals labeled with short-lived radionuclides. Table 8.1 summarizes some of the important radionuclides that are currently used in nuclear medicine; the predominant applications are in the field of diagnostic imaging (Freeman 1984).

Technetium 99m pharmaceuticals

The availability of short-lived radiopharmaceuticals, especially technetium-99m-labeled chemical complexes, has been responsible for the recent advancement in diagnostic clinical nuclear medicine. Technetium 99m has a half-life of 6 h, and it can be readily obtained (eluted with isotonic saline as sodium pertechnetate) from a generator system containing parent radionuclide (molybdenum 99 with a half-life of 66 h). This is used for brain, thyroid, and salivary gland imaging. The pertecnetate ion, when reduced to a cationic species, is capable of forming complexes with a variety of chemical compounds, although the precise chemical reactions are not fully understood. These chemical complexes can be divided broadly into several categories, primarily depending on the physical properties and the biological behavior. The most frequently used reducing agent is the stannous chloride. A number of "kits" are now available that contain stannous ions along with the desired

Table 8.1 Commonly used radionuclides in nuclear medicine

Radionuclide	Half-life	Transition	Production	Chemical Forms
Carbon 11	20.38 min	β^+	Cyclotron	3-N-methylspiperone
Fluorine 18	109.77 min	β^+	Cyclotron	Fluorodeoxyglucose
Phosphorus 32	14.29 days	β^-	Reactor	Phosphates
Chromium 51	27.704 days	EC	Reactor	Sodium chromate
Cobalt 57	270.9 days	EC	Cyclotron	Cyanocobalamin
Gallium 67	78.26 h	EC	Cyclotron	Citrate complex
Molybdenum 99	66.0 h	β^-	Reactor	Molybdate in column
Technetium 99m	6.02 h	IT	Generator	TcO$_4$ and complexes
Indium 111	2.83 days	EC	Cyclotron	DTPA and oxine
Iodine 123	13.2 h	EC	Cyclotron	Mainly iodide
Iodine 125	60.14 days	EC	Reactor	Diverse proteins
Iodine 131	8.04 days	β^-	Reactor	Diverse compounds
Xenon 133	5.245 days	β^-	Reactor	Gas
Thallium 201	3.044 days	EC	Cyclotron	Thallous chloride

chemical compound, such as (1) macroaggregated albumin for lung scanning, (2) albumin or sulfur colloids for liver and spleen scanning, (3) serum albumin for blood-pool imaging, (4) HIDA or an iminodiacetic acid derivative for gallbladder study, (5) a strong chelate such as DTPA for renal studies, and (6) methylenediphosphonate (MDP) for bone scanning. Simple addition of sodium ^{99m}Tc-pertechnetate solution to the kit provides the desired radioactive compound. Commercially available ^{99m}Tc generator and kits are pretested for pharmaceutical standards to reduce the need for time-consuming quality assurance tests for the radiopharmaceutical before administration to the patients.

Quality control in the development of any radiopharmaceutical is an important requirement, which starts from production of radionuclide and continues at every step of preparation and administration of the radioactive compound to the patient. It is based on the requirements for safety and efficacy of the radiopharmaceutical. The method of production of radionuclide should be such that it contains the smallest possible quantity of other contaminating radionuclides. The radiopharmaceutical should also be free from undesirable labeled compounds. The chemical agents must be nontoxic (usually not a problem because only small quantities are used). The radiopharmaceutical must be sterile, pyrogen-free, and safe for parenteral use. Improper handling of a radiopharmaceutical can generate significant amounts of degradation products. For example, most ^{99m}Tc-labeled compounds deteriorate with exposure to air or during storage for several hours. Storage of many compounds with very high specific activity generates impurities by radiolysis.

Application of radiopharmaceuticals

The design and development of new radiopharmaceuticals have been an integral part of nuclear medicine. Many have undergone significant changes in the progress of radiopharmacy. For example, formerly strontium 85 with a half-life of 64 days was used for bone scanning; later fluorine 18 with a half-life of 110 min had been utilized for the same purpose; then technetium 99m (half-life of 6 h), labeled *pyrophosphate,* was used; and now ^{99m}Tc-labeled diphosphonate is routinely used. Chemical structure is an important consideration in designing radiopharmaceuticals. Not only the structurally similar diphosphonates but also those without any phosphorus, substituted with arsenic, behave in a similar manner (Hosain and Wang 1981). The behavior of a radiopharmaceutical may be modified by interventional approaches. Interventional nuclear medicine is not necessarily an invasive procedure; mostly it entails the use of another chemical compound before, during, or after the use of a radioactive compound to increase the efficacy of a radiopharmaceutical (Hosain 1984). Similarly, an optimal result may not be obtained because of interaction of certain medication (Hladik et al. 1982).

There has been a considerable interest in using biochemicals labeled with short-lived positron emitters along with the positron tomographic system. It has been possible to visualize regional glucose metabolism, especially in the brain, using ^{18}F-fluorodeoxyglucose (a labeled analog of glucose). This technique is increasingly used in neurological and behavioral studies (Alavi and Reivich 1984). Recently, dopamine and serotonin receptors have been measured in the living human brain by positron tomography with ^{11}C-labeled 3-*N*-methylspiperone (Wong et al. 1984). However, the cost of having a cyclotron and positron tomographic system has restricted widespread use of radiopharmaceuticals labeled with short-lived positron emitters. Gallium 67, indium 111, and thallium 201 are the three cyclotron-produced radionuclides used routinely in nuclear medicine. They have half-lives of about 3 days and decay by electron capture. Iodine 123, a useful cyclotron-produced radionuclide with potential for single-photon tomography, has restricted

Table 8.2   Frequently Used procedures in nuclear medicine

Procedure	Radionuclides	Chemical Forms
Plasma/blood volume estimation	^{125}I, ^{131}I	Radioiodinated serum albumin
Red cell mass and life estimates	^{51}Cr	Labeled red blood cells
Vitamin B_{12} absorption	^{57}Co	Labeled cyanocobalamin
Thyroid function test	^{123}I, ^{131}I	Sodium iodide
Tumor and abscess imaging	^{67}Ga	Citrated complex
Thrombus imaging	^{111}In	Labeled platelets via oxine
Cerebrospinal fluid imaging	^{111}In	Chelated complex with DTPA
Myocardial imaging	^{201}Tl	Thallous chloride
Cardiac blood pool imaging	^{99m}Tc	Labeled blood pool
Brain imaging procedures	^{99m}Tc	Pertechnetate
Renal imaging procedures	^{99m}Tc	Chelated complex with DTPA
Bone imaging	^{99m}Tc	Methylenediphosphonate
Liver/spleen (RES) imaging	^{99m}Tc	Colloidal preparations
Liver/gallbladder imaging	^{99m}Tc	Iminodiaceticacid derivative
Lung perfusion imaging	^{99m}Tc	Macroaggregated albumin
Lung ventilation imaging	^{133}Xe	Gas
Thyroid therapy	^{131}I	Sodium iodide
Polycythemia vera treatment	^{32}p	Sodium phosphate

availability due to its relatively short half-life of 13 h. The majority of the nuclear medicine procedures in community hospitals depend on the use of generator-produced technetium 99m in conjunction with commercially available kits. Table 8.2 summarizes the frequently used radionuclide procedures at the present time.

Radiation Interaction and Dosimetry

We observe a process of energy transfer whenever ionization and excitation are induced in any medium. The energy absorbed within the medium can be expressed in terms of joules per kilogram or in units of gray. In a living biological system, the manifestation of direct and indirect effects of radiation varies greatly and depends on the level of exposure. Assessment of absorbed radiation dose has been very important in designing and developing radiopharmaceuticals. On the other hand, interactions of radiation with matter in various physical setups have been used for the detection and measurement of radiation and radioactivity. The nature of radiation encountered in nuclear medicine mostly falls into two broad categories: (1) charged particles and (2) photons. They essentially induce collision-type phenomena in any living or nonliving system composed of diverse materials.

Charged particles

The radiation consisting of charged particles (such as alpha and beta rays), while passing through a medium, usually ejects electrons from the outer shells. These ejected electrons, known as *delta rays*, usually have sufficient energy to cause further ionization in the medium. This phenomenon is known as *secondary ionization.* Sometimes, a fraction of the energy of the charged particle (primary or secondary) may be taken up by an orbital electron, which is not ejected but is pushed to a higher orbit (excited state). This would cause an emission of low-energy photons due to subsequent transition, depending on the difference of binding energies of the two shells involved (for example, fluorescence).

Occasionally, high-energy electrons are rapidly decelerated through a close encounter of the nuclear force leading to bremsstrahlung (gamma rays). The *bremsstralung,* or radiation losses, increase with high-energy beta particles interacting with a medium consisting of elements of high atomic number. The total loss of energy due to this process remains low, of the order of 5 percent for an upper limit, for beta particles emitted from radionuclides. The production of bremsstrahlung with accelerated electrons is most important in radiation therapy with an external beam. The probability of radiation loss (p) for a beta particle of maximum energy E_{max} in an absorber of atomic number Z is approximately represented by

$$p = ZE_{max}/3{,}000$$

The remaining energy of the charged particles is spent in inducing ionization and excitation. The secondary photons (gamma rays) also induce further ionization and excitation; these photons are often capable of ejecting electrons from an inner shell. This process would further lead to the production of characteristic x-rays and Auger electrons. A very small percentage of beta energy may be lost as Cerenkov radiation (bluish glow) in a medium such as water in which the charged particles (for example, 1 MeV beta) travel at a speed greater than that of light in the same medium.

Stopping power and range

The rate of loss of energy of the charged particles is expressed in terms of megaelectronvolts per centimeter and known as linear stopping power (S_l). The *linear energy transfer* (LET), which may be slightly less than S_l, represents the energy deposited along the track. The specific ionization (*SI*) gives the total number of ionizations per unit length of the track and is proportional to LET. The average energy expended per ionization ($W = LET/SI$) is independent of the type or the energy of the incident particle. This value ranges between 25 and 45 eV for a variety of gases (33.7 eV for air). The ionization potential (*I*) is the average energy required to produce an ion pair (10 to 15 eV for various gases). The difference of energy between W and I is spent in causing excitation.

An alpha particle, being a heavy charged particle, produces intense ionization on its relatively straight and short path. The mean range (R in centimeters in air) of alpha particles (of energy E in megaelectronvolts) can be approximately represented as

$$R = 0.325E^{3/2}$$

The beta particles (the negatrons as well as positrons), while passing through the matter, produce neither a straight path nor an intense ionization along the track as alpha particles do. They are deflected and follow rather a tortuous path. The negatrons, when slowed down, may produce an orbital electron. The positron, on the other hand, combines with an electron at the end and produces annihilation radiation (gamma rays of 0.511 MeV). The process of beta decay does not lead to the emission of monoenergetic particles. Thus, the maximum range in the medium corresponds to the maximum beta energy with respect to a radionuclide transformation. The range of the beta particles in an absorbing material is expressed in terms of milligrams per square centimeters. The following equation may be utilized for a range-energy relationship for negatrons as well as for positrons with a maximum energy ranging between 0.1 and 3 MeV:

$$X\tfrac{1}{2} = 41 \times E^{1.4}$$

where $X\tfrac{1}{2}$ is the half-value thickness of the absorber in units of milligrams per square centimeters.

Photons

Photons lose their energy mainly as a result of photoelectric effect, Compton scattering, and pair production. The most predominant factor is the Compton scattering, in which in every event the photon loses its energy and eventually is absorbed as a result of a photoelectric interaction. The phenomenon of pair production may occur with photons at higher energy, 1.022 MeV or more. The interaction of photons with matter is equivalent to collision with atoms without causing direct ionization. However, the electrons so produced or those ejected from the orbits are capable of producing ionization in the medium in the process of losing their energy.

The photoelectric effect becomes predominant at the lower end of photon energy. The photon, representing energy, is completely absorbed by an orbital electron, which is then either ejected or excited. The ejected electron acquires the kinetic energy equivalent to the difference between the incident photon energy and the binding energy of the corresponding shell for the ejected electron. Frequently such interactions occur with the electrons in the innermost shell. This creates vacancies and consequently produces characteristic x-rays or Auger electrons.

Compton scattering is the usual process by which a photon loses its energy in steps, finally being absorbed by a photoelectric effect. The incident photon interacts with an orbital electron of outer shell and loses a part of its energy. In this process, the electron is ejected from the orbit, and the photon is scattered at an angle. The loss of energy is equivalent to the binding energy of the corresponding shell and the acquired kinetic energy of the ejected electron.

Pair production provides a typical example in which energy is converted to mass. Sometimes, a photon of 1.022-MeV energy (equivalent to the rest-mass of two beta particles) or more may interact (usually with the nucleus) and transform to a positron-negatron pair. The difference between the photon energy and 1.022 MeV is shared by the pair as kinetic energy. Subsequently, these beta particles lose their energy by causing ionization and excitation. Finally within a very short time the positron collides with an electron, thereby producing a pair of 0.511-keV photons each moving in opposite directions.

Photon beam attenuation

The probability of interaction, or the absorption of radiation in matter, for photons depends on the energy of the incident photon and the thickness and density of the absorbing material. A simple equation can be set up to determine the intensity of the transmitted beam as

$$dI/dx = -\mu l x$$

where I is the intensity, x is the thickness, and μl is a constant (linear attenuation coefficient) for the material ($-$ve sign represents an absorption). This would give

$$I = I_0 \, e^{-\mu l x}$$

where, $I = I_0$ at $x = 0$. The transmission factor $T = I/I_0 = e^{-\mu l x}$ is true for a narrow beam of photons. For a broad beam, a build-up factor B, which is greater than 1, must be included. Then,

$$T = B \, e^{-\mu l x}$$

The half-value layer (HVL), or half-value thickness (HVT), or $X^{1/2}$ can then be determined by substituting $I = I_0/2$, approximately

$$X1/2 = \ln 2/\mu l = 0.693/\mu l$$

To express the absorption coefficient in a more general term, it is convenient to consider a mass attenuation coefficient ($\mu m = \mu l/\rho$), in terms of grams per square centimeter. This is an important consideration in designing radiation shielding. Most radionuclides emit gamma rays that consist of several components of different energy at varying intensities. If the absorbing material is not very thick, more of the lower-energy components are absorbed, leading to a beam hardening.

Radiation dosimetry

Radiation dose estimations are essential whenever a new radiopharmaceutical is to be introduced for clinical studies. Initially, an accurate assessment of radiation dose to patient is difficult because of the lack of precise biodistribution data of the radiopharmaceutical in humans. Biodistribution data are normally obtained in several animal species and extrapolated for the calculation of dose to a 70-kg normal human. Human data are accumulated over years. The biodistribution of a radiopharmaceutical may become significantly different from the accepted average values as the result of the influence of a disease or a drug. Special consideration must be made for children of different age groups, the fetus, and the embryo (Kereiakes and Rosenstein 1980). A small amount of radiation dose at a cellular level involving deoxyribonucleic acid (DNA), known as *microdosimetry,* is far more damaging than an overall absorbed dose to the tissue.

The classical method of dosimetry has been replaced by a modern method of radiation dose calculation through the effort of the Medical Internal Radiation Dose (MIRD) Committee (Mitchell 1969). The internationally accepted unit for radiation dose to tissue is the gray (Gy); 1 Gy is equivalent to the absorption of an energy of one joule per kilogram of the tissue under consideration. Previously the radiation absorbed dose was expressed as radiation absorbed dose (rad); 1 rad is equivalent to the absorption of an energy of 100 ergs per gram or 0.01 J per kilogram, which is equal to 0.01 Gy. Thus, an expression of 1 rad per millicurie (mCi) is equivalent 0.27027 milligray per megabecquerel (mGy/MBq), or 1 mGy per megabecquerel is equivalent to 3.7 rad per millicurie. Most of the compilations on radiation dosimetry that are available for nuclear medicine procedures have been expressed in terms of rads.

The modern method of calculation of radiation dosimetry depends on the availability of the biological data and the utilization of various tables published by the MIRD Committee, especially the table containing the values of specific absorbed dose constants (S-factors) for various radionuclides and different target-to-source combinations (Snyder et al. 1975). In general, the radiation dose estimates can be divided into one major and one minor component. The former is the radiation dose to the target organ when the same organ is the source of radioactivity. The latter is the combined doses to the target from the surrounding organs or tissues, where the contributions from the nonpenetrating radiation (such as beta particles) become negligible. However, sometimes this minor component may become the more significant one, such as the radiation dose to the ovaries from the urinary concentration of the radioactivity in the bladder. The total dose to target is the contribution from all components, and each component can be represented by

$$D_\alpha(T \leftarrow S) = Ac \times Sf$$

where

D_α = dose to target (T) from source (S)
Ac = cumulative activity in the source
Sf = sp. abs. dose const. (S-factor for T-S pair)

The total radiation dose to the target organ depends on the cumulative activity in the source organ, which is a time-activity integral. This can be obtained by

$$Ac = \int_o^\alpha A(t)\, dt$$

(either by integration or by graphical extrapolation). Under simplified conditions, it may be taken as

$$Ac = 1.443 \times Te \times A_o$$

where Ao is the maximum uptake in the source organ, which is assumed to occur soon after the administration of the radiopharmaceutical and clear in a single exponential fashion with an effective half-life of Te hours ($1/Te = 1/Tp + 1/Tb$, $Tp = T\frac{1}{2}$ and Tb = biological clearance half-time).

The value of Sf can be obtained from the table (Snyder et al. 1975) for a large number of radionuclides relevant to nuclear medicine for various target-source pairs. This factor can, however, be calculated as

$$Sf = 2.13 \times \Sigma\, n_i E_i \phi_i / m$$

where

n_i = *fractional yield of ith component of radiation*
E_i = *average energy (MeV) for the corresponding component*
ϕ_i = absorbed fraction of radiation in target tissue
m = mass of target tissue (g)

The values of ϕ_i depend on the size of target and the energy of gamma radiation. For nonpenetating radiation it is normally equal to 1 (if the source is within the target) or 0 (if the source is away from the target).

Radiobiology and radiation safety

Exposure to a high level of radiation to living organisms, mammals in particular, induces pathological conditions and even death. This feature is utilized in therapy for malignant diseases, where the intention is to deliver a localized high radiation dose to destroy the undesirable tissue. Exposure to lower levels of radiation may not show any apparent effect, except some chromosomal breakage, but it increases the risk of cancer as a long-term effect. It also increases the probability of genetic defects, if the gonads are exposed. This imposes the need for minimization of radiation exposure to the worker, as well as restrictions in medical applications. In case of therapy, a compromise is necessary, with due consideration for life expectancy and future risk. Assessment of risks at low levels of radiation is not easy. Recently, the American Association of Physicists in Medicine has addressed the questions involving legal, social, and scientific aspects of biological risks of medical irradiations (Fullerton et al. 1980).

The United States Nuclear Regulatory Commission (NRC) has adopted a philosophy of implementation of principles and practices for keeping occupational radiation exposure at medical institutions as low as reasonably achievable. Regulatory maximum exposure limit for the general public has been set aside as 0.5 sievert (Sv) (Rem) per year. Limits for occupational exposure are 1.25 Sv/3 mo for the whole body, and 18.75 Sv/3 mo for the extremities. Thus, one of the most important radiation safety procedures is to monitor both the personnel and the work area. The activities of a radiation safety officer involve (1) routine assessment of personnel exposure, (2) monitoring of radioactive contamination in work area, (3) evaluation of radiation shielding arrangements, and (4) arrangements for appropriate disposal of radioactive waste. The routine personnel monitoring is usually done with TLD film badges and ring-type finger badges. Radiation survey and wipe tests are carried out at certain intervals, and at times of incidental/accidental contamination. The common shielding material is lead, the thickness depending on the energy of gamma rays. Further, radioactive wastes are stored at assigned areas with appropriate shielding. The measure for radioactive waste disposal depends on the nature and half-life of the waste. All require a temporary storage facility; they are finally disposed locally according to prescribed rules or shipped in barrels to a permanent site. At the present time a vast majority of radioactive materials used in nuclear medicine are relatively short-lived. Shipment of waste to disposal sites can be avoided by having an in-house facility of storage of the waste for some time, usually equivalent to 10 to 20 half-lives. If the waste does not contain any environmentally toxic substances, it is incinarated or disposed as a regular waste product.

Instrumentation and Imaging Devices

There has been great advancement in nuclear instrumentation in recent years, especially for radionuclide imaging of organs and tomographic studies. Further, computers are increasingly used in medical science (Bronzino 1982). The systems for radiation analysis have two major components: the detector and the electronics. The design of the detectors depends on the utilization of the interaction of radiation with matter. A number of devices that utilize the ionization and excitation of atoms to measure radioactivity have been developed. Operation of all these devices requires certain electronic aids, such as high-voltage supply, preamplifier, linear amplifier, pulse-height analyser, and scaler or ratemeter. These electronic components can be housed in one unit to provide the necessary requirements for the operation of a radiation detector. They can also be obtained in various standardized modules known as nuclear instrument modules (NIMs) so that necessary units can be combined for a specific purpose. A general schematic is shown in Figure 8.2.

The development of radionuclide imaging devices has led to complex instrumentation and incorporation of computers for on-line data acquisition and analysis (Hine and Sorenson 1974). The most extensively used device in the current practice of nuclear medicine is the gamma camera, which is capable of obtaining images of the distribution of radioactivity in the body after the administration of a radiophamaceutical. These images are, however, two-dimensional representations of a three-dimensional distribution of radioactivity. Sometimes, it is not possible to identify small localized abnormal distribution at certain depth of the tissue. This has led to the development of tomographic systems, with which virtual slicing of the organ is possible by computer-assisted reconstruction of images (Ell and Holman 1982).

Gas-filled detectors

Gas-filled detectors use gases (air, helium, argon, and so on) as a medium for radiation interaction, enclosed in a chamber containing two electrodes. A voltage difference between the electrodes (anode and cathode) is set up to direct the electrons toward the anode. The radiation induces ionization in the gas. Ions are detected either as electrical current or pulses with the aid of electronics. Gas-filled detectors include ionization chambers, proportional counters, and Geiger-Müller (GM) counters. Their detection efficiency for photons is low. Earlier, GM counters were used extensively, especially the end-window GM counter for the measurement of beta activity (Figure 8.3).

Presently, the application of the gas-filled counter in nuclear medicine is limited. It is, however, utilized in radiation survey meters. The ionization chamber is routinely used for assaying the radioactive doses prior to the administration to the patient. Solid-state detectors, such as lithium-drifted germanium (Ge-Li) or lithium-drifted silicon (Si-Li), are occasionally used. These are solid-state analogs of gas-filled detectors.

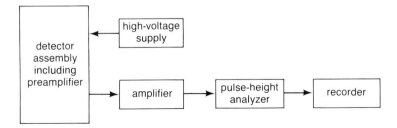

Figure 8.2 Schematic representation of a radioactivity-measuring device consisting of the detector and the basic electronic modules.

Scintillation counters

The major components of a scintillation counter are (1) a radiation absorbing medium in solid or liquid phase, (2) photomultiplier (PM) tubes, and (3) the necessary electronic devices. The most commonly used scintillation counter consists of a thallium-activated sodium iodide crystal coupled with a photomultiplier tube. The processes of excitation, due to absorption of radiation in the NaI(Tl) crystal and deexcitation in the crystal lattice, cause luminescence. The crystal is sealed in an aluminum cover, except on one side, for optical coupling to a photomultiplier tube. The whole unit is sealed against any external light (Figure 8.4). The PM tube is then connected to electronic devices to form a basic scintillation detector. The PM tube consists of a photosensitive cathode and a series of ten dynodes that are activated by applying a graded high voltage. A fraction of the light that is produced in the crystal falls on the photocathode. Photoelectrons that are ejected

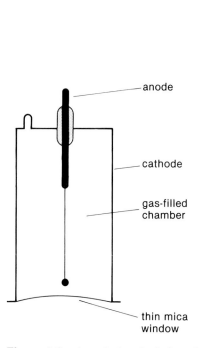

Figure 8.3 A typical end-window Geiger-Müller counter for the measurement of beta particles.

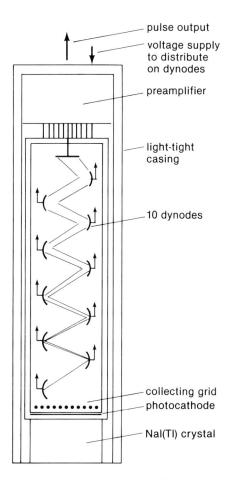

Figure 8.4 A typical scintillation detector consisting of a NaI(Tl) crystal optically coupled with a photomultiplier tube.

from the cathode are accelerated toward the first dynode, and secondary emission of electrons takes place. This process is repeated with successive dynodes. Ultimately an electric pulse that is proportional to the original number of photoelectrons ejected at the cathode is formed. These electrical pulses are then amplified and detected by an appropriate electronic device. The principle of liquid scintillation counting is similar, except that it utilizes organic molecules in liquid phase to produce scintillation. This system is most useful for assaying beta emission from small, colorless samples.

The NaI(Tl) scintillation counters are extensively used in nuclear medicine in one form or the other. They are highly efficient for the detection of gamma rays and are used in designing simple instruments as well as imaging devices. Scintillation probes and well-type scintillation counters remain the basic equipment in nuclear medicine for the detection and measurement of radioactivity from gamma-emitting radionuclides. Probes are routinely used for the measurement of radioiodine uptake in the thyroid, usually with tracer doses of iodine 131. Well-type scintillation counters are widely used for measuring radioactivity in small samples (such as blood and urine) obtained from individuals after administration of tracer doses of radioactive compounds. They are also used to assay radioactivity in a variety of procedures (such as radioimmunoassay) using iodine 125–labeled proteins. A number of such assays also utilize tritium- or carbon 14–labeled compounds, and the liquid scintillation counters measure the low-energy beta emissions in these in vitro diagnostic tests. Both the liquid scintillation counter and the well-type scintillation counter have been automated for changing the samples and printing out the results.

In most cases of radionuclide transformation, the photons emitted are not a single group of monoenergetic photons, but they have certain discrete energy levels. Moreover, other photopeaks are likely to be created by scattering and other processes. It is desirable to isolate the predominant photopeak and to use it for measuring radioactivity with better accuracy. The photopeak represents a Poisson or Gaussian type of distribution. The energy resolution can be represented by the full width at half-maximum amplitude. With a single-channel pulse-height analyser, one may obtain counts over a range of energy by using a narrow window. However, it is far easier to obtain the gamma ray spectrum with a multichannel analyzer (Figure 8.5).

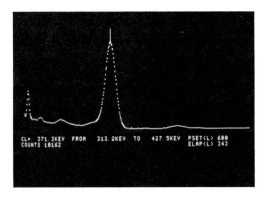

Figure 8.5 Spectrum of gamma rays of iodine 131 obtained by a multichannel pulse-height analyser.

The efficiency of a counting set-up is an important consideration. The overall counting efficiency, however, depends on diverse factors, such as intrinsic efficiency of the radiation detector, geometric relationship between the detector and the source, and absorption and scattering of radiation within the source. Errors in counting may also arise from any of these factors. At high count rates, one may lose counts because of dead time or pulse resolving time, which depends on the detector as well as on the associated electronics. At low levels of counts, the background counts and the statistical fluctuation in counting become significant in defining the accuracy.

Rectilinear scanners

The introduction of rectilinear scanners in 1960s was a major step in the advancement of diagnostic nuclear medicine. These scanners are essentially large scintillation detectors, generally with NaI(T1) crystals 2 in. thick and 5 in. in diameter. They consisted of one or two opposing probes, and a focused collimator could be attached. The lead collimators were designed with multiple tapered holes arranged in a hexagonal pattern and separated by septa suitable for low-, medium-, or high-energy gamma rays. The detector unit was capable of moving back and forth (along the x axis) with small increments in forward motion (along the y axis) between each pass, covering a rectangular area of interest. The system includes all the electronic devices required to operate a scintillation counter, plus others to display the distribution of radioactivity over the rectangular area. Initially a dot-making device represented the radiation intensity. Subsequently, photoscanning devices were used to expose an x-ray film with a narrow beam of light, the amount of exposure being proportional to the amount of radioactivity detected over a region. The developed x-ray film offered better gray scale. The image, or the scan, represented relative distribution of detected radioactivity.

Gamma cameras

The most important instrumentation in present-day nuclear medicine is the Anger camera, commonly known as the gamma camera. The basic principle behind gamma camera is NaI(Tl) scintillation counting, but it has to incorporate complexity of locating the site of scintillation event. It requires a large flat single crystal (normally 0.5 in. thick and 12 to 20 in. in diameter) that is optically coupled to an array of PM tubes (usually 37 tubes). An electronic logic circuit determines the location of each scintillation event within the crystal in terms of X, Y position as shown in the simplified diagram (Figure 8.6). Further, the output of all the tubes combines to form a Z signal that is subjected to pulse-height analysis. If the amplitude of this signal falls within the range defined by the selected energy window, the electron beam in a cathode-ray tube (CRT) produces a flash of light corresponding to X, Y location. A large number of events (100,000 to 500,000) have to occur in a relatively short time to represent the image of the distribution of radioactivity in the region. A collimator, with several thousand parallel holes covering the face of the flat crystal, plays the most important role in defining the location of radioactivity in rela-

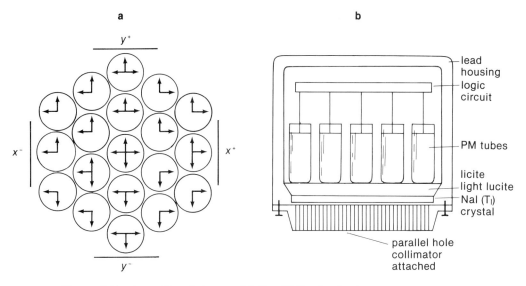

Figure 8.6 Assembly of photomultiplier (PM) tubes in the form of concentric rings with connections for X or Y output (a). These photomultiplier tubes are optically coupled to a flat slab of NAI(T$_l$) crystal (b).

tion to the scintillation event in the crystal. It establishes an approximate point-to-point relationship between the source and the scintillation event for the photons. The PM tube nearest to the event receives maximum luminescence, and the logic circuit determines the location.

An important issue in the design of collimators is the compromise between sensitivity and resolution. It is important to use a material of high density for efficient absorption of unwanted gamma rays. Gold is ideal but too expensive, tungsten is good but too hard; lead is the compromise used extensively in the manufacture of various types of collimators. For gamma cameras, the number and size of the holes covering the area of the crystal depend on the specific design to accomplish higher sensitivity or higher resolution. The size of the hole and the septa, and consequently the total number of holes, also depends on the intended use of gamma rays of particular energy range. Low- and medium-energy collimators are commonly used with the gamma cameras. Collimators with slanted holes have been designed to cover larger or smaller areas than the flat surface of the crystal could cover. A pinhole collimator, used sometimes for imaging small organs, offers the best compromise between sensitivity and resolution against a large area of background tissue activity. It is generally used for thyroid imaging with ^{99m}Tc-pertechnetate. It also gives an inverted image. Seven-pinhole and slant-hole collimators that offer certain tomographic capabilities with conventional gamma cameras have been designed. The procedures of imaging with gamma cameras are known as *static* and *dynamic studies.* The dynamic images are a series of static images obtained at short intervals during a given period of time.

Advanced systems

A simple gamma camera system, at the present time, is the most important as well as the most basic instrument for diagnostic nuclear medicine. It imposes a limitation in cardiac studies. Interfacing with a digital computer makes the system more versatile. Digital image-processing systems perform data collection, storage, and analyses. Data acquisition requires digitization of the image by an analog-to-digital converter (ADC), which divides a rectangular image area into small elements, or *pixels,* usually a 64 by 64, 128 by 128, or 256 by 256 matrix. One can select a particular region of interest to obtain certain quantitative information. The ADC improves dynamic studies in particular. The regional rate of uptake and clearance pattern can be obtained from the serial images for any particular region. Interfacing of a computer with a gamma camera is essential for fast dynamic studies (such as cardiac wall motion studies).

The gamma camera systems are large and heavy and cannot be moved easily. They are regarded as stationary cameras. However, relatively mobile versions are available with computer interface specially for cardiac studies. The gamma cameras often have capabilities for obtaining whole-body images by linearly moving either the camera head or the patient bed. Often called *scanning cameras,* they have replaced rectilinear scanner systems. A major innovation in gamma camera design has been the addition of an extra camera head with rotational capabilities (Figure 8.7), which is used with a computer system known as *single photon emission computered tomography* (SPECT) for carrying optional tomographic work. The technique is known as computer-assisted reconstruction tomography and is similar to x-ray computed tomography (CT) scanning. Tomograms represent the images of isolated cross-sectional slices of the body. They facilitate identification of abnormalities that are otherwise difficult or impossible to identify in a two-dimensional image covering overlying and underlying tissues.

Positron imaging

The positrons emitted through transformation of a radionuclide can travel only a short distance in a tissue (a few millimeters), and then are annihilated. A pair of 511-keV photons that travel at 180° to one another is created. A pair of scintillation detectors can sense positron emission by measuring the two photons in coincidence. Annihilation coincidence detection provides a well-defined cylindrical path between the two detectors. Multihole collimators to define the position are unnecessary in a positron camera because electronic collimation accomplishes the task. Positron cameras have limited use; however, they have attained great importance in a highly modified form in *positron-emitting transaxial tomography,* or *positron emission computed tomography* (PET scanning). A large number of small NaI(Tl) detectors is arranged in an annular form so that annihilation photons in coincidence at 180° permits detection of positron. Tomographic images are, however, obtained by computer-assisted reconstruction techniques. Several large centers use positron emission tomography in conjunction with cyclotron-produced short-lived radiopharmaceuticals (mainly carbon 11, nitrogen 13, and fluorine 18) to provide structural as well as metabolic information.

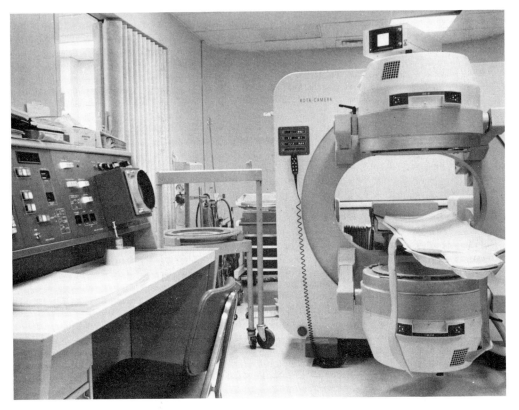

Figure 8.7   Modern dual-head gamma camera, which can obtain tomographic images by single photon emission computed tomographic principle.

CLINICAL APPLICATION OF NUCLEAR MEDICINE TECHNIQUES

With the discovery of artificial radionuclides, the "modern era" of nuclear medicine began. The availability of these radioactive elements increasingly encouraged the pioneers of this discipline to employ radioactive tracer techniques to gain information regarding biological and physiological systems. One of the first physiological systems to be studied in both animal and man was the metabolism of phosphorus. Using the cyclotron-produced tracer ^{32}P, several investigators observed the great efficiency with which the body absorbed inorganic phosphorus and preferentially utilized it in rapidly multiplying tissues, such as those associated with malignancies. In 1936, John Lawrence, recognizing the therapeutic implications of these findings, acted. He used ^{32}P in the treatment of leukemia and in the process inaugurated the therapeutic employment of artificial radionuclides (Wagner 1975).

Although the early uses of radioactive materials in medicine were chiefly in radiation therapy, today most radioactive materials are used to provide useful diagnostic information. These radionuclides can be monitored within the patient (in vivo) or in various bodily fluids removed from the patient (in vitro). For example, it is possible to inject a patient with a radioactive substance that is "taken up" by a particular organ such as the kidney. By placing a detector over the kidneys, the amount of radioactive material accumulated by the kidney can actually be measured. This *uptake test* allows the clinician to monitor the activity of specific organs and determine whether they are functioning properly. Another example of an in vivo study involves imaging the distribution of a radionuclide within an organ. This can be extremely important, especially since it has been demonstrated that abnormal tissue tends to accumulate more or less of the radionuclide administered than the normal tissue surrounding it. In this way, in vivo measurement can help the clinician delineate the presence of these tissue abnormalities.

The in vitro category, on the other hand, includes tests made outside the body. These tests are used to study various chemical, as well as physiological, processes. Today, in vitro tests are capable of detecting extremely small amounts of various hormones and chemicals in the blood and have been used to determine (1) insulin dosage in diabetics, (2) whether individuals are immune to specific diseases such as hepatitis, and even (3) the proper dosage of digitalis required by cardiac patients. Recent developments in this area have indicated that this is an area of application that will continue to grow in importance over the next decade.

The major thrust of the current application in nuclear medicine lies primarily in the use of radioactive tracers in both in vivo and in vitro studies to evaluate various physiological systems within a patient. *The key to success in this application is the specificity of the radioactive material utilized.* That is, the more closely the radionuclide can be tied to a specific function, then the easier it is to examine the dynamic physiological system under study. It is beyond the scope of this text to provide a complete outline of all the possible applications presently available; however, several important applications will be discussed.

Lungs

As discussed in Chapter 4, the two lungs serve as the locale for bringing together venous blood and air. The blood comes from the right side of the heart (output of the right ventricle); although the vessel carrying the blood is termed the *pulmonary artery,* it is actually a vein and transports blood that is low in oxygen and high in carbon dioxide (see Figure 8.8A). This blood is delivered to progressively smaller vessels until it reaches the level of capillaries. It has been estimated that there are about 2 billion capillaries in the lungs (2×10^9). The general scheme of blood arrival at the lung and air delivery involves *perfusion,* the distribution of blood, and *ventilation,* the pattern of delivery (see Figure 8.8B). Usually ventilation/perfusion in a region of the lung is "matched": blood is delivered to capillaries around air pockets (alveoli) that are ventilated.

In a clinical sense one of the important questions that arise is, How can the spatial distribution of perfusion, and of ventilation, be measured during life? Let us consider initially the case of perfusion. Figure 8.8A indicates that the output of the right side of the heart is usually entirely to the lungs. The lung capillaries are

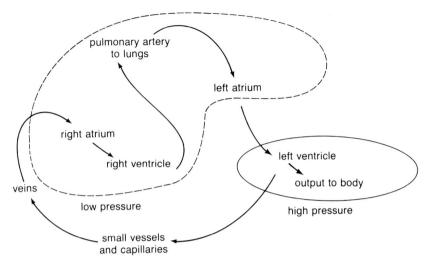

Figure 8.8A Schematic outline of pulmonary circulation, which is a low-pressure system.

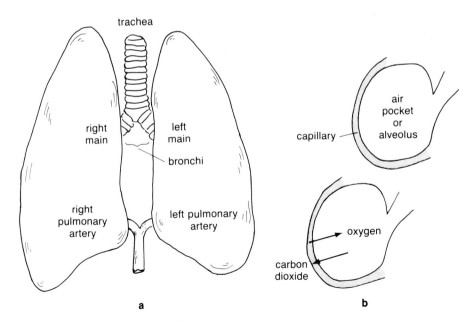

Figure 8.8B (a) Schematic representation of delivery of blood and air to the lungs. (b) Events occurring in the air pockets or alveoli.

about 10 micrometers (μm) in diameter (and red blood cells are 7 μm across). Introduction of particles larger in diameter than the capillaries into the right side of the heart delivers them to the pulmonary capillaries and results in embolization, or "hang-up." The crucial point is that particles to be used must be acceptable to the biological system. That is, they must be readily degraded and nontoxic. The first particulates used were made from human serum albumin labeled with [131]I. The protein solution was brought to the isoelectric point and heated. Small particulates precipitated; those greater that 10 μm in diameter were suitable for embolizing (blocking) capillaries. A few particles that were smaller in size passed through the lung capillaries, to be picked up by the reticuloendothelial system. Some of the particles were larger than 50 μm and embolized precapillary vessels. A useful advance in producing particulates of uniform size was projecting a solution of human serum albumin into a lipid bath. The 15-μm-diameter particles (referred to as *microspheres*) can be radiolabeled with [99m]Tc. Hence, a short-lived radionuclide could be used in a radiopharmaceutical to explore pulmonary vasculature. Once the particles lodge in the lung capillaries, they are subject to the mechanical action of the pulsatile blood and to enzymes in the circulation. Half the particles are degraded to a size small enough to pass through the capillaries in about 3 h. How many particles are injected intravenously? A usual number is about 200,000 (2×10^5). This is necessary in order to produce a distribution throughout both lung fields. Since 2×10^5 capillaries are blocked (if each particle goes into a separate capillary), then $(2 \times 10^5)/(2 \times 10^9)$, or 1 capillary in 10,000, is obstructed for several hours. There are likely three relative contraindications to the use of the microparticulates:

1 Patients who are cyanotic (blue, as a result of the presence of a high concentration of unoxygenated blood), probably cannot afford to lose the use of even a small number of capillaries for several hours.

2 A small number of individuals have a defect in the heart wall between the major pumping chambers (an interventricular septal defect). If the radiolabeled particles are injected into an arm vein, they travel to the right side of the heart. Some may pass into the left pumping chamber if there is a hole between the chambers. Once the particles are in the left ventricle, they can be pumped into the body and lodge in capillaries in the brain and other organs.

3 In pregnancy, use of any radioactive material may deliver a radiation exposure to the fetus. This effect must be weighed against the needed diagnostic information on the mother and the potential adverse reactions due to other diagnostic methods.

When a blood clot arrives in the right side of the heart, it is pumped into the vessels of the lungs and produces a pulmonary embolus. Blood cannot pass beyond the clot. When the radiolabeled microparticulates are injected intravenously, they also travel to the right side of the heart and then to the lungs. Since they cannot pass through the obstructed point, it appears as an area of reduced perfusion and a "negative" defect (less radioactivity than surrounding regions). A perfusion defect (Figure 8.9) can be caused by a pulmonary embolus, or by a variety of disorders that reduce blood flow. Each perfusion lung scan has to be interpreted with the patient's chest x-ray in hand.

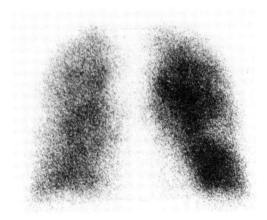

Figure 8.9 Anterior perfusion lung scan (right is to the viewer's left). The right lung has less perfusion than the left. In addition, a wedge-shaped defect is present in the left lung.

It was remarked earlier that ventilation and perfusion in the lungs are usually matched, in that blood is perfused only through regions of the lungs that are ventilated. What happens if an airway is obstructed? The corresponding lung region is underoxygenated, or *hypoxic,* and blood flow shifts away from the hypoxic area. How can this be differentiated from a pulmonary embolus? Information is needed about the distribution of air flow into the lungs; it is obtained by use of a radioactive gas that is inhaled or of small (less than 2-μm) radiolabeled particles that are carried in the air stream.

If a radioactive gas is used (such as radioxenon,[133] Xe), the patient is placed on a closed circuit and breathes via a mouthpiece into a system containing oxygen and an absorbent for carbon dioxide. When the radioactive xenon gas is introduced into the system, the inhalation phase and entry into the lungs are monitored by a gamma camera. Rebreathing is performed through the closed system, to allow entry into all parts of the lung, and washout from the lung is monitored by admitting room air into the rebreathing system and routing the expired air through charcoal to trap radioxenon that is breathed out.

In a pulmonary embolus, the blood vessel is blocked, but the airway is initially open in the region. That is, the perfusion scan shows a defect, but the ventilation scan does not. This condition is a ventilation/perfusion mismatch. A mismatch is presumed to be caused by a pulmonary embolus. In airway disease, the ventilation scan is abnormal in the region, and the perfusion scan is also abnormal (since blood is shifted away from the hypoxic area). Since the ventilation and perfusion scans are both abnormal, there is no mismatch.

Another interesting use of lung imaging uses a soluble radiotracer. Consider a diagram of the entry and disappearance of a tracer in the lungs, after injection into the vein of an arm (Figure 8.10). Entry represents blood coming into the lungs from the right side of the heart. Blood then exits from the lungs by passage into the left side of the heart. What occurs when there is a defect (hole) in the wall between the right and left ventricles? Some of the radiolabel in the blood reenters the right ventricle from the left ventricle through the defect in the wall. Activity reenters the lung, and the curve of radioactivity versus time falls less rapidly than normally (Figure 8.10[b]). Computers can analyze the curves and use them to calculate the extent of the shunting from the left ventricle to the right.

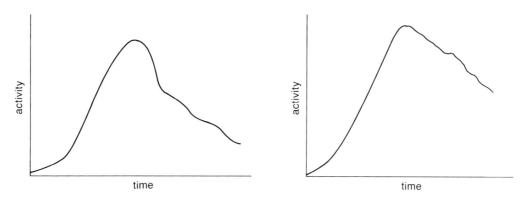

Figure 8.10   Left: time-activity curve of blood passing through the lungs after intravenous administration of a soluble radiotracer into an arm vein. Right: curve from a patient with a defect in the wall between the ventricles.

Liver and Spleen

The liver is the largest internal organ. In addition to importance in terms of size, it has a variety of essential metabolic functions. To understand the activities of the liver, two facts have to be recognized.

1   The liver has a dual blood supply (Figure 8.11). Blood from an arterial source (hepatic artery) is high in oxygen content but relatively small in quantity. The hepatic artery contributes about 30 percent of total blood flow to the liver. As liver damage develops, the venous blood supply is affected, rather than the arterial. The arterial flow is under high pressure. The venous inflow (portal vein) contributes about 70 percent of the blood, and is a low-pressure system. All of the outflow from the spleen (splenic vein) and from the intestine (mesenteric vein) merges together to form the portal vein. The portal inflow, under low pressure, is reduced as the liver is damaged by alcohol or other toxins.

$$\frac{\text{Fractional liver flow}}{\text{from portal vein}} = \frac{\text{portal vein}}{\text{portal vein } + \text{ hepatic artery}}$$

The fraction of liver blood flow from the portal vein decreases in liver damage.

2   The liver has two distinct functional cell types: the *hepatocytes* (also referred to as *parenchymal cells*) and *phagocytic cells* (termed *reticuloendothelial* or *Kupffer's cells*).
a   The hepatocytes perform a variety of metabolic activities and are also involved in the transfer of substances into the bile. A number of compounds follow the following sequence:

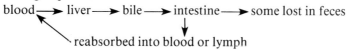

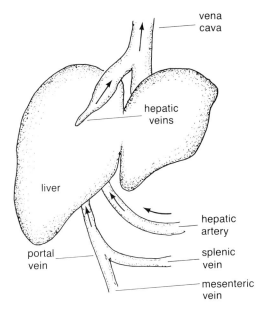

Figure 8.11   Blood flow to the liver (there are two inflows). The venous drainage is into the vena cava or major vein in the abdomen.

This pattern is referred to as the *enterohepatic pathway*. The internal circulation can be probed by bile acids radiolabeled with radioactive carbon (^{14}C, a beta particle emitter) or by a small quantity of selenium 75 as in ^{75}Se-selenocholic acid. Selenium 75 has $T_{1/2}$ of 120 days and emits a gamma ray. Some compounds follow part of the enterohepatic pathway (blood $\longrightarrow$ liver $\longrightarrow$ bile $\longrightarrow$ intestine $\dashrightarrow$ all into feces). These *hepatobiliary agents* probe liver extraction (from the blood) and excretion into the bile. Because they are in motion, the quantity in the liver is changing.

b   The reticuloendothelial (RE) cells extract particulates from the bloodstream; however, most are retained within the liver and do not leave. Since RE cells are not present in most liver tumors, agents (such as radioactive colloids) extracted by RE function are used when studying the liver for contained tumors.

Hepatobiliary agents (Figure 8.12) are utilized to examine extraction from the bloodstream by the liver and subsequent passage into the bile. A major use is in patients with suspected obstruction of the bile excretory system. The most frequently employed compounds for exploring this pathway are ^{99m}Tc adducts of analogs of hepatic iminodiacetic acid (HIDA).

$$R - N \Big\langle \begin{matrix} CH_2 . COOH \\ \\ CH_2 . COOH \end{matrix}$$

The two carboxyl groups bind the ^{99m}Tc. The R grouping is large and imparts *lipophilicity* (fat solubility). Upon intravenous administration, about 90 percent of the

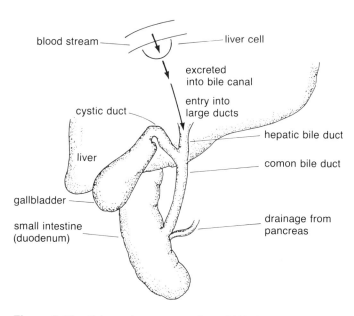

blood stream ——— ——— liver cell

excreted
into bile canal

entry into
large ducts

cystic duct

hepatic bile duct

liver

comon bile duct

gallbladder

small intestine
(duodenum)

drainage from
pancreas

Figure 8.12   Schematic representation of bile flow.

^{99m}Tc-HIDA is extracted by the normal liver in less than 10 min. The remainder passes out through the kidneys.

If the extraction function of the liver is damaged, ^{99m}Tc-HIDA requires more time to concentrate within hepatic tissue. Once in the liver, the hepatobiliary agents then undergo outward transport into bile canals. Sometimes the outward transport system is damaged, and the radiopharmaceutical stays in the liver for a prolonged period. Normally, movement of the ^{99m}Tc-HIDA agents is rapid, and collecting ducts within the liver can be delineated. If the ductal system is open, then the column of radioactivity passes outward from the liver into the hepatic bile duct. A portion enters the gallbladder via the cystic duct (Figure 8.12). The main column enters the *common bile duct* (the portion below the confluence of the cystic and hepatic ducts). From the common duct, activity then enters the small bowel. When the small bowel is obstructed, some of the ^{99m}Tc-HIDA can reflux upward into the stomach.

A major use of hepatobiliary studies has been in searching for acute inflammation of the gallbladder (acute cholecystitis). In 95 percent of the cases of acute cholecystitis, the duct to the gallbladder (cystic duct) is obstructed by a gallstone or other cause (Figure 8.13). Since most of the obstructions are due to gallstones, patients often have ultrasound examinations to determine the presence and extent of the stones. However, not all patients with gallstones present (cholelithiasis) experience acute gallbladder inflammation (cholecystitis).

If the gallbladder fills with the ^{99m}Tc-HIDA compounds, then 95 percent of the time, the patient is not having an acute gallbladder attack. If the gallbladder does fill, and the suspicion of an acute gallbladder attack is still high, the patient can be given a stimulus to induce the gallbladder to contract.

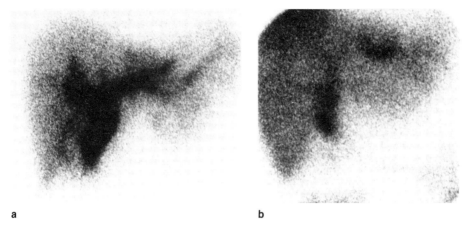

a   b

Figure 8.13 Two hepatobiliary studies. (a) Retracer is draining into the ductal system. (b) There is clearly radioactivity outside the liver, where it has drained into the small bowel.

If the wall of the organ is inflamed, it does not respond to appropriate stimuli. The usual stimuli are an injected peptide (cholecystokinin) that stimulates contraction or a fatty meal (which releases neural and endocrine stimuli for gallbladder contraction). Contraction of a gallbladder that has filled with the hepatobiliary agent virtually rules out acute cholecystitis. This strategy is useful when the gallbladder is inflamed but a stone has not occluded the cystic duct. In this *acalculous cholecystitis,* ^{99m}Tc-HIDA can enter the gallbladder, but the wall does not respond to stimuli to contract.

Radiocolloid

Reticuloendothelial cells have the ability to filter out particulates circulating in the bloodstream. This ability is tested by intravenous injection of radioactive colloid. The most commonly used material is ^{99m}Tc-sulfur colloid, which has a particle size of about 1 μm (the size of a bacterium). When given intravenously, ^{99m}Tc-sulfur colloid is cleared rapidly from the bloodstream.

1 The patient is positioned under a gamma camera and receives the radiocolloid intravenously. Since the major liver blood flow is from the portal system (and not from the hepatic artery), normally little entry occurs on the first pass (Figure 8.14) Tumors within the liver almost invariably obtain their blood supply from the arterial side. Thus, they have a "blush" on first pass of radiocolloid.

2 The usual distribution pattern of the radioactive ^{99m}Tc-sulfur colloid is liver, 80 percent; spleen, 10 percent; bone marrow, 10 percent. When the liver is damaged (for example, through the effects of alcoholism), the radiocolloid is

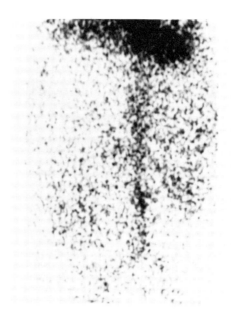

Figure 8.14   Anterior hepatic dynamic study.

significantly extracted by splenic reticuloendothelial cells and those in the bone marrow; this phenomenon is referred to as a *shift of radiocolloid.*

Radiocolloid images allow estimation of liver size. The liver is approximately 8 cm in length (L) at birth and grows about 0.5 cm in length up to age 16 (A):

$$L = 8 + 0.5A$$

In adults, the liver is $17 \pm {}^2$ cm in length. A small liver in an adult (13 cm or smaller) represents either a liver that never grew or one that was of normal size and then contracted as the result of disease. In infants, an inflammation of the umbilical vein can produce obstruction of the portal vein (chronic portal vein obstruction). In such a case, the liver obtains blood from the hepatic artery only, is barely able to function, and does not grow very large. More common is the liver that has been of normal size and then contracts through disease such as alcoholism (Figure 8.15).

The large liver (21 cm in length or greater) can result from fatty infiltration, from tumors or cysts, or from infiltrates. Tumors and cysts present focal defects in the liver (areas with less uptake of radiocolloid); these can be single or multiple (Figure 8.16). Following radiation or chemotherapy, radiocolloid images can be used to determine whether the lesions are becoming smaller.

The adult liver weighs about 1,500 g. The spleen weighs only 150 g. By weight, the liver/spleen ratio is about 10:1, as is the relative extraction of radiocolloid by the liver and spleen. Relatively greater extraction by the spleen occurs when the liver is damaged. Reduced splenic uptake of radiocolloid can be observed when the organ has been infiltrated by tumor or damaged by reduced oxygen. In some diseases, such as sickle cell anemia, blood flow to the spleen is impaired. The sickle cells assume half-moon and other shapes that block capillaries in the spleen. As the

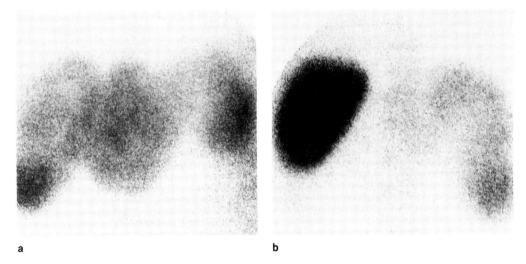

a   b

Figure 8.15 (a) Anterior image. (b) Posterior image.

Figure 8.16 Radiocolloid image of the liver, showing defects.

oxygen content falls, the splenic ability to extract radiocolloid decreases. *Functional asplenia* is the anatomical presence of the spleen, with an inability to concentrate radiocolloid from the bloodstream.

At birth, the spleen is about 5 cm in length; its growth with age (up to 16 yr) is described by $S = 5.7 \pm 0.31A$.

Lymphomas or other tumors can involve the spleen. A particularly important use of radiocolloid imaging of the spleen has been to search for splenic trauma. When the spleen is damaged, radiocolloid images may show intrasplenic defects, subcapsular irregularities, or splitting of the spleen into two or more fragments. Because of the importance of the spleen in filtering out bacteria and in producing antibodies, efforts are made to save the organ rather than to remove it surgically after trauma.

Tumors and Infections

A majority of studies in nuclear medicine depend upon deposition of radiopharmaceutical into a organ. Agents that "search out" a tumor or a site of infection would be useful and are gradually being developed.

Radiogallium

When given intravenously, radiogallium 67 (^{67}Ga-citrate) has some of the properties of radioactive iron; that is, much of it binds to transferrin in the bloodstream. White blood cells also contain transferrin-related proteins and take up a portion of the radiolabel. In a radiogallium image (Figure 8.17), the liver is the principal organ of uptake. Bone contains some of the radiopharmaceutical. Because a significant portion exits into the intestinal tract, radiogallium cannot be employed to determine whether inflammation of the intestine is present.

Why does radiogallium accumulate in tumors or sites of infection? There are likely several mechanisms involved.

1 White blood cells pick up radiogallium (probably because of the protein lactoferrin, which is related to transferrin). These white cells are chemically attracted to sites of infection (and, to a lesser extent, to certain tumors).

2 A direct protein-to-protein transfer occurs; that is, from transferrin in the bloodstream radiogallium shifts to lactoferrin. Receptors for transferrin plus iron (or gallium) are present on cells, and lactoferrin like proteins exist in many tumors. Some bacteria also have iron receptors and can take up radiogallium.

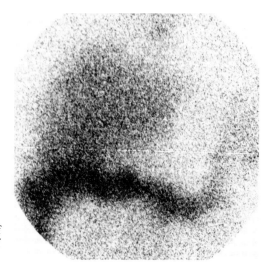

Figure 8.17   Radiogallium image of the abdomen, also showing the tip of the sternal bone, liver, and colon.

A major use of radiogallium is in searching for hidden infections. When ^{67}Ga-citrate is given intravenously, it probably localizes in lesions during the first several hours. However, the significant quantity ("high background") in the bloodstream makes early detection difficult. Thus, 1 to 3 days may elapse before a site of inflammation becomes apparent. Radiogallium is very effective in detecting inflammatory locals (usually due to infection). Exceptions can occur when the typical response to infections is not present. For example, in some instances of anaerobic bacterial infections (bacteria that do not use oxygen) and in infections with ameba, the usual white blood cell response does not occur. In such cases, radiogallium may not pinpoint the lesion.

The ability of radiogallium to detect tumors and their spread varies widely. Among the tumors with good avidity for the radiopharmaceutical are lung malignancies (bronchogenic carcinoma), lymphomas, and liver tumors (hepatomas). Other tumors have lesser uptake. This is likely related to the content of transferrin-iron receptors. Radiogallium can be used to stage tumors, that is, to detect the tumor and the extent of its spread locally or to regional tissue or lymph nodes. If the primary tumor accumulates radiogallium, then the metastases usually also take up the radiotracer.

An interesting use of radiogallium is in the subtraction technique. A bone infection reveals accumulation of bone imaging agents (such as the ^{99m}Tc-phosphonates). Since radiogallium also goes to many of these lesions, in each image (by means of weighting factors) the bone image can be subtracted from that of radiogallium. In a bone infection, excessive radiogallium is present in the lesion (it is incongruent).

Labeled white cells

It has been pointed out that a problem with radiogallium imaging is that the agent was excreted by the intestine and hence the material cannot be used for studying intestinal infections. What of labeling white blood cells? Radioactive indium (^{111}In) can be complexed to the compound 8-hydroxyquinoline (oxine). The ^{111}In oxine complex is relatively stable. When it is incubated with white blood cells, some of the radiopharmaceutical enters the cells. Inside the white cells, indium transfers to intracellular proteins; the oxine then leaves and in essence has the role of a carrier or shuttle. When the ^{111}In white cells are injected intravenously, a portion enters the spleen, liver, and bone marrow. A portion of the remaining labeled cells circulate and may concentrate at sites of inflammation. Since no excretion occurs through the bowel, ^{111}In white blood cells can be employed for studying inflammation of the intestinal canal.

Monoclonal antibodies

The development of monoclonal antibodies opened the way to searching for a number of tumors during life. That is, such antibodies can be radiolabeled by use of ^{111}In, ^{131}I, or other radionuclides and employed in the search for tumors.

When administered intravenously, labeled antibodies have the opportunity to bind slowly to the appropriate antigen; this is the basis for radioimmunoimaging. Although of great potential, the method has a number of practical problems.

1   The rate of disappearance of the antibodies (produced by cleaving the immune globulins by means of digestive enzymes). These labeled fragments disappear from the bloodstream at a more rapid rate than the intact antibody.

2   To correct for radiolabel still in the blood stream, two approaches have been utilized:

a   Antibodies to the first labeled antibody can speed disappearance from the blood.

b   A second label can be placed into the blood and a subtraction performed to correct for the blood content.

The specificity of monoclonal antibodies makes them very attractive for radioimmunoimaging, but further development will depend on solving the problem of slow blood disappearance.

Endocrine System

Multiple organs of the body produce secretions that exit via canals or ducts. For example, the secretory glands near the mouth, which produce saliva, have a well-developed series of drainage canals for delivering the fluids to the mouth cavity. Since their ducts carry the secretions outside the organ into a lumen, the organs are referred to as *exocrine,* or outwardly secreting. By contrast, a variety of other organs send their secretions inward to the body (usually via the bloodstream) and are termed *endocrine,* or inwardly secreting. Their secretions are termed *endocrine* or *hormonal.* The endocrine organs comprise two large groups, depending upon the regulation of their secretions. Some of the endocrine glands have a feedback relationship with the pituitary gland (which is located deep in the brain), for example, the thyroid gland.

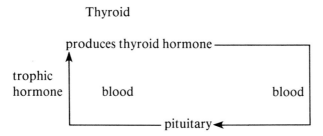

The system is a negative feedback between pituitary and thyroid. That is, if the circulating blood level of thyroid hormone is low, the pituitary secretes thyroid stimulating hormone (TSH), which induces the thyroid to make and secrete thyroid hormone. By contrast, if the blood level of thyroid hormone is high, the pituitary secretion of TSH is reduced (the negative feedback). The following is a partial listing of endocrine organs.

Endocrine Organs under Pituitary Control	Endocrine Organs Not under Pituitary Control
Thyroid	Parathyroid
Testes	Pancreas
Ovary	Adrenal (medulla)
Adrenal (cortex)	Intestinal hormones

One approach to studying the endocrine organs has been to measure the quantity of circulating hormone in the bloodstream. This is accomplished by means of radioimmunoassay (RIA). The principle of RIA is as follows: We are trying to measure the quantity of hormone H. To do so, we add a known amount of radiolabeled hormone H^*. To the mixture of H and H^* is then added an antibody, which binds a percentage of both H and H*. Use of a separatory column or other procedure separates the quantity of H^* bound to the antibody from the unbound H^*. The ratio of H^* bound to H^* unbound is calculated. If much hormone (H) were present, the antibody would principally bind to H and not to H^*. Therefore, with much H, the ratio of H^* bound to H^* unbound would be low. A standard curve of H^* bound to H^* unbound, versus amount of hormone present, is constructed.

Overactivity of an endocrine organ elevates the blood level of the hormone. In such a situation, the blood concentration of the pituitary trophic (stimulatory) hormone is usually depressed. The following chart may be helpful for understanding the relationship between the circulatory (blood) levels of the secretion of an endocrine organ and of the pituitary.

	Blood Level	
	Pituitary Hormone	Endocrine Secretion
Endocrine organ overactivity	Decreased	Increased
Endocrine organ underactivity	Increased	Decreased

Usually the feedback system works well. Sometimes, a portion or all of an endocrine organ fails to respond appropriately to the pituitary signal; this condition is referred to as becoming *autonomous*. In such cases, the endocrine organ continues to secrete hormone into the bloodstream despite low circulating values of the pituitary trophic hormone. On quite rare occasions, the pituitary develops a tumor that oversecretes the trophic hormone. This condition is characterized by elevated blood levels of both the trophic hormone and the endocrine organ's secretion.

Thyroid

One of the origins of nuclear medicine was in studies of the thyroid gland because the thyroid is relatively large (20 to 30 g in an adult) and is located superficially in the neck with little overlying tissue. In addition, the thyroid possesses a great avidity for iodide and radioiodide. The results of many years of study can be described as follows.

The initial keys are the ability of the thyroid to concentrate iodide (I^-) from the bloodstream and the availability of radioactive iodine (in the form of iodide).

Radionuclide	Half-life	Gamma Ray Energy (MeV)	Comments
^{131}I	8.1 days	364	This had been the most commonly utilized radionuclide of iodine for studies during life. However, the long physical half-life and the beta emissions contribute to a significant radiation exposure.
^{123}I	13.1 h	159	The half-life and gamma ray energy are well suited to clinical studies. The material is somewhat expensive and, since it is cyclotron-produced, less readily available in a pure form.
^{125}I	60 days	35	^{125}I is no longer used for imaging the thyroid during life, since the low-energy gamma ray is absorbed by soft tissue. However, ^{125}I is one of the most used radionuclides for test tube (in vitro) assays, such as radioimmunoassay.
^{99m}Tc	6.0 h	140	In the form of pertechnetate ($^{99m}Tc\text{-}O_4-$) the ionic charge and radius appear to resemble iodide; hence pertechnetate is used as an iodide analog for thyroid imaging. However, although pertechnetate is transported by the thyroid gland, it is not made into thyroid hormone (organified).

Before proceeding, it is important to note that assays of the blood levels of the hormones are the first approach to evaluating endocrine organs because such in vitro studies may answer most questions and do not involve radiation exposure. The use of radionuclides in vivo (direct administration to a patient) is justified when morphological (anatomical) information must be obtained in addition to functional data, or when there is a discrepancy between the in vitro tests.

The patient swallows a capsule containing a small amount (microcuries) of radioactive iodide containing several micrograms of I^-. The amount of iodide administered is not enough to perturb the body's iodide stores. At various time intervals, the quantity of radioiodide accumulating in the thyroid is determined by a probe that detects the gamma rays emitted by radioiodide:

1 The neck area is counted at a distance from the probe. Counts recorded are the sum of thyroid contributions, radioactivity in muscles and other neck structures (small but real), and background "noise." These are all part of the neck (N) counts.

2 A body area approximately as large as the neck, such as the lower thigh, is counted to correct for activity in soft tissue and background ($T + B$). The geometry of counting used for assaying the neck is employed (that is, the distance and configuration are unchanged).

3 Again using the identical geometry, the standard is counted; it is equal to the quantity that the patient ingested. These counts are due to standard plus background ($S + B$).

4 The standard is removed and a background count (B) obtained for the same time period.

The following calculation determines the quantity of radioiodide in the thyroid at each point in time:

$$\text{Percentage uptake in thyroid} = \frac{N - (T + B)}{(S + B) - B} \times 100$$

In hyperthyroidism (thyroid overactivity), the quantity of iodide taken up in the gland is usually elevated. In hypothyroidism (thyroid underactivity) the uptake of radioiodide in the thyroid is most often reduced. However, this assumes that the overall size of the iodide pool is the same. If the iodide pool is greatly expanded, as after intake of a significant amount of I^- from food, medicine, or x-ray contrast agents, then radioactive iodide is diluted into a larger pool. The sequence of events in the thyroid can be schematized as follows:

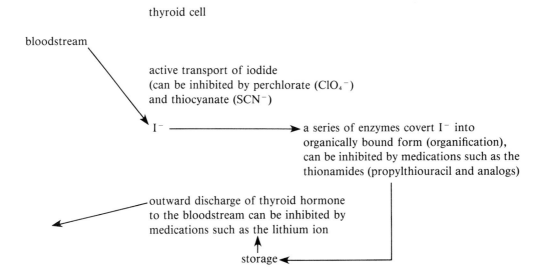

A way to analyze part of the thyroid's activities is to attempt to quantify the amount of iodine in the gland. One of the several possible approaches is fluorescence scanning. A beam of gamma rays is directed at the thyroid. If the energy of the photons is sufficient to displace an inner shell electron, other electrons transit inward to fill the vacancy. The resulting *fluorescence x-ray* (the electron transition from L to K shells) is detected by a solid-state device such as a SiLi detector. The number of emissions is proportional to the quantity of stable iodine present. The distribution of iodine can be "mapped" by moving the fluorescent scanner (activating beam and detectors) back and forth a line at a time. This produces an image that looks like a rectilinear scan. However, the patient does not receive any radioactive material.

A few comments on fluorescence scanning of the thyroid are appropriate:

1   Since the device is expensive and often difficult to maintain (some models require that the detector be kept at the temperature of liquid nitrogen), relatively few of them are in use.

2   However, on some occasions a fluorescence scan (Figure 8.18) is of assistance:

a   It is one of the few imaging modalities that can be used for thyroid evaluation during pregnancy because there is no internally administered radiopharmaceutical and hence no fetal radiation.

b   Fluorescence scanning can be used to monitor compliance in taking thyroid hormone medication. If the patient is prescribed exogenous thyroid medication, endogenous production of TSH (from the pituitary) is suppressed. The thyroid gradually loses its contained hormone and, hence, its iodine content. If the patient has complied in taking the medication, the iodine content of the thyroid should be gradually decreasing.

c   A frequent use of fluorescence scanning is to determine whether a thyroid nodule (lump) contains iodine. If iodine is present, then the nodule is either benign or a well-developed and functioning malignancy that can be treated with radioiodide. The reverse, however, is not true: lack of iodine in a thyroid mass does not prove that it is malignant. Many thyroid benign lesions (cysts and areas of bleeding, for example) also do not contain significant amounts of iodine.

More commonly employed is thyroid emission imaging. The patient receives a radiopharmaceutical that at least partially localizes within the thyroid. The emissions are then detected externally, hence the term *emission imaging*. An emission thyroid scan is a road map of that part of the gland that is transporting radioiodide or an analog. If ^{99m}Tc-pertechnetate is used, images are made about 15 min after the substance is injected intravenously. This means that only the transport system for the iodide analog is being visualized (in addition, pertechnetate cannot be organified). When radioiodide is utilized, the material is given orally, and imaging of the thyroid is performed several hours later. These emission images represent the net effect of both transport and organification with storage.

Thyroid imaging usually demonstrates uniform distribution of radiotracer in the gland (Figure 8.18b). The right lobe is, 90 percent of the time, slightly longer than the left and begins slightly higher in the neck. Intrathyroidal areas having lower uptake of radiotracer are referred to as *cold* (Figure 8.18b); those having increased concentration of the radiopharmaceutical are referred to as *hot*. Thyroidal hot spots are most frequently benign.

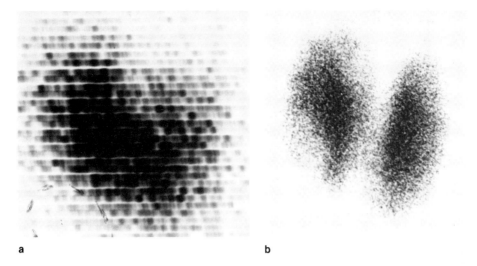

a   b

Figure 8.18 (a) Right anterior oblique fluorescent scan of the thyroid. (b) Anterior emission scan of the same patient, obtained after intravenous administration of ^{99m}Tc pertechnetate.

Radioiodide therapy of hyperthyroidism

A small, but important part of the use of radiopharmaceuticals is in therapy. The most common of these therapeutic applications is in treating the overactive thyroid (hyperthyroidism). The three techniques for reducing thyroid overactivity are antithyroid medication, surgery, and use of radioactive iodine. Antithyroid drugs must be taken each day and have a high incidence of allergic responses or depression of the white blood cell counts. When drugs are taken each day as prescribed, about 60 percent of the cases of hyperthyroidism are in remission after 1 yr. Surgery can be used but only after the overactive gland is brought under control. Surgical removal of part or most of the thyroid, although often successful in treating hyperthyroidism, carries with it the risk of anesthetic-related problems, of damage to nerves to the vocal apparatus, and of removal of the parathyroid glands (small endocrine organs concerned with calcium metabolism, which are usually located in or near the thyroid; these are discussed in a later section).

The third type of therapy for hyperthyroidism is use of radioiodide. Here we are considering quantities about a thousand times greater than that employed for the diagnostic studies. Radioiodide ^{131}I, $T_{1/2} = 8.1$ days) emits gamma rays used for uptake or imaging purposes. The radionuclide also emits beta particles; these weak electrons contribute to the radiation burden of the thyroid but cannot be detected externally (since all their energy is deposited into a small volume of tissue). Current Medical Internal Radiation Dose (MIRD) calculations consider each emission individually. Using the assumption of uniform distribution of the radionuclide within the tissue, one determines the fraction of the total energy that is deposited. For gamma rays, much of the energy escapes the area, and the absorbed fraction is a number much less than 1 (a value of 1 indicates total absorption). For most beta rays with low energy and numerous local interactions, the absorbed fraction approaches 1; that is, nearly all energy is deposited in the tissue.

It is often simpler to revert to the calculations of the "classical method." Consider the beta particles separately from the gamma rays. For *weak* beta particles (low energy and short path length in tissue), we assume that all of the energy is deposited within the thyroid. This is a reasonable assumption, since each lobe of the thyroid gland is about 4 cm in length, and the path length (of the betas from ^{131}I) is a fraction of a millimeter in tissue. The radiation dose is directly proportional to the following:

1   The quantity of radioiodide deposited in the tissue, expressed as C, the concentration, and given in microcuries deposited per gram of tissue.

2   The average beta ray energy, E_B, in terms of million electron volts (MeV). If a radionuclide with a lower beta ray energy is used, less energy would be deposited. For ^{131}I, the emitted beta rays have an average beta ray energy of 0.19 MeV.

3   The effective half-life (because of biological turnover as well as physical decay, the quantity of radioactivity in the thyroid gland decreases with time), $T_{1/2 \text{ eff}}$, expressed in days. The usual value is about 6 days.

The equation for the radiation dose in the thyroid due to the beta emissions is expressed as

$$D = KCE_B T_{1/2 \text{ eff}}$$

When the radiation dose is in units of rads, the constant K has a value of 73.8. These calculations assume uniform distribution of radiotracer and do not compensate for variations in radiation sensitivity.

Let us try a hypothetical case. A patient with an overactive thyroid receives 8 mCi of radioiodide (^{131}I-sodium iodide) orally. The thyroid gland takes up 70 percent of the quantity within 24 h. The thyroid thus has 8 mCi × 70 percent, or 5.6 mCi (5,600 μCi) within its tissue. By serial counting over the thyroid, we find that the effective half time is 5 days. The missing bit of information is the weight of the thyroid, so that we can determine the concentration of ^{131}I (in microcuries per gram). There are formulas for estimating thyroid weight from its appearance on the scans. In this case, the thyroid was about twice normal size, or 40 g:

$$D = (73.8) (5,600) \, \mu\text{Ci}/40 \text{ g}) (0.19 \, \text{MeV}) (5 \text{ days})$$
$$= 9,815 \text{ rads}$$

This is the beta particle contribution to irradiation of the thyroid. There is also a gamma ray contribution, but it is usually only about 10 percent as much. Radioiodide is also used in irradiation of thyroid cancer when the tissue shows the ability to concentrate and retain the iodide.

Skeletal System

Bone is the supporting structure of the body (in the cavity of bone is the marrow, the site of production of blood cells). Three aspects of bone can be investigated by the techniques of nuclear medicine: density of bone, functions of the bone marrow, and activity of the bone matrix (or "hard stuff").

Density of bone

The outer part of bone is composed of a protein (collagen) and large amounts of calcium and phosphorus. The presence of the minerals imparts strength to bone and also gives it a density that is apparent on an x-ray of an extremity. A number of diseases can compromise the density of bone, making it less supportive of the body's weight. That is, when bone mineral is lost, bone is more likely to fracture. One type of loss of bone mineral, *osteoporosis,* occurs in a number of situations and is particularly noted in women after the menopause. The combination of aging and declining estrogen contributes to loss of bone mineral and often debilitating collapse of vertebrae or fracture of other bones. Programs designed to prevent and treat osteoporosis thus have national significance.

The measurement of bone density employs a monoenergetic beam of photons (such as the 35-keV gamma rays from ^{125}I or the 60-keV gamma rays from ^{241}Am). Refer to Figure 8.19 for an idealized diagram of the principle involved in

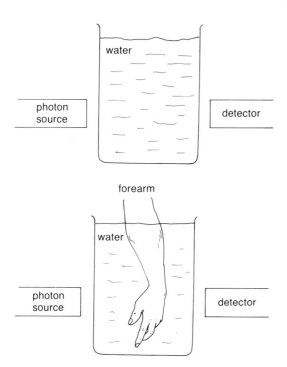

Figure 8.19   The principle of measuring bone density by a monoenergetic photon beam.

bone densitometry. A photon source faces a detector, with an interposed water source. When the forearm is placed into the water, the number of photons passing through to the detector decreases. The forearm consists of water-equivalent tissues (muscle and skin) and denser material (bone). Since water has been displaced, the additional absorption of photons is due to bone mineral. The intensity of photons detected (I) is related to the original intensity (I_0) by

$$I = I_0 e^{-ud}$$

Here u represents the absorption coefficient and d is the distance, or thickness of bone. The equation is solved by placing it into logarithmic form:

$$ud = -\ln \frac{I}{I_0}$$

Bone densitometers have built in the photon source, the detector, and the circuitry for solving the equations. If the thickness of bone is known, then the absorption (density) per unit thickness can be determined.

Single-photon absorptionmetry works well for the forearm bones (radius and ulna) because the tissues are either water-equivalent or bone. However, the procedure does not function appropriately for measurement of the density of the vertebral bodies(lumbar vertebrae).

Why measure the density of the lumbar vertebrae? There is frequently not a good correlation between the density of bones of the forearm and that of the vertebral bodies. Fractures of the vertebrae, with their pain, limitation of motion, and possible damage to the spinal cord, are of greatest concern.

Why is the single photon technique ineffective with the lumbar vertebrae? In addition to water-equivalent tissues and bone, there is also fat present, as the beam goes through the vertebrae and internal tissues before exiting. To compensate for this, two distinct photon beams are required (that is, two photons each with a different energy). For example, some of the dual beam or dual energy bone densitometers utilize radioactive gadolinium (^{153}Gd) as the source. This radionuclide has two photons, which have 44-keV and 100-keV energy. The differential absorption of these two different gamma rays allows the calculation of both bone mineral and fat content.

Bone marrow

The central cavity of most bones contains cells of two types: phagocytic cells (reticuloendothelial) and precursors of red blood cells (erythrons).

Bone marrow imaging can be performed by using radioactive colloids (such as ^{99m}Tc-sulfur colloid). This material is distributed as follows: about 80 percent to the liver, 10 percent to the spleen, and 10 percent to the bone marrow. Thus a small amount is distributed over a large volume of bone marrow (an imaging thus takes a longer time since the count rate is low). Some other radiocolloids have a smaller particle size, such as technetium-antimony colloid (about 0.1 μm in diameter, versus 1 μm for ^{99m}Tc-sulfur colloid). These smaller agents go to the bone marrow in larger amounts; however, they are also cleared from the bloodstream more slowly. The assumption that the distribution of the phagocytic cells is the same as that of the erythrons is usually valid; however, in some diseases one of the cell types may be affected more than the other.

The unusual property of red cells is their iron content. Indeed, about 90 percent of iron within the body is contained in circulating red blood cells. Theoretically, radioactive iron can be used to follow uptake into the red cell precursors. However, nature has not provided a readily usable radionuclide of iron. The available ^{59}Fe has a long half-life (45 days) and energetic emissions. However, in small amounts, about 10 μCi, radioiron can be injected intravenously and used to follow blood disappearance, sites of deposition, and eventual incorporation into red blood cells. Radioiron usually enters the bloodstream as a ferrous salt. It binds to a protein in the plasma, transferrin. From transferrin, the radioiron is deposited into regions that are either storing iron or using it for making red blood cells. By placing probes over various regions, serially, one can plot the time-activity relationship. An area of effective erythropoiesis (red cell production) shows uptake of radioiron, followed by slow discharge into red cells that then enter the bloodstream.

Since there are no readily available iron radionuclides with desirable imaging characteristics, can an iron analog be used? Indium is such an element, and a number of indium radionuclides are available. For example, ^{111}Indium has a physical half-life of 2.8 days, and gamma ray emissions of 173 and 247 keV. When administered intravenously as indium chloride, the metallic ion binds to transferrin. However, some of the indium also forms a colloid that deposits in the liver and spleen. The presence of radioindium in the liver or spleen can, therefore, not be used as evidence that sites of unusual red cell production are present in those organs.

Bone scans

One of the most frequently called upon procedures in nuclear medicine is the bone scan (Figure 8.20). To look at the metabolic activity of bone, analogs of calcium or phosphorus have to be employed (since there are no acceptable radionuclides of Ca or P that can be used for imaging). Compounds presently in use bind radioactive technetium to analogs of pyrophosphate:

$$
\begin{array}{ccccc}
O & & & O & \\
\| & & & \| & \text{Pyrophosphate} \\
P & - & O & - & P \\
| & & & | & \\
(OH)_2 & & & (OH)_2 &
\end{array}
$$

One of these is methylenediphosphonate (MDP):

$$
\begin{array}{ccccc}
O & & & O & \\
\| & & H & \| & \text{Methylenediphosphonate (MDP)} \\
P & - & C & - & P \\
| & & H & | & \\
(OH)_2 & & & (OH)_2 &
\end{array}
$$

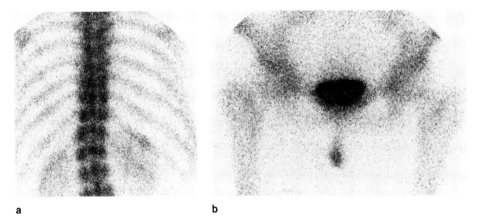

a   b

Figure 8.20   Bone scans. (a) Gamma camera faced the patient's back. (b) Gamma camera faced the front of the pelvis.

When ^{99m}Tc-MDP is administered intravenously, it is rapidly cleared from the bloodstream, with about one half of the material excreted in the urine (the kidneys and bladder can be evaluated) and the other half deposited in bone. More pertinently, deposition apparently represents metabolic activity in bone. When a bone is fractured, deposition of the bone imaging material does not increase immediately. A number of hours later, if the bone-avid agent is injected intravenously, it deposits in large amounts in the fracture site. That is, increased activity does not occur at first. Bone scans to search for microfractures after an accident (if an x-ray of the area is negative) require that a sufficient interval (up to 48 h in some cases) elapse to produce results.

The major application of bone scans has been in searching for the spread of malignant tumors to bone (usually by transport through the bloodstream). For example, cancers of the breast in women and of the prostate in men frequently metastasize to bone. Early in bone spread of these tumors, x-ray indicates no evidence of change. However, the bone scan can reveal areas of increased uptake where metastases are located. If we consider x-rays of an area and a bone scan of the same region, there are four possibilities. In box 1, both the x-ray and the bone scan are positive. The lesion is metabolically active and visible on the x-ray. In box 4, the x-

		X-ray	
		+	−
Bone scan	+	① + +	② − +
	−	③ + −	④ − −

ray and bone scan are both negative. This is not to say that no lesion is present; it simply denotes that it is not possible to detect anything by these two powerful procedures. What of the two boxes in which the x-rays and bone scans do not agree? Box 3 denotes positive x-rays and negative bone scans.

This condition occurs in only about 5 percent of bone scans and has two principal causes: (1) Some tumors dissolve bone and yet do not produce a bone-forming (osteoblastic) response. One reason is that certain tumors, for example, multiple myeloma, produce chemicals that inhibit the osteoblastic reaction. (2) Another reason for a positive x-ray but a negative bone scan is that the metabolic response may have occurred some time ago and then decreased with time. For example, when a vertebral body fractures, there is an intense metabolic response. Over a period of months, this decreases. Bone scans can indicate whether a fracture site is metabolically active.

Box 2 (x-ray negative, bone scan positive) demonstrates is the reason that bone scans are performed. Many lesions can be detected by use of bone scans, prior to any major changes on x-rays:

1 Osteomyelitis is an infection in bone. The bone scan can show an area of increased uptake at the site of infection. If the bone scan is not positive, it can be repeated in 1 or 2 days, or a radiogallium study may be considered.

2 Stress fractures are microscopic fractures that develop along the medial surface of bones after unusual stress (such as long marches). The bone scan can show these before any x-ray changes are apparent.

3 Metabolic changes result when any of a number of hormones is overproduced in the body. The response in bone may be exaggerated, for example, when a calcium-regulating hormone (parathyroid hormone) is produced in excessive amounts. The outer part of bone (periosteum) has a diffuse and increased uptake of the technetium-phosphate. Some diseases also produce areas of decreased deposition of the bone imaging radiopharmaceutical. When blood flow to a portion of bone is absent, the bone imaging agent cannot be deposited. This occurs when a major vessel to bone is blocked (avascular necrosis) and the region of bone becomes nonfunctional.

Urinary System

The production and transit of urine can be readily followed by the use of radioactive pharmaceuticals. That is, kidney accumulation of radiolabel from the bloodstream, excretion into urine, passage down the ureters into the bladder, and finally passage out the urethra can all be monitored. The study does not have the elegant anatomical resolution of radiographic studies of the kidneys. Why then are the nuclear medicine images of the urinary system so useful? There are a number of reasons:

1 The radiopharmaceutical-based studies are functional evaluations. That is, they examine a specific function of the urinary system.

2 These studies can be made quantitative. Data are acquired and then computer-processed to derive such quantities as relative blood flow to each kidney and concentrating ability of each side.

3 Such radionuclide studies give only a small radiation exposure. This can be an important consideration when serial studies are to be performed over a period of time.

4 The nuclear medicine studies of the urinary system do not give an allergic response and do not load the system with an osmotic burden.

The purpose of these studies is thus to obtain data about the function of the urinary apparatus and not on its fine anatomical structure. Thus such radionuclide-based assays have a distinct role.

Urine is made by blood passing through loops of capillaries, the *glomeruli*. This glomerular filtrate is the first part of the fluid and solutes that form the urine. The glomerular filtrate is then processed (added to or subtracted from) by active events in the kidney tubules. Tubular secretion or absorption thus modifies the glomerular filtrate. For example, glucose and most nutrients are "pulled out" of the glomerular filtrate by the renal tubules. On the other hand, the tubules actively secrete a number of chemical species from the blood into the exiting fluid. To give meaning to urine production, there are thus several steps to assay.

The material most frequently utilized for radionuclide evaluations of the kidneys is a glomerular agent (one filtered out by the glomeruli) that is not appreciably augmented or decremented by the tubules. The radiopharmaceutical ^{99m}Tc-DTPA is a chelate and biologically inert. Upon intravenous administration, it is carried by the bloodstream to the kidneys. The patient is positioned so that the back and hence the kidneys are close to the gamma camera. Information generated is fed to a computer-compatible system.

In the first several seconds, as blood and its contained radioactivity arrives at the kidneys, the relative amount entering each kidney (background corrected) can be ascertained: that is, the relative blood flow to each kidney is determined. This does not give a value such as flow in terms of volume per minute; it indicates what portion of blood going to the two kidneys is arriving at the right and the left. In some cases of hypertension (high blood pressure), the cause is related to reduced blood flow to one kidney. The origin can be a blood clot partially occluding the vessel to the kidney or a constriction of the muscle around the vessel wall. In either case, however, the result is the same: reduced flow to one kidney and renovascular hypertension. The diagnosis is important, since the vessel may be potentially repaired by surgery (with cure of the hypertension). The radionuclide study uses ^{99m}Tc-DTPA and measures relative flow of the kidneys during the first pass of blood down the aorta into the renal vasculature.

Once blood, with its contained ^{99m}Tc-DTPA, arrives at the kidneys, the radiopharmaceutical begins to undergo filtration via the glomeruli. That is, the radiolabel begins to enter into the process that will make the urine. Renal function is studied in terms of clearance (*C*): a certain volume of blood is cleared of a particular substance per unit time. The formula for clearance is as follows:

$$C = \frac{U \cdot V}{P}$$

Where U is the urine concentration of the material, P is its plasma concentration (since they have the same units, they cancel), and V is the urine volume during the study period. Hence, clearance represents the volume of blood cleared of an agent. Since ^{99m}Tc-DTPA leaves the body only via the urine, it can be used to measure the glomerular filtration rate (GFR). There is another interesting way to measure GFR with the radiolabel: the ^{99m}Tc-DTPA molecule is small and is widely distributed in the body, entering almost all of extracellular water. Since the kidneys are the only route of excretion of ^{99m}Tc-DTPA, the rate of disappearance from a site such as the thigh must reflect kidney function. As long as the volume of extracellular fluid is normal, the clearance of ^{99m}Tc-DTPA from body sites can be employed to indicate kidney function. Usually, 0.8 to 1.0 percent of the extracellular fluid is cleared of ^{99m}Tc-DTPA per minute after it has been widely distributed. In kidney disease, this percentage can be drastically reduced.

As the radiopharmaceutical is cleared from the bloodstream, the kidneys become more prominent on the images, and the "background" falls. After the blood or perfusion phase and the entry of activity in the kidneys, urine is secreted and enters the collecting system. From there, it usually quickly passes down the ureters, toward the bladder. Only when there is obstruction the ureters become quite apparent. If there is delayed exit of the activity from the kidneys, two possibilities must be considered: reduced wash-out related to a small urine flow and true mechanical obstruction. To distinguish between these the diuretic assisted renogram is used. That is, at about 20 min into the study, a diuretic (an agent that increases urine production) is given intravenously. Movement of activity downward shows that mechanical obstruction is not present.

Figure 8.21(a) shows the two kidneys from the posterior, after intravenous administration of ^{99m}Tc-DTPA; the left (slightly higher) and right kidneys are clearly visible. Several minutes later (Figure 8.21[b]), activity should be moving downward as additional ^{99m}Tc-DTPA is filtered and that in the kidneys exits. However, two focal collections are apparent. There is slight retention in the right kidney and major retention on the left. Further, low on the left a collection of activity is visible outside the kidney; it is due to retention in the ureter or a pouch off the ureter. Figure 8.21(c) is a lateral view of the left kidney, ureter, and bladder, some minutes later.

Additional radiopharmaceuticals can probe other functions of the kidneys. Active tubular section can be monitored by means of orthoiodohippuric acid (carrying radioiodine), which is usually rapidly secreted by the tubular system and quickly exits. The technetium-based compound dimercaptosuccinic acid binds to the renal tubules transiently and can be used for examining relative tubular mass. This compound binds ^{99m}Tc; when given intravenously, it attaches to the renal tubules.

$$
\begin{array}{l}
\mathrm{COOH} \\
\quad | \\
\mathrm{HS-C-H} \\
\quad | \\
\mathrm{HS-C-H} \\
\quad | \\
\mathrm{COOH}
\end{array}
\qquad
\begin{array}{c}
\text{dimercaptosuccinic} \\
\text{acid}
\end{array}
$$

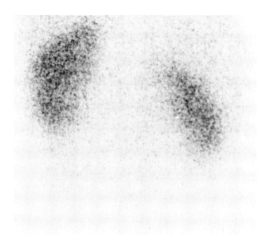

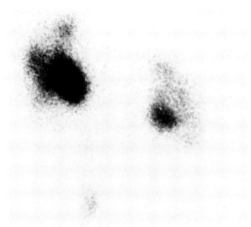

a

b

Figure 8.21   Images from a ^{99m}Tc-DTPA renal evaluation. (a) Posterior view of kidneys (left kidney higher). (b) Image obtained some minutes later. (c) Left lateral view (anterior to the viewer's left).

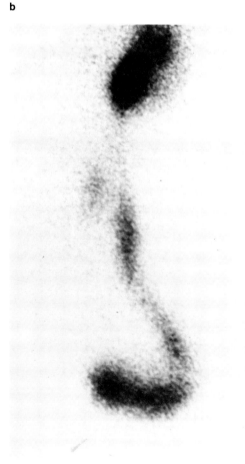

c

One use of these studies has been in following renal transplants. The initial question to be answered is whether the surgical site of joining the renal artery from the transplanted kidney into the patient's own blood vessels is still open. This, and subsequent evaluation of function, can be determined by use of the radiotracers. It is also used after surgery on the urinary tract, when serial evaluation of function is needed.

Central Nervous System

The *central nervous system* comprises the brain and spinal cord. Radionuclide studies played an important role in the initial evaluation of these sites. Subsequently, computerized tomographic studies nearly entirely replaced the radiopharmaceutical examinations, since they could evaluate not only brain density but that of the contained cerebrospinal fluid canal as well. The dramatic resurgence of radionuclide studies has been due to a "new generation" of compounds that enter into the brain and map specific functions. Hence, we will examine both the classical approach to brain scans and the recent methodology.

First we will focus on the fluid that circulates through the center of the spinal cord and the brain, the *cerebrospinal fluid* (CSF). Production of CSF occurs in portions of the brain referred to as the *choroid plexus,* which secretes both fluid and other consituents such as electrolytes and drugs. Passage of the CSF is due entirely to secretion of additional material within the brain and its outward migration with absorption occurring over the convexity of the brain. A radiopharmaceutical introduced into the CSF at any of a number of points (usually in the lumbar [low back] region) is carried upward by bulk flow (or by a mixture of convection and flow). Usually passage proceeds readily, with a block suggesting a mechanical or functional obstruction of CSF circulation. Upon reaching the level of the brain, the radiolabel can pass inward via connections or communications between fluid within the brain and that outside. *Hydrocephalus* (literally "water head") is the build-up of fluid within the brain; if the radiolabel can pass across the communications, it is called *communicating hydrocephalus.* In some cases, the passages are closed by scarring or infection. Since the therapies for these two types of hydrocephalus differ, the functional information is of great importance.

The foundation for brain scans was the observation that although most foreign materials injected intravenously had wide distribution on the body, they entered into the brain. It is recognized that brain capillaries differ from those in most other locales and prevent foreign molecules from entering the brain; the functional exclusion is called the *blood-brain barrier* (BBB). When the blood-brain barrier is damaged, for example, by stroke (blood vessel obstruction) or tumor, then molecules previously not permitted to enter can go into the brain. In a brain scan, the usual image is of regional structures but not of the brain.

Refer to Figure 8.22(a), which is an anterior view of a brain scan, taken 1 h after intravenous administration of approximately 15 mCi of a soluble ^{99m}Tc compound (such as DTPA or glucoheptonate). The outer rim of the skull is visible, as are inner major vessels that have radioactivity in the blood (such as the midline

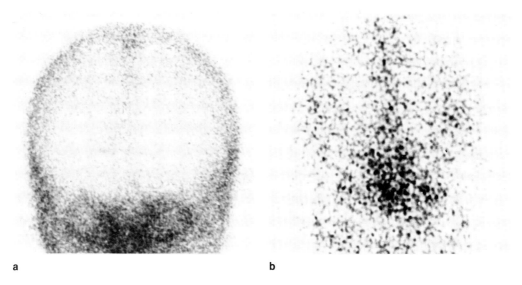

a   b

Figure 8.22   (a) Anterior view of a brain scan. (b) Sequence
from an anterior cerebral dynamic study.

structure, which is the draining vein or sinus). The brain itself has little radioactivity. Only when there has been disruption of the barrier are major amounts of the radiolabel found in the brain. A preliminary part of the study, the *cerebral dynamic study*, was often quite helpful: In it the passage of radioactivity into the brain was followed to determine whether disruption of any of the major vessels had occurred. A soluble radiolabel injected into an arm vein passes to the heart (right side), lungs, left side of the heart, and then into the general circulation and the arteries going up the neck (the common carotids).

Figure 8.22(b) is an anterior view of the common carotid arteries as they pass up the neck. Just before entering the skull, the common carotid gives off the external carotid branch; it then continues to the brain as the internal carotid artery. The central "hot" area on the image is the switching point or junction for cerebral circulation known as the *circle of Willis*. Coming up the two sides are the main blood supply for the brain, the middle cerebral arteries. In the midline, two anterior cerebral vessels supply the midline. The posterior cerebral blood vessels are not apparent on this view as they are posterior structures. From this *arterial phase*, blood enters a capillary phase and finally into the venous channels that drain the area. The cerebral dynamic study was thus a time sequence analysis of the major blood flow to and from the brain. It can be useful in blood vessel obstruction, in outpouchings or aneurysms of the great vessels, and in the abnormal passage of blood to tumors or to arteriovenous shunts.

Although a major step forward, radionuclide brain scans were largely replaced by computerized tomographic studies, which could delineate many abnormalities due to subtle differences in the density of lesions (and the CSF) as compared with the normal brain. However, brain scans are again useful because of materials that readily cross the blood-brain barrier. For example, it is known that the brain uses glucose as its principal metabolite. The compound 2-deoxy-2-fluoroglucose has been synthesized with the positron-emitting [18]F (half-life of 1.7 h). This agent crosses the blood-brain barrier, is phosphorylated as though it were glucose, and then does not undergo any additional steps of glucose metabolism. It is said to be *metabolically trapped* and can be imaged by suitable devices such as the positron emission tomograph (PET) scanner. The significance is that a map can be developed of glucose metabolism in each area of the brain. As various regions of the brain are activated, their metabolism of glucose changes, and this change can be observed. In instances of localized abnormal discharge of brain activity (focal epilepsy) the regions demonstrate reduced glucose consumption during the period between seizures and elevated glucose use during and just after the seizure.

Other positron-emitting radionuclides such as ^{11}C ($T_{1/2}$ of 20 min) and ^{13}N ($T_{1/2}$ of 10 min) can be synthesized into organic compounds that cross from the bloodstream into the brain, allowing estimation of regional brain metabolism. This has been called a "window on the brain"; for the first time in history, it is feasible to delineate the location and extent of brain metabolic functions in health and disease.

Other measurements are feasible using the "conventional," or single photon emitting, radionuclides. For example, after labeling of red blood cells with ^{99m}Tc, cross-sectional images of the brain can delineate the regions of the brain that have a blood pool and have been deprived of blood (as following obstruction of a blood vessel in the area). It has been demonstrated that a series of amines readily crosses from the blood to the brain. Labeled amines, extracted from entering blood on the first pass, are thus indicators of the efficacy or more likely patency of blood flow. A series of iodine-labeled amphetamine analogs are known and have been employed in examining blood delivery to areas of the brain. There are other radionuclide techniques for looking at brain blood flow. One involves administering a radioactive inert gas such as xenon 133 by injection or inhalation; the rate of wash-out of the gas from the brain substance is proportional to blood leaving the region.

Radionuclide studies of the brain have gone full cycle from use, through disuse, to rebirth with a variety of agents, from those that focus on metabolism to those that measure blood flow.

Evaluation of the Heart

Diseases of the heart and blood vessels are the leading cause of death in the United States. Noninvasive procedures for evaluating these structures are therefore of considerable importance. Nuclear medicine has several procedures available for examining the heart wall (myocardium) and heart function.

Probes of abnormal myocardium

Radiopharmaceuticals that localize in the abnormal or damaged (usually oxygen-deficient) heart wall are useful in diagnosis. One of these is ^{99m}Tc-pyrophosphate.

It was a chance observation that this bone imaging agent localized in heart wall damaged by oxygen deprivation (as during a heart attack). At about 6 h after a portion of the heart wall is deprived of oxygen by obstruction of the blood vessel, sufficient changes have occurred that subsequently injected intravenous ^{99m}Tc-pyrophosphate localizes in the damaged portion of the heart wall. Not only does bone take up this technetium-phosphate, but the damaged myocardium also shows localization. This peaks at about 48 h after the blood vessel has been blocked. Persistence after about the fifth day is thought to represent continuing damage to the heart by extension of the infarct (the dying zone of heart tissue). Uptake of ^{99m}Tc-pyrophosphate also occurs in the heart, but to a lesser degree and in a more diffuse pattern, in inflammation of the heart (myocarditis) and in some cases of involvement of the sac around the heart (pericarditis).

A second probe of the abnormal myocardium uses a labeled monoclonal antibody that is directed against an intracellular component (it is an antibody against the muscle protein myosin; normally, myosin is located entirely intracellularly). Usually, the antimyosin cannot bind to myosin, since the heavy antibody molecule can not penetrate into intact living cells. When antimyosin labeled with ^{131}I or other radionuclide is given intravenously, it does not show any appreciable uptake by the heart. In a "heart attack" or damage of part of the wall via blood vessel obstruction, oxygen deprivation results, and the cells in the region become abnormally permeable. Hence, the labeled antimyosin can bind to myosin in or leaking from cells in the damaged region. Uptake of labeled antimyosin both signals that the heart has been damaged and shows which portion is involved.

Probes of normal myocardium

The principal positive ion within muscle is potassium. When radioactive potassium is given intravenously, it is widely distributed in the body and largely passes intracellularly. However, no readily available potassium radionuclide emits gamma rays suitable for imaging. A potassium analog, thallium 201 (^{201}Tl) does have emissions that are readily detected. When about 2 mCi of ^{201}Tl-thallous chloride is injected intravenously, some localizes in the heart, viscera, and other structures. More can be directed to the heart, and less to the viscera, by exercising the patient. That is, the patient exercises (for example, on a treadmill) while the heart signal is monitored with an electrocardiogram. At the peak of exercise, the radiothallium is injected intravenously, and exercise continues for another minute. The patient is then placed under a gamma camera, with imaging performed anteriorly and at various angles around the chest to examine the left ventricle adequately. That part of the heart, which does most of the pumping of blood, is much thicker and more metabolically active then the right ventricle. Hence, considerably more ^{201}Tl enters the left heart wall than the right. Radiothallium images (Figure 8.23) are metabolic maps of the left side of the heart. The left ventricle usually has rather uniform distribution of radiothallium, except for thinning near the tip or apex. What is the significance of a defect in the myocardium on a radiothallium study? There are two possibilities: First, the defect could represent a region of infarction (tissue deprived of oxygen and essentially nonviable). Second, the area of reduced radiothallium uptake may represent a region transiently lacking in oxygen (ischemia

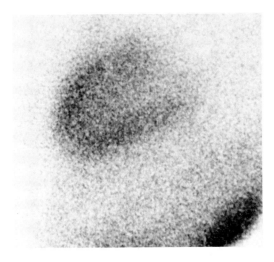

Figure 8.23   Left side of the chest after intravenous radiothallium.

during exercise) but still viable. How can the two situations be distinguished? The patients are allowed to rest for three h and then brought back for reimaging. If the region were infarcted, it would show little change after 3 hours; the infarcted area does not show increased potassium exchange after rest. However, if the region were simply low on oxygen during exercise but could regain viability during rest, then it would again show the ability to exchange potassium (and radiothallium). Hence, the delayed or reperfusion images are of importance in distinguishing low-oxygen (hypoxic) regions from those that have become nonviable.

Functional analysis of the heart

Up to this point, we have been focusing on the heart wall; another perspective is provided by heart function, rather than the appearance of the wall. We can examine the efficiency with which heart is functioning by the way it pumps the contained blood. The images will be of the contained blood pool and not of the heart wall. What is injected is either human serum albumin labeled with ^{99m}Tc or labeled red cells (tagged by first injection of stannous phosphate and then ^{99m}Tc-pertechnetate). We can then image the blood pool in the heart and great vessels. When this occurs as the blood is rushing through after injection into an arm vein, it is a *first pass study*. More commonly, the blood pool is examined after the tagged plasma or red cells have equilibrated.

   If images of the beating heart are made continuously, a blurred view of the area results. What is needed is a signal to turn the gamma camera off and on so that the contained blood pool is visualized in well-defined stages of cardiac contraction or relaxation. We wish somehow to "gate" the views. The gating device is the electrocardiogram (Figure 8.24). The signal produced is marked by the R wave or signal for the ventricle to contract. After the R wave the heart is fully contracted; some time later it relaxes, and an image taken for a few microseconds will show the blood pool of the fully dilated or filled heart. The electrocardiogram signals the gamma camera when to acquire images. The procedure can be taken one step fur-

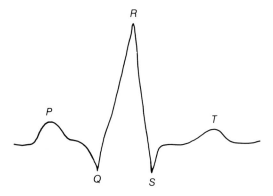

Figure 8.24 Idealized output of an electrocardiogram. R wave is the electrical signal for the ventricles to contract.

ther: The interval between one R wave and the next is divided into 24 time intervals. As the R wave is recorded, counts coming in are sorted into the correct storage area in the computer. As the next R wave comes along, it resets the system so that the following counts are correctly sorted out by the time that they appeared after the R wave trigger. Many heart beats are processed to provide enough information for each time slot. Once the information is played back in cinemode or continual motion, a continuously moving image of the intracardiac blood pool appears. Areas that are moving normally are referred to as *normokinetic;* underactive areas are *hypokinetic;* those not moving at all are *akinetic.* Finally, some areas of the heart (as inferred from the motion of the contained blood pool) are moving "the wrong way" (while the heart is contracting, they are bulging out, indicating either an aneurysm or a region that is not receiving the contraction signal on time).

In addition to estimation of cardiac function during rest, cardiac function can also be assessed during exercise. The *ejection fraction* is the percentage of blood within the ventricle that is squeezed out as the heart contracts. The ejection fraction is a number between 0 and 1; it reflects the efficiency of the heart as a pump. The two ventricles are considered separately. The left ventricle is the chamber that pumps blood through the high-resistance area of the body. The left ventricular ejection fraction (LVEF) is 0.55 or greater (an efficiency of 55 percent or more in health). The right ventricular ejection fraction (RVEF) can be 0.45 or greater. It is often less than LVEF since the right ventricle is larger, and the same quantity of blood can be moved through the low-resistance (pulmonary or lung) circuit with a lower pumping efficiency.

As a patient exercises, for example, lying supine and pumping a bicycle, two events occur: The heart rate increases; the LVEF also increases. That is, the heart pumps more blood during exercise because of a more rapid pump rate and because of greater efficiency of the pump. Normally the LVEF increases by 0.05 (5 percent) or more during exercise. If the heart is damaged and just making its way at rest, function may markedly deteriorate during exercise. That is, the heart may appear to be functioning adequately during rest; when the heart is stressed but blood flow to the coronary arteries cannot increase (coronary vessel disease), then heart function can markedly deteriorate and LVEF may decrease. Also during exercise, abnormalities of wall motion may develop. To monitor the degree of exercise, the *double product* is used. If the heart rate is 80 beats per minute at first and blood pressure (systolic/diastolic) is 120/80, then the double product is the product of heart rate and systolic pressure ($80 \times 120 = 9,600$). The double product is related to oxygen consumption and increases as exercise becomes more strenuous. When the heart rate climbs to 130 and the blood pressure to 150/90, the double product is $130 \times 150 = 19,500$. When clinically possible patients exercise to maximal tolerance to bring the double product close to 20,000. The heart can, of course, be monitored both before and after coronary artery bypass surgery to determine whether functional improvement has occurred.

SUMMARY OF CLINICAL STUDIES

Many other studies are used in nuclear medicine, to measure functional indices such as gastrointestinal absorption, passage of food, and working of internal structures. Since they can be readily performed and give clinically useful data, their use may expand. However, the majority of present tests are summarized in Table 8.3 beginning on page 342. In addition, several studies have incorporated interventions with medications or physiological techniques. Whichever way medicine may evolve, it is likely that radiotracer studies will provide clinically significant data.

FUTURE DEVELOPMENT

From the present perspective, there appear to be only two techniques that can probe the chemistry of the body during life. These methodologies are magnetic resonance imaging and nuclear medicine. Hence, if information about chemistry and function prove to be paramount in the development of medicine, then these two disciplines will have a major role to play.

Evolution of nuclear medicine will depend on three factors. The first is the availability of radiopharmaceuticals that can take advantage of unique metabolic pathways. For example, analogs of nutrients (bearing a suitable radiolabel) might be employed to probe pathways of intermediary metabolism. Radiolabeled monoclonal antibodies may be fashioned to mark the boundary layer of cells; whether such large molecules will be able to penetrate cells without some "opening" of the membrane is conjectural. The second factor is the development of new instrumentation for providing both dynamic and tomographic aspects of the studies in nuclear medicine. Cross-sectional images, and their change with time, may give detailed information on binding and release of probing molecules. The third factor is the ability to process data. That is, more development is needed in the software for nuclear medicine, so that processing can be done faster and with equal or greater precision.

Table 8.3   Major clinical procedures in nuclear medicine (by organ system)

Organ or Function	Radiopharmaceutical	Procedure
Adrenal, cortex	Iodocholesterol-^{131}I	Adrenal cortex uses cholesterol to make its hormones. Functional tumors take up more of the radiolabel than surroundings.
Adrenal, medulla	meta-iodobenzylguanidine-^{131}I	The central part of the adrenal makes epinephrine-like chemicals. m-IBG enters this process. It can delineate tumors of the adrenal medulla (pheochromocytoma) and related tumors (such as neuroblastoma).
Bone, density	Single beam, forearm: ^{125}I or ^{241}Am external sources Dual beam, lumbar vertebrae: ^{153}Gd	Differential absorption of single photons by bones in forearm can be used to measure density of radius, and ulna. With lumbar vertebrae, fat is present in the path length, and a second energy photon beam must be used for correction (^{153}Gd has photons of 44- and 100-keV energy).
Bone, marrow	Radiocolloids (e.g., ^{99m}Tc-sulfur colloid) Iron and its analogs, (e.g., indium 111) to study uptake in red cell precursor areas	Bone marrow has 2 major cell types. One is the phagocytes, which take up radiocolloid. The other cell type (red cell precursor or erythrons) accumulates radioiron. Radioindium transfers to the bone marrow but does not incorporate into red cells.
Bone, matrix	^{99m}Tc-diphosphonates	Delivery to bone is by blood flow. Uptake is likely to the surface of the matrix, in areas of bone cell (osteoblast) activity.
Brain, blood-brain barrier	^{99m}Tc-DTPA	This chelate usually does not accumulate in the brain. Damage to the blood-brain barrier, by tumor, vascular accident, or trauma, allows entry.
Brain, perfusion	^{123}I-iodoamphetamines	Several compounds cross the blood-brain barrier and are extracted by the brain in proportion to blood flow or perfusion to the area.
Brain, receptor sites	^{11}C or ^{18}F nutrients	These are cyclotron-produced and positron-emitting radionuclides, which can be made into nutrients and drugs of biological importance.
Esophagus, aberrant cells	^{99m}Tc-pertechnetate	Stomach-like cells are present in the esophagus which can be detected by their uptake of the radiolabel.
Esophagus, reflux	^{99m}Tc-DTPA	A liquid acidified load is given orally with radiolabel present. If reflux occurs spontaneously or after pressure on the stomach, upward movement can be detected.

Table 8.3   Major clinical procedures in nuclear medicine (by organ system)
continued

Organ or Function	Radiopharmaceutical	Procedure
Esophagus, transit	^{99m}Tc-sulfur colloid	Upon swallowing in the standing position, the bolus usually clears from the esophagus in 5–6 s. There is only slight prolongation on lying flat. Diseases of the esophageal muscle greatly prolong transit.
Gastrointestinal bleeding	^{99m}Tc-red blood cells	The radioactive cells are given intravenously, and imaging of the abdomen is performed. If there is active bleeding, a site of accumulation of radiolabel is noted; motility of the gut may propel this away from the initial site.
Heart, function	^{99m}Tc–red blood cells or ^{99m}Tc–human serum albumin	Function of the heart is inferred from its ability to pump contained red cells or plasma. The *ejection fraction* is the percentage of blood in the ventricle that is pumped out.
Heart, wall (myocardium)	^{201}Tl-thallous chloride	This material is a potassium analog and localizes in the heart wall when given intravenously. During exercise, more accumulates in the heart and less in the intestinal area.
Liver, partition of blood flow	^{99m}Tc–red blood cells or ^{99m}Tc–human serum albumin	The appearance of an intravascular label in the liver is monitored and computer-processed. The initial component is from the hepatic artery; portal vein flow appears some seconds later.
Liver, hepatobiliary function	^{99m}Tc-iminodiacetic acid derivatives	These compounds are rapidly extracted from the bloodstream by the liver; they then exit in the bile, allowing delineation of the pathway and the gallbladder.
Liver, pump flow	^{99m}Tc-macroaggregated albumin	Some patients have an implanted pump that delivers chemotherapy to tumors in the liver, via the hepatic artery. The large particles (15 μm) are injected into the system to observe whether flow is to the tumor and whether any shunts through to the lungs.
Liver, reticuloendothelial function	^{99m}Tc-sulfur colloid	This radiocolloid (particle size about 1 μm) is extracted from the bloodstream by liver, spleen, and other sites of reticuloendothelial function.

Table 8.3   Major clinical procedures in nuclear medicine (by organ system)
continued

Organ or Function	Radiopharmaceutical	Procedure
Muscles, striated	^{99m}Tc-diphosphonates ^{201}Tl-thallous chloride	In rhabdomyolysis (breakdown of muscles) uptake of the bone imaging agents occurs. Radiothallium enters muscle and can be used to compare usually symmetrical groups of muscle.
Parathyroid	^{201}Tl-thallous chloride ^{99m}Tc-pertechnetate	When given intravenously, the potassium analog (radiothallium) distributes to thyroid, parathyroid, and other neck tissues. Upon subtracting out the thyroid (by its uptake of pertechnetate), the parathyroids can often be delineated.
Red blood cell, production	^{59}Fe-ferrous citrate	When given intravenously, the radioiron binds to transferrin and is then deposited in bone marrow. The radioiron is then incorporated into newly forming red cells and appears in the circulation.
Red blood cells, destruction	^{51}Cr-sodium chromate	This is a random label in that cells of all ages are radiolabeled. The tag is lost when the cell is destroyed; some is also eluted (washed off the cells).
Skin, blood flow	^{133}Xe in saline	This is injected into the skin; the rate of wash-out is proportional to blood flow.
Spleen	^{99m}Tc-sulfur colloid	The spleen also has phagocytic or reticuloendothelial function (as does the liver).
Stomach emptying	Liquid: ^{99m}Tc DTPA Solid: ^{99m}Tc-sulfur colloid in food	Liquids empty faster than solids from the stomach. If distinguishable labels are used (such as ^{111}In and ^{99m}Tc) differential emptying can be determined.
Thyroid, function	^{123}I; sometimes ^{131}I	Iodide is concentrated from the blood stream by the thyroid. Longer-lived ^{131}I is used when serially following thyroid content.
Thyroid, imaging	Radioiodide (^{123}I, or ^{131}I for thyroid cancer) ^{99m}Tc-pertechnetate	Both radioiodide and pertechnetate are actively transported by thyroid cells. Iodide incorporated into thyroid hormone; pertechnetate is not.
Testes, blood flow	^{99m}Tc–red blood cells	A variety of radiolabels have been used to determine whether blood flow to the testes is compromised in torsion (twisting).
Vitamin B_{12} absorption	^{57}Co-vitamin B_{12}	Absorption is measured by flushing out part of the quantity absorbed and counting urinary radioactivity.

REFERENCES

Alavi, A., and Reivich, M. 1984. Functional imaging of the brain in central nervous system disorders. In Spencer, R. P. (ed.) *Interventional nuclear medicine,* Orlando Fla.: Grune & Stratton. pp. 187–215.

Bronzino, J. D. 1982. *Computer applications in patient care.* Reading, Mass.: Addison-Wesley.

Ell, P. J., and Holman, B. L. (eds.) 1982. Computed emission tomography. Oxford: Oxford University Press.

Freeman, L. M. (ed.). 1984. *Freeman and Johnson's clinical radionuclide imaging.* Vol. 2. Orlando Fla.: Grune & Stratton.

Fullerton, G. D., Kopp, D. T., Waggener, R. G., and Webster, E. W. (eds.). 1980. *Biological Risk of Medical Irradiations.* New York: American Institute of Physics.

Goodwin, P. N., Quimby, E. H., and Morgan, R. H. 1970. *Physical Foundations of Radiology,* ed. 4, New York: Harper & Row.

Hine, G. J., and Sorenson, J. A. (eds.). 1974. *Instrumentation in nuclear medicine,* vol. 2. New York: Academic.

Hladik, W. B., III, Nigg, K. K., and Rhodes, B. A. 1982. Drug-induced changes in the biologic distribution of radiopharmaceuticals. *Semin Nucl Med* 12:184–218.

Hosain, F. 1984. Interventions in radionuclide therapy. In Spencer R. P. (ed.) *Interventional nuclear medicine.* Orlando Fla.: Grune & Stratton. pp. 557–575.

Hosain, F., and Hosain, P. 1978. Selection of radionuclides for therapy. In R. P. Spencer (ed.) *Therapy in nuclear medicine,* New York: Grune & Stratton, pp. 33–43.

Hosain, P., and Wang, T. S. T. 1981. Bone imaging compounds with special reference to structure-affinity relationship. In Spencer, R. P. (ed.) *Radiopharmaceuticals: Structure-activity relationship.* New York: Grune & Stratton. pp. 521–537.

Kereiakes, J. G., and Rosenstein, M. 1980. *Handbook of radiation dose in nuclear medicine and diagnostic x-ray.* CRC Press: Boca Raton.

Lebowitz, E., and Richards, P. 1974. *Radionuclide generator systems.* Semin. Nucl. Med. 4: 257–268.

Mitchell, T. G. 1969. Radionuclide dosimetry. *Radiol Clin North Am* 7:195–205.

Myers, W. G., and Wagner, H. N., Jr. 1974. Nuclear medicine: How it began. *Hosp Pract* 9:103–113.

Palmer, A. J., Clark, J. C., and Goulding, R. W. 1977. The preparation of fluorine-18 labelled radiopharmaceuticals. *Int J Appl Radiat Isot* 28:53–65.

Snyder, W. S., Ford, M. R., Warner, G. G., and Watson, S. B. 1975. "S", absorbed dose per unit cumulated activity for selected radionuclides and organs. MIRD pamphlet no. 11. New York: Society of Nuclear Medicine.

Sorenson, J. A., and Phelps, M. E. 1980. *Physics in nuclear medicine,* New York: Grune & Stratton.

Spencer, R. P., and Hosain, F. 1976. Radionuclide generators with equal decay constants for parent and daughter. *Int J Appl Radiat Isot* 27:57–58.

Wagner, H. N., Jr., 1975. *Nuclear Medicine,* New York: HP Publishing.

Wong, D. F., Wagner, H. N., Jr., Dannals, R. F., Links, J. M., Frost, J. J., Ravert, H. T., Wilson, A. A., Rosenbaum, A. E., Gjedde, A., Douglass, K. H., Petronis, J. D., Folstein, M. F., Toung, J. K. T., Burns, H. D., and Kuhar, M. J. 1984. Effects of age on dopamine and serotonin receptors measured by positron tomography in the living human brain. *Science* 226:1393–1396.

CHAPTER **9**

Principles of Diagnostic Ultrasound

Robert A. Peura, Ph.D.

Professor of Biomedical Engineering
Worcester Polytechnic Institute
Worcester, Massachusetts 01609

INTRODUCTION

Diagnostic ultrasound has found wide acceptance within the medical community for routine examination of patients. It has become the method of choice in many situations, such as evaluation of the fetus and of carotid artery disease, to name only two. In addition, diagnostic ultrasound has found significant applications in the fields of neurology, ophthalmology, and cardiology.

It is interesting to note that ultrasound was discovered by Strutt (1877) 12 years before x-rays, which found comparatively immediate medical use. However, the radiological application of ultrasound began in the 1920s. The main reason for this delay was the availability of appropriate technology that would generate the desired ultrasonic field, detect the resultant attenuated signal, and process the information to display meaningful results.

The technique uses *ultrasound,* or high-frequency sound waves that the human ear cannot hear. These sound waves in the megahertz range can image body organs and thus provide information concerning the structure and function of body tissues. The information derived from this approach is directly related to the acoustic or ultrasonic properties of the tissues under study and is distinct from that supplied by other diagnostic techniques in use today, such as x-ray, computerized axial tomography, isotope imaging, and nuclear magnetic resonance imaging. The clinical application of ultrasound has the additional advantage that the technique is completely noninvasive, using nonionizing radiation without reported negative side effects.

Real-time ultrasonic imaging techniques, outlined in this chapter, give the ultrasonographer an opportunity to modify the scan plane to examine body tissues from a number of views in order to differentiate normal from abnormal tissue. The dynamic function of a tissue or organ can be visualized by real time imaging, i.e., the heart can be viewed during the cardiac cycle. Ultrasonic scanning is used routinely to identify cysts and tumors in many organs including uterus, liver, kidney and breast. Blood flow can also be measured noninvasively using Doppler ultrasonic techniques.

The medical application of ultrasound for diagnostic testing grew out of the work of Firestone (1946) and Desch and collaborators (1946), who used pulse-echo techniques for the nondestructive testing of metallic structures. Howry and Bliss (1952) designed the first two-dimensional ultrasonic scanner and made the first cross-sectional pictures in 1950. Howry (1957) continued the work and constructed a two-dimensional compound scanner using surplus World War II military equipment, in which the patient was immersed in a water-filled tank. Figure 9.1 shows a two-dimensional ultrasonic scan through the neck. Later this system was modified to one in which the patient was positioned outside the water tank, against one wall of the tank that was a flexible plastic membrane.

Ludwig and Struthers (1950) demonstrated a pulsed echo technique for the detection of gall stones. Wild and Reid (1955), beginning with a World War II radar trainer, developed an ultrasonic imager that successfully showed a tumor in excised brain and subsequently in a brain of a living patient through a craniotomy. Wild and Reid (1952) published the first paper on the ultrasonic differentiation of normal and malignant breast tissue.

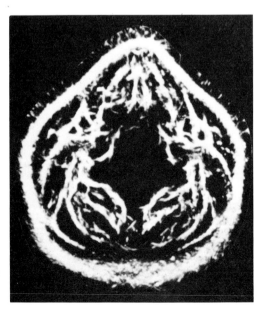

Figure 9.1   Two-dimensional horizontal ultrasonic scan through the neck (after Howry, DH, Bliss, WR 1955. *J Lab Clin Med* 40: 579, 1952).

Leksell (1956), using a British industrial flaw detector, demonstrated ultrasonic echoes from the brain through the intact skull. The development of echocardiography for ultrasonic studies of the heart was originated by Edler (1961) with Hertz, who showed ultrasonic echoes from cardiac structures. Mundt and Hughes (1956) were the first to apply ultrasonic locating techniques to ophthamology. Donald (1964) developed the first direct-contact two-dimensional ultrasonic scanner. This work was based upon his earlier visit to a boiler-making factory where he used industrial ultrasonic flaw detector probes to examine fibroids and ovarian cysts. Wells (1964) was the first to use two articulating arms for a two-dimensional scanner that continually tracked the position of the ultrasonic probe.

The Doppler shift in the back-scattered ultrasound from moving cardiac structures was first described by Satomura (1957). Callagan and coworkers (1964), using Doppler techniques, first demonstrated the fetal heart movements. McLeod (1964) reported on a Doppler ultrasonic physiological flowmeter. Shortly thereafter, Strandness and associates (1966) demonstrated a transcutaneous Doppler flowmeter for occlusive arterial disease. Three independent groups reported on the development of pulsed Doppler systems, Flaherty and Strauts (1969), Peronneau and Leger (1969) and Wells (1960). Mozersky and collaborators (1971) extended the Doppler technique to the development of two-dimensional images of blood vessels using pulsed Doppler.

This chapter deals with physical properties of ultrasound and its propagation and attenuation in the soft tissue of the body. The characteristics and design of an ultrasonic transducer are presented. Doppler blood flowmeter principles and associated circuitry, including pulsed Doppler systems, are presented. The design of real-time scanners and their clinical applications in various medical specialties are included. The future applications of diagnostic ultrasound are discussed in the final section.

PHYSICAL PROPERTIES

Sound waves are similar to light waves in that they can be reflected, refracted, and absorbed by a medium. The speed of transmission of sound is a function of the wavelength λ and the speed of propagation of sound in the medium

$$\lambda = C/f \qquad (9.1)$$

where C = speed of sound in the medium
f = frequency of the applied sound

Light and sound waves differ in that light particle motion is transverse to the wave motion, whereas with sound the particle and wave motion are both longitudinal. Figure 9.2 summarizes longitudinal wave motion. As can be seen the ultrasonic wave is sinusoidal in both time and space. The particles of the medium oscillate forward and backward about the mean position so that sound energy is propagated in the same direction as the particle vibrations. The wavelength can be calculated

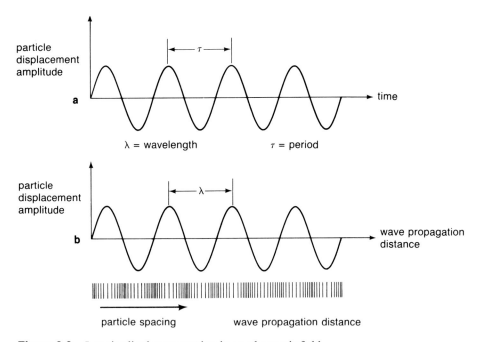

Figure 9.2   Longitudinal wave motion in an ultrasonic field. (a) Distribution of a wave in time; particle displacement amplitude is at a particular instant in time. (b) Distribution of a wave in space; particle displacement amplitude is at a particular point in space.

given the speed of ultrasound propagation in a specific medium. Table 9.1 summarizes ultrasonic properties for some important materials (Wells 1983). This table is based on the premise that for practical purposes the speed of sound in any given material is independent of the ultrasonic frequency.

Example: Given an ultrasonic signal at 2 MHz, what are the period and wavelength of the ultrasound wave in water?

Solution:
   Period $\tau = 1/f = 0.5 \; \mu s$
Wavelength $\lambda = C/f,$ where $C = 1{,}520 \; m/s$ (from Table 9.1)
Thus, $\lambda = 1{,}520 \; m/s \quad 0.5 \times 10^{-6} \; s \quad = 0.76 \; mm$

From Table 9.1 it is noted that the sound travels faster through a more dense material, such as a solid, than it does through a less dense medium such as water. It travels even more slowly in air. The acoustic impedance (or characteristic impedance) of a medium, which is given in the third column of Table 9.1, is defined by

Table 9.1 Ultrasonic properties of important materials

Material	Propagation Speed ($m\ s^{-1}$)	Density ($g\ mL^{-1}$)	Characteristic Impedance ($kg\ m^{-2}\ s^{-1}$)	Absorption Coefficient at 1 MHz ($dB\ cm^{-1}$)	Frequency Dependence of Absorption Coefficient
Air	330	0.0012	0.0004	1.2	f^2
Aluminium	6,300	2.7	17	0.018	f
Blood	1,530	1.06	1.6	0.1	$f^{1.3}$
Bone	2,700–4,100	1.38–1.81	3.7–7.4	10	$f^{1.5}$
Fat	1,460–1,470	0.92	1.4	0.6	f
Lead zirconate titanate	4,000	7.7	30	—	—
Lung	650	0.40	0.26	40	$f^{0.6}$
Muscle	1,540–1,630	1.07	1.7	1.5–2.5	f
Polyethylene	2,000	0.92	1.8	—	—
Water	1,520	1.00	1.5	0.002	f^2

*Source: Wells, P.N.T. 1983. Ultrasound imaging. In Rolfe, P. (ed.) *Non-Invasive Physiological Measurements* (2d ed.). London: Academic, chap. 9.

$$Z = \rho C \tag{9.2}$$

where

ρ = density

C = sound propagation speed of the medium

ULTRASOUND PROPAGATION

As mentioned, sound waves pass through media similar to light; thus the laws of geometric optics apply. That is, the amount of reflection and refraction at a boundary between two media is directly related to the difference in the bulk properties of the two media. If a sound wave impacts the boundary between two media at 90°, it is propagated along the same axis into the second medium. It should be noted that since some biological interfaces are irregular, some energy will be reflected back even when the incident beam is normal to the surface. However, if the angle of incidence is not 90°, then the sound wave is refracted unless the speed of sound in both media is the same. The relationship between the angle of transmission, Θ_t, and incident, Θ_i, is given by

$$\frac{\sin \Theta_i}{\sin \Theta_t} = \frac{C_1}{C_2} \tag{9.3}$$

where

C_1 = velocity of sound in medium 1

C_2 = velocity of sound in medium 2

It should be noted that

$$\Theta_i = \Theta_r \quad \text{angle of reflection} = \text{angle of incidence}$$

Figure 9.3 illustrates the behavior of sound waves at the boundary of two different media; this phenomenon is known as *specular reflection*.

The reflection coefficient R, a measure of the fraction of the total energy reflected at the boundary of two media, is given by the equation

$$R = [(Z_2 - Z_1)/(Z_2 + Z_1)]^2 \tag{9.4}$$

where

$$Z_n = \text{characteristic impedance of medium } n$$

It is clear that when the characteristic impedances are equal ($Z_1 = Z_2$), then $R = 0$, and there is no reflection at the boundary. At soft tissue boundaries, where the characteristic impedances of tissue are very similar (see Table 9.1), only small reflections occur. However, on the other extreme, when there is a large mismatch between the characteristic impedances, $R = 1$, and complete reflection occurs with no energy transmission.

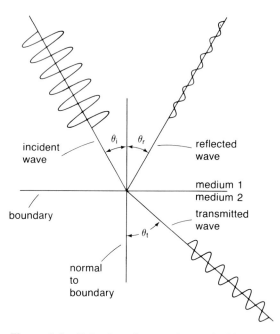

Figure 9.3 Behavior of a sound wave incident on the plane boundary between two media, θ_i = angle of incident, θ_r = angle of reflection, and θ_t = angle of transmission.

Example: Calculate the reflection coefficient R at the interface between soft tissue and air.

Solution: From Table 9.1 the characteristic impedance of muscle, $Z_1 = 1.7$, and the characteristic impedance of air, $Z_2 = 0.0004$.

Then

$$R = [(0.0004 - 1.7)/(0.0004 + 1.7)]^2 \doteq 1$$

or complete refraction occurs.

Similar calculations would show that 0.0013 of the incident energy is reflected at the blood-muscle interface and one-third to one-half of the energy is reflected at the interface between muscle and bone. These factors are used to advantage in outlining body organs by using B mode ultrasound (discussed later). We see that bone and other structures containing calcium produce strong echoes. Parenchymal organs are less well defined. Further, the use of acoustic coupling gel between ultrasound transducer and skin minimizes reflections from the skin surface. This facilitates ultrasonic transmission to deeper tissues of the body.

The specular reflection calculations detailed do not apply to characteristic impedance discontinuities due to small particles or rough interfaces. In cases in which the wavelength is large with respect to the size of the reflecting body, Rayleigh scattering occurs. Sound energy is scattered uniformly as spherical waves in all directions. The intensity of the returning wave is inversely related to the fourth power of the wavelength.

Example: Do red blood cells act as Rayleigh scatterers for Doppler ultrasound, when the frequency f = 5 to 10 MHz?

Solution: The longest dimension of a red blood cell is approximately 8 micrometers (μm) (1 μm = 0.008 mm).

Wavelength of the ultrasound $\lambda = C/f$

where

$$C = 1530 \text{ m/s}, \qquad f = 5\text{-}10 \text{ MHz}$$

Thus

$$\lambda = 0.31\text{-}0.16 \text{ mm}$$

Red blood cells act as Rayleigh scatterers for Doppler ultrasound since the size of the red blood cell is small with respect to the wavelength.

Scattering centers exist in other tissues as well. Hill (1978) has indicated that these centers exist in liver, spleen, muscle, and brain. The echo intensities from these "diffraction scatterers" vary significantly with the angle of the sound beam to the tissue. Figure 9.4 illustrates Rayleigh scattering.

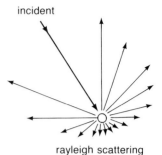

Figure 9.4 Rayleigh scattering occurs when the sound wave strikes a reflector that is small in relation to the length of the sound wave. Part of the incident energy is refracted, and part is reflected.

ATTENUATION

As an ultrasonic wave travels through biological tissue its intensity is exponentially attenuated. This intensity loss is due to scattering (discussed previously), divergence of the ultrasonic beam, and absorption. *Absorption* is the conversion of the acoustic energy to heat.

$$\text{The attenuation coefficient } \alpha = af^b \quad \text{(db/cm tissue)} \qquad (9.5)$$

where

a and b = coefficients varying with the medium

f = frequency in MHz

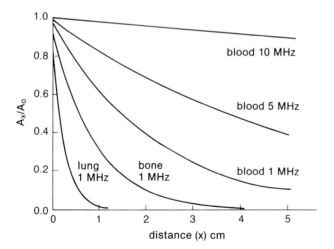

Figure 9.5 Attenuation, A_x/A_0, represents the ratio of the sound amplitude at different frequencies in various media, at a distance x to that at the source (after Sumner, DS: Ultrasound, in Kempczinski, R, and Yao. *Practical Noninvasive Vascular Diagnosis*. Chicago: Year Book).

Table 9.1 gives the absorption coefficient (*a*) of various materials used in diagnostic imaging as well as frequency dependence of each absorption coefficient (*b*). Wells (1983) notes that these data are actually values of attenuation, but often the literature is not clear enough to make a distinction between attenuation and absorption. He further states that the tissue temperature and "freshness" are often not specified.

The effect of ultrasound frequency on the attenuation of the sound intensity, for various media, is shown in Figure 9.5. Since the absorption coefficient is frequency-dependent, the depth of penetration is determined by the source frequency. As frequency is increased, the greater is the ultrasound attenuation. Thus, to reach deep tissues, the 1- to 2-MHz ultrasound should be used. For superficial tissues, higher frequencies of 5 to 10 MHz can be used with greater resolving power. The *resolving power* is the capability to distinguish objects or interfaces that are close to each other. To reflect ultrasound from an object, the size of the object should be at least one fourth the wavelength of the ultrasound.

TRANSDUCER

The ultrasound transducer consists of a *piezoelectric,* or pressure electric, crystal. The piezoelectric crystal changes its shape when excited by an electric field. Mechanical vibrations of the crystal produce pressure waves consisting of alternate regions of compression and relaxation. These sound waves propagate through the medium by vibrating it. Tissue boundaries reflect some of the incident beam's intensity. The piezoelectric transducer is also used to transduce returning ultrasonic echoes (mechanical vibrations) into a voltage output.

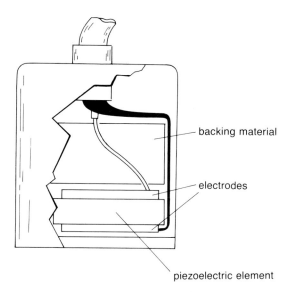

Figure 9.6 Main components of an ultrasonic transducer.

Commercial ultrasound piezoelectric transducers are built by using polycrystalline ceramic materials such as barium titanate, lead titanate, zirconate, or lead metaniobate. Figure 9.6 illustrates the basic components of an ultrasonic transducer. The transducer backing material determines the property of the emitted ultrasonic signal. If air backing is used, as in the case of a continuous signal Doppler (described later), there is a large impedance mismatch between the piezoelectric crystal and the air. Thus, most of the energy is transmitted in the forward direction in which there is a more favorable acoustic impedance match. The disadvantage with air-backed crystals is the relatively long ringing period. To reduce this ringing, the crystal is backed with resin, which absorbs sound energy in the backward direction.

An ultrasound transducer produces two distinct zones, a near field and a far field, as shown in Figure 9.7. The near field, or *Fresnel zone,* is close to the transducer. In this zone the longitudinal sound waves are essentially parallel. These waves begin to diverge in the far field, or *Fraunhofer zone.* The lateral resolution becomes poor in the far field such that objects appear larger because of the diverging beam. The effect of the far field divergence can be improved by using an acoustic lens to focus the sound waves.

The near field length, *l,* can be calculated from

$$l = r^2/\lambda \qquad (9.6)$$

where

r = transducer radius

λ = wavelength

The angle of beam divergence in the far field, Θ, is given by

$$\Theta = \text{arc sin} (0.61\ \lambda/r) \qquad (9.7)$$

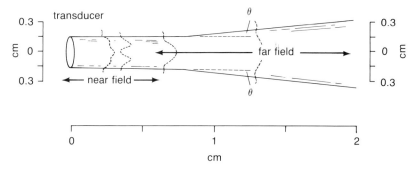

Figure 9.7 Dimensions of an ultrasound beam produced by a 3-mm circular crystal that vibrates at 5 MHz. No divergence exists in the 0.7-cm near field. Divergence (θ) in the far field is 7.2°. Relative sound energy intensity is indicated by the dashed lines in the plane through the center of the beam.

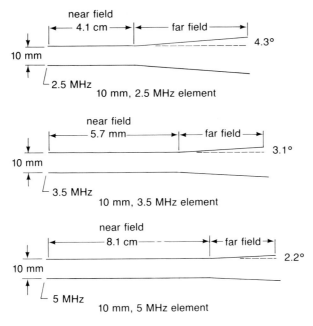

Figure 9.8   Increase in the transducer frequency results in an increase in the length of the near field.

As can be seen from the equation, the near field is lengthened by increasing the diameter of the transducer. Figure 9.8 shows the effect of frequency of the length of the near field.

Example: Given a 10-mm-diameter transducer and a 2.5-MHz source of excitation, calculate the length of the near field and the angle of beam divergence in the far field.

Solution:
$$\lambda = c/f = 1,540 \, \text{m/s}/2.5 \, \text{MHz} = 616 \times 10^{-6} \, \text{m}$$
$$1 = (5 \, \text{mm})^2/616 \times 10^{-6} \, \text{m} = 4.1 \, \text{cm}$$
$$\Theta = \text{arc sin} \, (0.61) \, (616 \times 10^{-6} \, \text{m})/5 \times 10^{-3} \, \text{m} = 4.3°$$

DOPPLER FLOWMETER

The Doppler principle is a very useful technique for measuring blood flow. Most individuals associate the Doppler principle with the changes in train whistle pitch: as an observer listens to an approaching train, the pitch or frequency is higher or lower than the true frequency as the train approaches, and then recedes with distance, respectively.

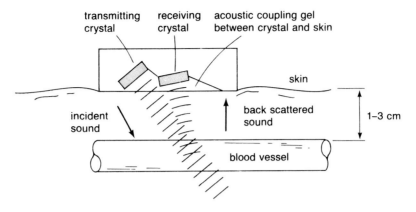

Figure 9.9 Operation of a transcutaneous Doppler flowmeter (after Rushmer R. F., Baker, D.W., Stegan, H.F. 1966. *J Appl Phys* 101:554-566).

Blood flow can be measured by using the Doppler technique either transcutaneously or by placing a transducer directly on a vessel. The principle of operation is the same in both cases. Figure 9.9 illustrates the transcutaneous application. Two piezoelectric crystals are positioned on the skin surface. An ultrasonic signal between 5 to 10 MHz is beamed into the blood stream, and part of the signal is back-scattered and excites the receiving crystal. The difference between the transmitted and detected frequencies is the Doppler shift due to the back-scattered sound. This Doppler frequency shift is a measure of blood velocity.

The basic diagram for calculating the Doppler frequency shift is given in Figure 9.10. This assumes that the transducer is placed around the blood vessel. The frequency of the source is f_s, C is the speed of sound in blood, V = blood velocity, and Θ is the angle the piezoelectric crystal makes with the flow axis. The relative sound velocity with respect to the source is $(C - V\cos\Theta)$ when the sound is emitted upstream. Conversely, the relative velocity of sound at the receiver is $(C + V\cos\Theta)$ when the sound is traveling in the same direction as flow. The sound wavelength λ is the same in both cases; thus

$$\lambda = (C - V\cos\Theta)/\text{fs} = (C + V\cos\Theta)/\text{fr} \tag{9.8}$$

Solving for fr we get

$$\text{fr} = [\,(C + V\cos\Theta)/(C - V\cos\Theta)\,]\,\text{fs} \tag{9.9}$$

The frequency shift $\Delta f = \text{fs} - \text{fr}$

or

$$\Delta f = \text{fs}\,\frac{C + V\cos\Theta - 1}{C - V\cos\Theta} = \text{fs}\,\frac{2V\cos\Theta}{C - V\cos\Theta} \tag{9.10}$$

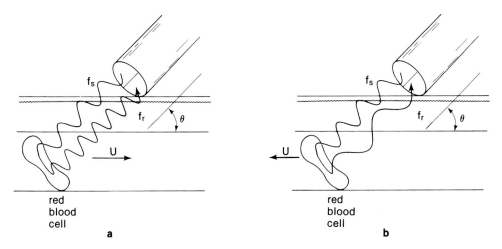

Figure 9.10 Doppler frequency shifts produced by a red blood cell. Frequency (f_s) transmitted is the same in parts *A* and *B*. The frequency (f_r) back-scattered increases when the cell moves toward the probe and decreases when the cell moves away from the probe (B). The angle (θ) of the sound beam and the velocity (U) of the red blood cell are illustrated intersecting the velocity vector.

or

$$\Delta f = fs \left[\frac{2V \cos \Theta}{C} \right]$$

since $C >> V$.

Example: Given a 5-MHz Doppler positioned at 45° to the flow axis, what is the frequency shift when the blood velocity is 30 cm/s?

Solution:

$$f = fs \frac{2V \cos \Theta}{C} = 5 \times 10^6 \frac{2 \times 30(\cos 45°)}{1.5 \times 10^5}$$

$$= 1414 \, \text{Hz}$$

The most common method of interpreting the Doppler signal is audible frequency analysis. The audible Doppler frequency shift is evaluated by an experienced technician. Doppler spectral frequency analysis is discussed in a following section.

DOPPLER CIRCUITRY

As mentioned previously, the output from a continuous wave Doppler flowmeter is an audio frequency. This signal can be further processed by means of a zero crossing detector circuit to produce an analog voltage proportional to blood velocity. Figure 9.11 shows this signal-processing system, in which a pulse is produced each time the input signal passes through zero. The detector output consists of large low-frequency waves with additive small-amplitude high-frequency signals. The low-frequency signal is due to blood vessel wall motion that is eliminated by high pass filtering, at approximately 100 Hz; this unfortunately eliminates low red blood cell velocity signals less than 1.5 cm/s, which may occur adjacent to the vessel wall. The output pulses from the zero-crossing detector are low pass filtered (0

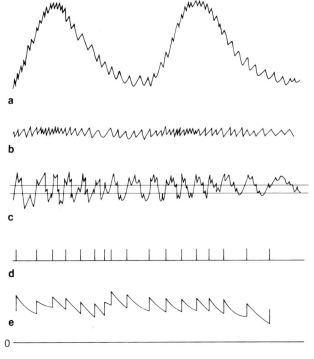

Figure 9.11 Continous-wave Doppler signal-processing waveforms. (a) Large low-frequency waves from detector output result from blood vessel wall motion. Low-amplitude, high-frequency signal is produced by the red blood cells. (b) High pass filtering by the AF amplifier eliminates wall-motion artifacts. (c) Zero crossing detector with adjustable hysteresis band (horizontal lines). (d) Zero crossing detector output produces equal area pulses. (e) Low pass filtering of zero crossing detector output produces a signal proportional to cell velocity (after Webster, J. G.: Measurement of Flow and Volume of Blood, in Webster, J. G. 1978. *Medical Instrumentation Application and Design.* Boston: Houghton Mifflin).

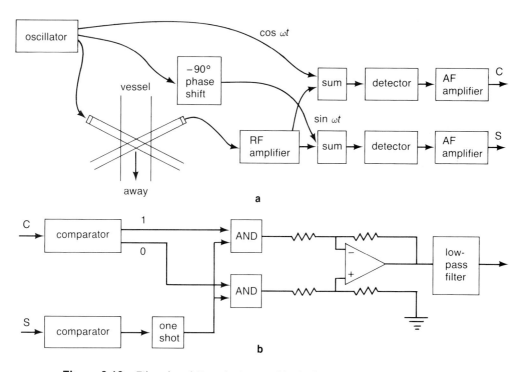

Figure 9.12 Directional Doppler system block diagram. (a) Carrier frequency sine and cosine signals are summed with the quadrature-phase detector. When the flow is toward the transducer, the output from the cosine channel C lags the output from the sine channel S and leads when the flow is away from the transducer. (b) Logic circuit uses two AND gates to indicate whether the flow is away from or toward the transducer. Bidirectional output pulses provided by the differential amplifier are then filtered (after Webster, J. G.: Measurement of Flow and Volume of Blood, in Webster, J. G. 1978. *Medical Instrumentation Application and Design.* Boston: Houghton Mifflin).

to 25 Hz) to remove high frequencies. The process produces an output signal related to cell velocity.

The major problem with this system is that positive and negative flow produce similar results, and the detection of flow direction is not possible. Quadrature detection techniques can be used to determine flow direction (McLeod 1967). Figure 9.12 illustrates a directional Doppler block diagram. A 90° phase-shift network separates the carrier into two signals separated by 90°. These signals are said to be in quadrature. The radio frequency (RF) signal is summed with reference cosine and sine waves to produce a RF enveloped as illustrated in Figure 9.13, with the assumption that the RF signal does not contain a carrier signal.

Blood flow in the forward direction, or away from the transducer, produces a Doppler shift frequency lower than the carrier. The phase of the Doppler wave lags behind the reference carrier. A phasor diagram of the reference carrier, sine,

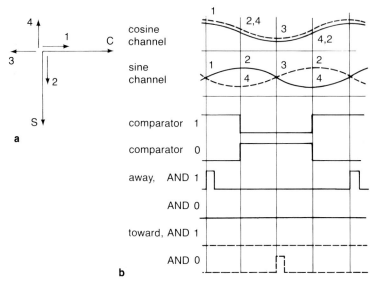

Figure 9.13   Directional Doppler signal waveforms. (a)
Vector diagram shows the carrier frequency sine wave, which
lags the cosine wave by 90°. Doppler frequency is lower than
the carrier frequency when flow is away from the transducer.
Doppler signal rotates clockwise and is represented by the
short vector (1, 2, 3, and 4). (b) Timing diagram shows the
single-peak envelope of the carrier plus the Doppler signal
before detection (top two channels). Comparator responds to
the cosine channel audio signal after detection. Sine channel
provides one-shot pulses that are gated through the
appropriate AND gate by comparator outputs. Flow toward
transducer indicated by the dashed lines (after Webster, J. G.:
Measurement of Flow and Volume of Blood, in Webster, J. G.
1978. *Medical Application and Design.* Boston: Houghton
Mifflin).

cosine, and Doppler signals can be used to interpret the results (Figure 9.13[a]).
Positive rotation in the clockwise direction is indicated by times 1 to 4. Figure
9.13(b) illustrates the detector signals as a function of time. At time 1, the reference carrier and Doppler are in phase and add, producing a larger output in the cosine output. Since the Doppler is 90° out of phase with the sine wave, the sine output remains the same. At time 2, the carrier and Doppler add, giving a larger sum
in the sine output. The rest of the cycle can be analyzed in the same way.

Blood flow in the reverse direction produces a Doppler frequency higher
than the carrier. In this case the Doppler vector rotates counterclockwise. The
dashed waveform in Figure 9.13 results in this case, and the sine and cosine phase
relationships are reversed. The direction of flow is thus determined by the sign of
the phase.

Figure 9.12 shows a diagram of the logic that detects the sign of phase and
thus indicates whether the flow is toward or away from the transducer. Figure 9.13

gives the logic timing diagram for the flow determination. Comparator 1, driven by the cosine signal, has an output that does not change with flow direction. Conversely, Comparator 2, driven by the sine signal, triggers a one-shot with a short pulse width. The direction of flow controls whether the one-shot triggers at the beginning or halfway through the period. The AND gates produce a pulse into either the top or bottom input of the differential amplifier. This bidirectional amplifier output thus gives a signal proportional to direction of blood velocity.

TRANSIT-TIME PULSED-SONIC FLOWMETER

An early method used for blood flow measurement through intact vessels is the *transit-time pulsed-sonic flowmeter* (Farrall 1959). This device consists of two piezoelectric crystals placed on a cylindrical probe such that they are diagonally across from each other when placed on the vessel lumen. Figure 9.14 illustrates this arrangement, in which each crystal serves alternately as the sonic transmitter and receiver. The frequency of direction change of the ultrasonic pulses is 400 Hz. The pulses take longer to travel upstream than downstream since the relative speed of sound is decreased by the blood velocity.

The relationship for the time difference, Δt, between upstream and downstream transit time is derived as follows:

$$t = \frac{l}{C \pm V \cos \Theta} \tag{9.12}$$

where

l = distance between the upstream and downstream piezoelectric crystals

C = velocity of sound

V = velocity of medium

Θ = angle between the ultrasound propagation and the flow axis.

$$\Delta t = t_{up} - t_{down}$$

$$\Delta t = \frac{l}{C - V \cos \Theta} - \frac{l}{C + V \cos \Theta} \tag{9.13}$$

or

$$= \frac{2lv \cos}{C^2 - V^2 \cos^2 \Theta}$$

$$= \frac{2lv \cos \Theta,}{C^2} \quad \text{since } C^2 >> V^2$$

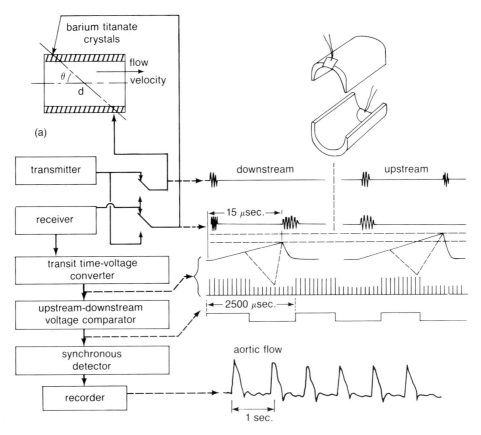

Figure 9.14   Ultrasonic flowmeter block diagram (after Farrell, W. 1959. Design consideration of ultrasonic flowmeters, IRE Transactions on Medical Electronics ME-6(4):201, used with permission IEEE).

The circuitry functions in the following way. The instant that a burst of ultrasound leaves the transmitting crystal, the transmitter turns on a flip-flop. The arrival of the ultrasound pulse at the receiver crystal turns off the flip-flop. During the flip-flop on-time a gate allows a ramp generator to run so that the final amplitude of the ramp is proportional to the transit time in one direction. Two similar circuits are used, one for upstream and the other for downstream transit time determinations.

Example: For a transit time ultrasonic flowmeter, calculate the time difference between upstream and downstream propagation if the distance between the crystals is 1 cm and the mean velocity of the blood is 1 cm/s. The angle of the crystals is 45° with respect to the flow axis.

Solution:

$$\Delta t = \frac{2lv \cos \Theta}{C^2}$$

$$= \frac{2(1\ \text{cm})\ (1\text{cm/s})\cos 45°}{(1.5 \times 10^5\ \text{cm/s})^2}$$

$$= 0.63 \times 10^{-10}\ \text{s}$$

Which is a small time difference, requiring complex electronics to achieve adequate stability.

ULTRASONIC SCANNER MODES

A number of different ultrasonic scanning modes are employed to examine tissue structure. A-scan devices were the first practical ones and led to the acceptance of ultrasonics for clinical diagnostic applications. The *amplitude mode,* or *A-mode,* measures the tissue discontinuity along the scan axis. Using this technique it is possible to study simple structures and measure dimensions from the ultrasonic echo sizes and shapes. Figure 9.15 shows the application of an A-mode scanning system to measure the position of the brain midline. The system includes a hand-held transducer, ultrasound driver, processing and display circuitry, and a camera for recording the scan. The rate generator initiates the scan by simultaneously triggering the ultrasonic transmitter, the time-base generator, and the sweep gain generator. The returning ultrasonic echoes are amplified by the receiver and displayed

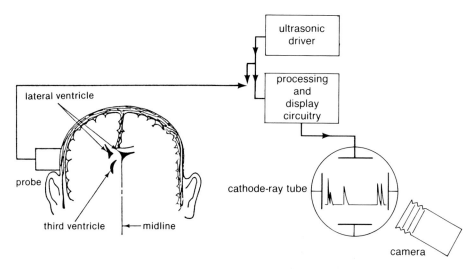

Figure 9.15 Block diagram of an A-mode system.

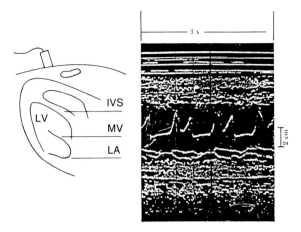

Figure 9.16   Ultrasound time-motion scan of mitral valve (MV) for three heart cycles (middle trace). Relatively static structures, interventricular septum (IVS), and left atrium (LA) also shown (after Sieband, M, and Holden, J: Medical Imaging Systems, in Webster, J. G. 1978. *Medical Application and Design.* Boston: Houghton Mifflin).

on the *y* axis. In this way, the strength and position of the echoes correspond to the ultrasonic echo-producing targets along the ultrasonic beam within the patient.

Tissue discontinuities between the two brain hemispheres produce echoes in the middle of the display. The measurement of the midline position is important clinically since a shift can be caused by pathological conditions due to to either severe head trauma or several disease states. Typical repetition rates of 2,000 times per second produce flicker-free displays.

The *time motion* (TM) *scan* is an extension of the A-mode approach, in which a single stationary transducer is used. The depth of the echo is displayed on the vertical axis. The brightness of the oscilloscope display is modulated by the echo amplitude. Figure 9.16 shows a TM ultrasound scan of the mitral valve of the heart. Effectively, the TM scan is just an A-mode scan that is continuously recorded, with the echo delay proportional to the depth of the structure and the beam intensity proportional to the strength of the echo. In this way the morphology of the tissue along the transducer axis is displayed as a function of time.

The time required to form a single *brightness scan* (B-scan) line is determined by the depth of ultrasound penetration. A 10-cm penetration takes 133 μs (Wells 1983). Body structures do not move a significant distance during this short time; thus with a sufficiently fast repetition rate it is possible to visualize the movement of tissue structures such as the heart valves.

The B mode produces a two-dimensional image of the tissue under study by combining A-mode signals from various directions by mechanical transducer scanning. The transducer position is determined by measuring the angle of the gantry arm with respect to a reference (see Figure 9.17). The echo amplitude can control the unblanking in a storage oscilloscope.

This scanning system utilizes the gantry relative angle and the elapsed echo-delay time to generate the two-dimensional image. In addition, the image bright-

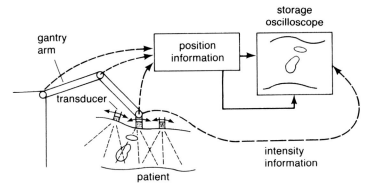

Figure 9.17   Multiple B-mode ultrasonic scans produce two-dimensional shape on storage oscilloscope.

ness at a given scan position is proportional to the echo intensity, in the same way as for the A-mode scan. The system is designed so that an increasing distance into the patient is given by a more downward vertical deflection, and time increases in the horizontal direction from left to right.

The early version of the two-dimensional B scan was used for static measurements in the visualization of abdominal cavity tissues. The requirements for cardiology are much more challenging in that to visualize valve action, a frame rate of at least 40 per second is necessary to visualize heart valve movements adequately. The frame repetition rate is limited by the speed of ultrasound in tissue (Wells 1983). The resultant time difference is in the nanosecond range, requiring complex electronics to achieve a sufficiently stable response.

Example :   Given a desired ultrasound penetration depth of 15 cm, what are the maximum pulse repetition rate and the number of lines per frame, assuming that the system can produce 40 frames per second?

Solution: $t = d/C = (30 \, cm/150,000 \, cm/s) = 200 \, \mu s$

The maximum repetition rate would be 5,000/s. Since the system can produce 40 frames per second, this gives 125 lines per frame. In many cases, these analog B-mode images are stored on a video storage tube or video tape. The signals can also be digitized for signal enhancement and for calculations of pertinent anatomical structure and physiological function by means of a dedicated microcomputer system.

PULSED DOPPLER SYSTEMS

The pulsed Doppler system illustrated in Figure 9.18 is unlike the continuous wave Doppler in that a piezoelectric crystal produces a burst of high-frequency sound. The piezoelectric crystal acting as a transmitter is deenergized, and the crystal is then connected to receiver circuitry to pick up the resultant returning echoes.

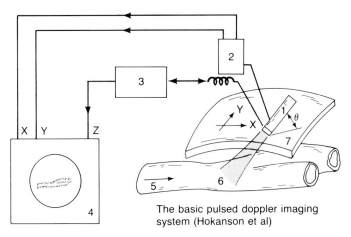

The basic pulsed doppler imaging
system (Hokanson et al)

Figure 9.18   Basic pulsed Doppler imaging system: (1) single
element transducer, (2) *X-Y* potentiometer, (3) Doppler signal-
processing transmit and receive unit, (4) storage oscilloscope,
(5) artery under examination, (6) ultrasonic beam, (7) skin
surface (after Hokanson et al. 1972. Ultrasonic arteriography:
A non-invasive method for arterial visualization. *Radiology*
102:435–436).

These systems are designed to detect blood flow selectively at specific distances
from the probe. Figure 9.19 illustrates the operation of a typical pulsed Doppler
flow detection system.

   Red blood cells are flowing in two blood vessels, 1.0 cm and 3.0 cm from the
ultrasonic probe, Figure 9.19. A pulsed Doppler flowmeter, with a frequency of 4
MHz, emits a burst of ultrasound once every 1/12,000 s, a pulse repetition rate of
12 KHz, such that the ultrasound lasts for 1.25 μs (or 5 oscillations). This 1.2-μs
burst of sound extends over 1.8 mm of tissue (1.2 μs $\times$ 1.5 $\times$ 10^4 cm/s = 1.8 mm)
There is a quiescent period of 82 μs (total period = 83 μs) in which the transmitter is
turned off. The receiver gate is adjusted to open at 13 μs and 38μs to pick up the reflected signal from the red blood cells inside vessels 1 and 2, respectively. These receiver windows only allow the Doppler system to detect and process return signals
from specific depths.

   The blood velocity profile can be approximated by varying the depth of the
range gate so that the blood velocity is sampled at various points across the vessel
diameter (Histand and associates 1973). Sumner (1982) has indicated that pulsed
Doppler flow measurements at the center of the flow stream yield valuable clinical
information.

SPECTRAL ANALYSIS OF DOPPLER VELOCITY SIGNALS

It has been found in clinical studies that good correlations result when frequency
spectra of Doppler signals are used to predict various blood vessel pathological

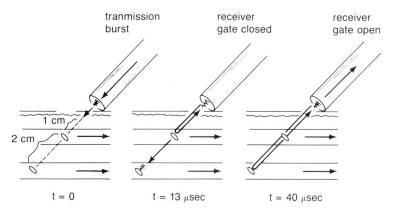

tranmission burst   receiver gate closed   receiver gate open

1 cm

2 cm

t = 0   t = 13 μsec   t = 40 μsec

Figure 9.19   Pulsed Doppler flow detector in operation. Red blood cells are moving in two vessels, 1.0 and 3.0 cm from the probe. Transmission of 1.0-μs burst, of 4 MHz sound with a repetition rate of 12 KHz is indicated. First, receiving gate is closed; then it opens at 40-μs permitting detection of the signal from the deeper vessel. No signals are detected from the superficial vessel.

conditions (Sumner 1982). Early Doppler spectral systems used mini- and large computer systems for their frequency spectrum analysis. More compact and specialized frequency spectrum analyzers have been developed for Doppler blood flow evaluations. Many Doppler instruments incorporate microcomputer systems for fast fourier transform (FFT) analysis of the Doppler waveforms.

Figure 9.20 shows a sound spectrum analysis from a human carotid artery. Frequency is displayed on the vertical axis and time on the horizontal for one cardiac cycle. The amplitude of the signal is indicated by a continuous gray scale: the darker the image the stronger the signal amplitude. The Doppler frequency shift envelope corresponds with the maximum blood flow velocity at any given time in the cardiac cycle. Brown and coworkers (1982) showed a higher correlation between spectral analysis of a continuous wave Doppler and the diameter of the internal carotid artery in patients.

Pulsed Doppler spectral analysis studies produce quite different spectra from the continuous wave Doppler studies. Figure 9.21 shows a typical real-time spectral analysis of a pulsed Doppler signal measured in the center of a normal human carotid artery. The spectra appear as a narrow band of frequencies in parallel to the maximum frequency spectra envelope. It is noted from Figure 9.20 that essentially all frequencies from zero to maximum value appear in the recording for the continuous wave Doppler system. The reason for these differences is that the continuous wave system insonates the total diameter of the vessel at the same time. Thus the full range of blood velocities is converted into proportional Doppler spectral frequency changes.

However, when the pulsed Doppler is used to measure laminar flow it produces frequency shifts in a narrow range since the blood velocities in the center of

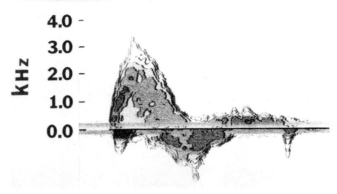

Figure 9.20   Doppler signal of sound spectrogram in a human femoral artery. Forward flow is positive; reserve flow is negative (below the horizontal line) (after Sumner, D. S.: Ultrasound, in Kempczinski, R., and Yao, J. *Practical Noninvasive Vascular Diagnosis*. Chicago: Year Book).

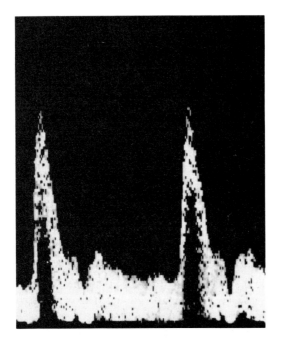

Figure 9.21   Real-time spectral analysis of a pulsed Doppler signal from the center of a human carotid artery. Peak frequency is 3080 Hz (after Kempczinski, R., and Yao, J. *Practical Noninvasive Vascular Diagnosis*. Chicago: Year Book).

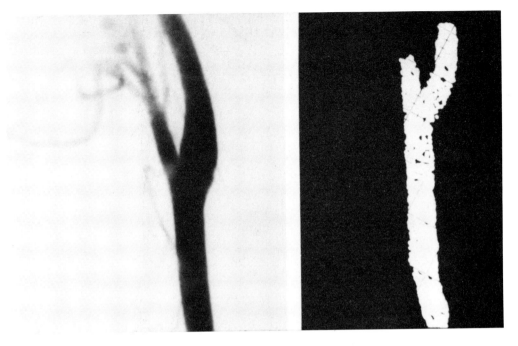

Figure 9.22   Pulsed Doppler image of carotid bifurcation
(right) and carotid angiogram (left). Individual has a stenotic
internal carotid artery.

the vessel are maximum and approximately the same value. St. Thomas (1984), using in vitro studies, has shown that with turbulent flow the distinction between the
results obtained from the pulsed and continuous wave Doppler are less distinct.

Pulsed Doppler systems can image arterial lumen by successive mapping of
the position of flow. These instruments are similar to the B-scan imaging devices in
that a position-sensing device determines the x–y coordinates on a storage oscilloscope. In this way a skilled operator can "paint" the inside of a blood vessel by
sensing the locations in which velocity is above a minimum value. Simultaneous
spectral analysis of the velocities at various positions in the flow stream can be processed on a number of commercial instruments. Figure 9.22 shows pulsed Doppler
and angiographic images from a carotid bifurcation in which the internal carotid
artery is stenosed.

REAL-TIME SCANNERS

A *real-time scanner* processes the ultrasonic information as it is received rather
than storing it for future use. These systems are mechanical or electrical B scanner
systems that can scan 15 to 60 frames per second. The transducer can be moved

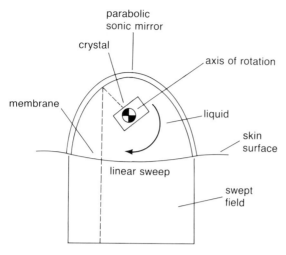

Figure 9.23   Rotating crystal transducer including a liquid path and a reflecting, parabolic mirror.

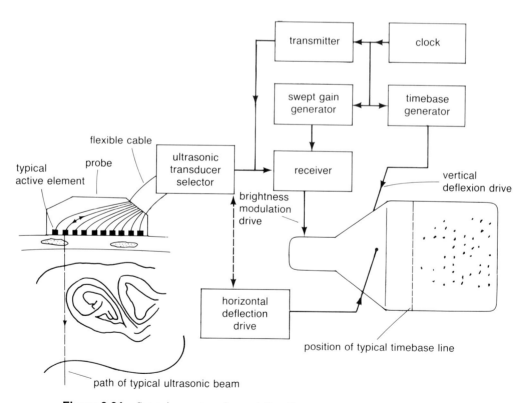

Figure 9.24   Scanning system for real-time linear array: ten separate transducer elements addressed in sequence to form a two-dimensional image.

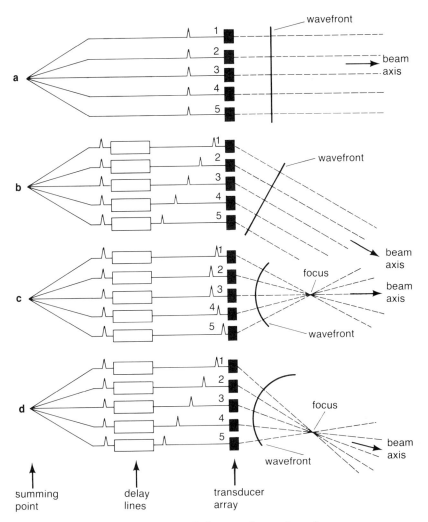

Figure 9.25 Electronically steered ultrasound transducer in a five-element array. (a) Simultaneous excitation produces parallel beam. (b) Excitation in sequence deviates parallel beam. (c) Spherical time grading focuses beam. (d) Combined linear and spherical time grading focuses beam off axis.

and angled to visualize tissue structures in three dimensions, giving the operator direct visual feedback.

A mechanical scanner is illustrated in Figure 9.23; in it three single-element ultrasound transducers are mounted on a rotating wheel. An image sector is swept as each transducer contacts the patient. These systems normally use water, oil, or gel inside the transducer housing to improve the transducer-patient interface.

The ultrasonic beam can be steered by electronic means. There are two basic types of electronic scanners, the linear array and the electronic beam steering systems. The linear array is shown in Figure 9.24. Each element is addressed sequentially to produce individual scan lines to produce rectangular image formats. This

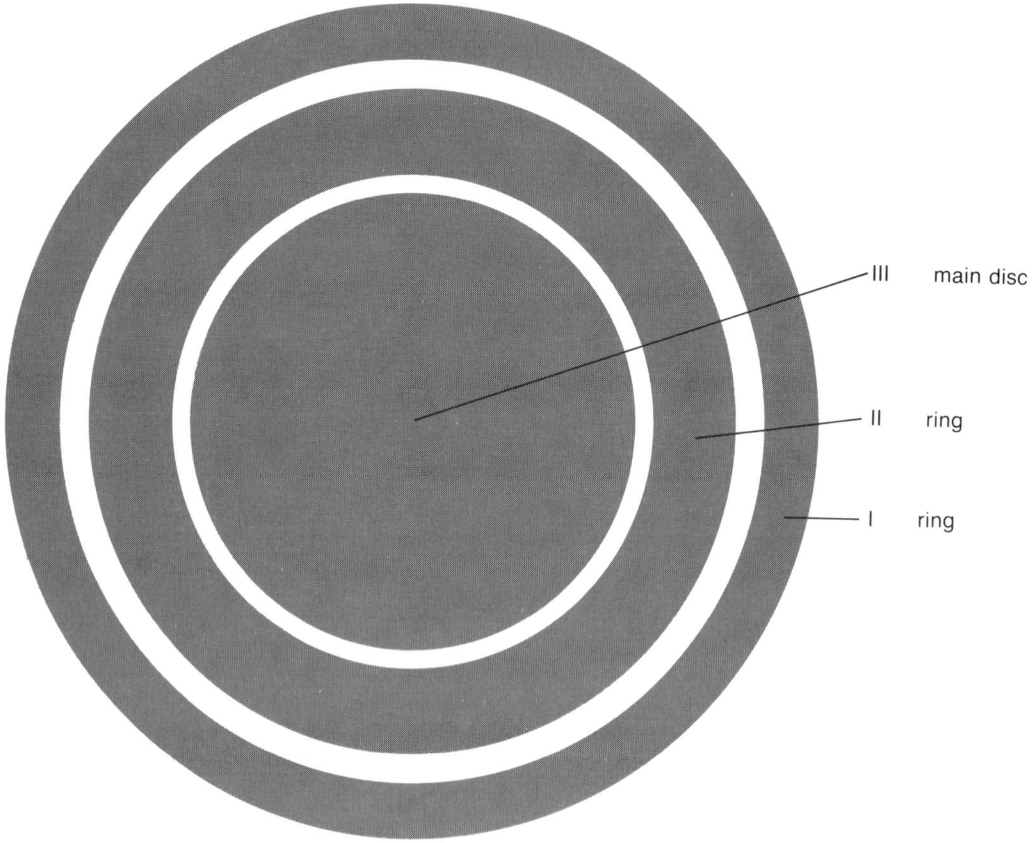

Figure 9.26 Basic concentric ultrasound transducer element (enlarged ten times) (after Hajjar W. M. 1981. Multi-focus multi-elements matrix ultrasonic transducer for real-time Doppler imaging design, construction and evaluation. Ph.D. Dissertation, Worcester Polytechnic Institute).

nonsegmental array produces an ultrasonic field with high divergence. A smaller divergence and a longer near field can be produced if several elements are tied together in overlapping groups.

Further improvements in real-time scanners are realized with electronic beam steering systems. An ultrasonic beam can be focused by electronic switching of arrays of small piezoelectric crystals, arranged in various geometric patterns. Figure 9.25 illustrates the way a phased array of transducers can focus the ultrasonic beam. The wave front is composed of the individual wavelets produced from the individual crystals. By controlling the firing times for the individual elements it is possible to shape the wave front. By first firing the outside elements, 1 and 5, and then elements 2 and 3, and finally 4, it is possible to cause the wave front to converge or focus at a point, in the same way as an acoustical lens does. This approach, known as a *phased array*, allows for dynamic changes in the ultrasound focus point.

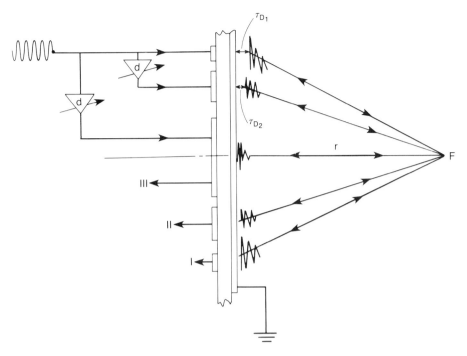

Figure 9.27 Focusing technique for concentric ultrasonic elements; excitation pulse is time-delayed to ring II and the main disc III. Constructive interference occurs at point F (after Hajjar W. M. 1981. Multi-focus multi elements matrix ultrasonic transducer for real-time Doppler imaging design, construction and evaluation. Ph.D. Dissertation, Worcester Polytechnic Institute).

Phased array elements can be constructed in the form of circles or series of rings; these are known as *annular-phased array systems* and are used in some ultrasonic imaging systems. An annular-phased array system is shown in Figure 9.26. The basic focused element consists of two concentric rings and a main disk. Focusing is achieved by delaying the excitation pulse to the inner ring by a given time and that to the main disk by an additional amount. This results in constructive interference or focusing at point F. Figure 9.27 illustrates the way an ultrasonic pulse can be "steered" by a phased-array system.

AN ULTRASOUND IMAGING SYSTEM

The following material deals with the design of the Hewlett-Packard (HP) HP77020A Ultrasound Imaging System (Banks 1983). This is a real-time phased-array system with a 90° sector image. The system has the ability to image and display in real time (30 Hz). This allows the cardiologist to visualize the heart, especially the valves. Figure 9.28 shows a sonographer imaging a patient's beating

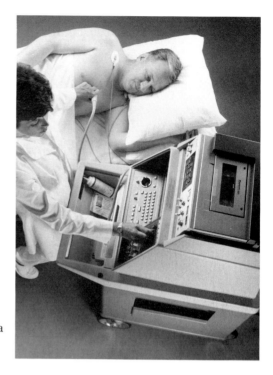

Figure 9.28   Sonographer imaging a patient's heart (courtesy of Hewlett Packard, Andover, Mass.).

heart. A phased array system is used in that a small transducer transmits ultrasound between the ribs. In this way a large field of view shows the full adult heart.

Figure 9.29 is a block diagram of the 77020A in which a phased array transducer is used. The pulser and timing section of the scanner generates 64 different transmit pulses at the appropriate phase to steer the acoustic beam in the desired direction. The transducer can be changed from a real-time scanner to an M mode.

The return echoes are detected by the transducer, fed to the 64 preamplifiers, and combined in the phasing delays to generate the video signal. The video signal is processed and sent to the controller in which it is interfaced with the strip chart recorder. This is normally used for paper recordings of the M mode signals. The controller also processes other analog physiological data such as the ECG and provides control signals for the video camera and videocassette recorder (VCR) circuits.

The system communication interface provides a high-speed bus from the scanner A/D converter output to the R-Theta circuit. This conversion algorithm remaps the data from polar coordinates to raster-output Cartesian coordinates. In addition, a HP-IB system bus allows the communication of three 16-bit MC5 microprocessors.

The acoustic signal is available for analysis before the scan conversion and subsequent video conversions with associated modifications of the signal. Tissue identification studies could be performed at this point on a larger computer system.

The data are stored in a 480 by 640 5-bit display memory and is gray scale-mapped. Using a bit map, the data are summed with graphic/character data and converted to video for display in any of the following modes: high-speed display in

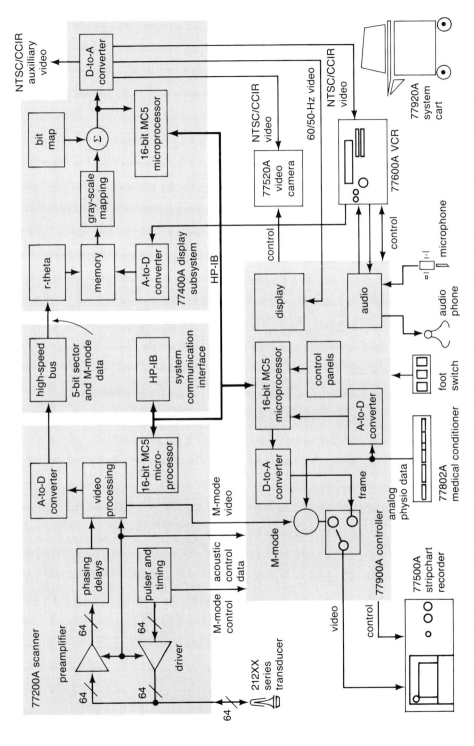

Figure 9.29 Block diagram of the 77020A Ultrasound Imaging System (courtesy of Hewlett Packard, Andover, Mass.).

the controller, VCR storage, transmission to any standard video auxiliary device, or transmission to the video camera for hard-copy output.

The system is designed to allow full gray-scale control of the video playback for the VCR. This is accomplished by first converting the image from analog to digital data and then reading it back into the memory. Audio data such as heart sounds or physician's verbal comments can also be stored and played back through this system.

A fiber-optic oscillographic recorder is required to handle the gray-scale data, which are normally used for the M-mode hard-copy output. A full-frame image can be added to the M-mode strip chart recorder by routing the data via the HP-IB from the digital scan converter memory through the controller to the strip chart recorder. Physiological data such as the ECG can also be added to the real-time image or hard copy for timing and additional diagnostic information.

CLINICAL APPLICATIONS OF REAL-TIME SCANNERS

Real-time ultrasonic examinations of moving tissue are being used diagnostically in many areas of the body to characterize normal and abnormal anatomical structures accurately. In addition, more importantly, normal and abnormal anatomy are delineated in any desired scan plane. It should be noted that the results are operator-dependent. Proper interpretation requires knowledge of tissue pathology and the characteristics of ultrasonic images. This section will summarize some of the significant applications of ultrasonic imaging.

Ultrasonic images of the fetus can be realized by real-time scans of the mother's abdomen. Ultrasound is especially useful in fetal examinations since there is no electromagnetic radiation danger. Nuclear magnetic resonance imaging cannot be used since the fetus would not remain in one position long enough. Ultrasound can guide a needle to harvest ovary material for pathological tests. It is estimated that from one-half to two-thirds of the pregnant women in the United States have at least one fetal ultrasound scan. It is required by law that all pregnant women in Great Britain and West Germany have it. Fetal ultrasound scans are used to view the fetus and to determine whether the fetus is normal. Figure 9.30 shows a normal fetus at 25 wk sucking its thumb. Fetal anatomical features including the width of the fetal head, size of brain ventricles to monitor possible hydrocephalus, crown-to-rump length to determine the age of the fetus, spinal examination to check for abnormalities, the femur length to correlate with biparietal diameter to assess proper physical development of the fetus, and detectable fetal anomalies can be determined.

Real-time ultrasound has been used to perform interventional therapeutic techniques on the fetus in utero *Fleischer & James, Jr. (1984). Fetal transfusions have been performed using real-time ultrasonic visualization. Also ultrasonic guidance has been used to drain hydrocephalus, posterior urethral valves and chylothorox in utero.

The introduction of ultrasonic examinations of the heart has had great impact on the field of cardiology. The original one dimensional M-mode examination

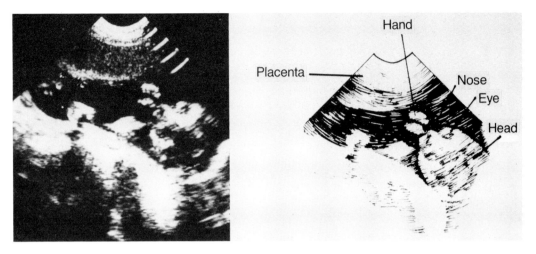

Figure 9.30   Real-time scan at 25 wk of a normal anterior placenta, showing the fetus sucking its thumb (after Fleischer, A., and James, Jr., A. E. 1984. *Real Time Sonography.* East Norwalk, Conn.: Appleton-Century-Crofts).

of the heart required highly trained users. The present real-time two dimensional ultrasound images or echocardiograms provide an almost unlimited number of cross sectional image planes. Figure 9.31 shows a normal real-time ultrasound image of both ventricles and atria. An abnormal cardiac ultrasound scan is shown in Mitral valve disease was first studied by clinical ultrasound using M-mode. The addition of the second dimension, with the use of real-time scanners, has resulted in

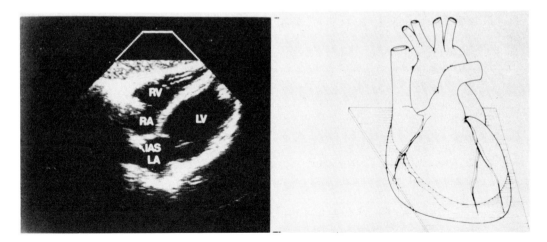

Figure 9.31   Real-time scan (subcostal view) showing the interatrial septum (IAS) with both ventricles (RV and LV) and atria (RA and LA) (after Fleischer, A., and James, Jr., A. E. 1984. *Real Time Sonography.* East Norwalk, Conn.: Appleton-Century-Crofts).

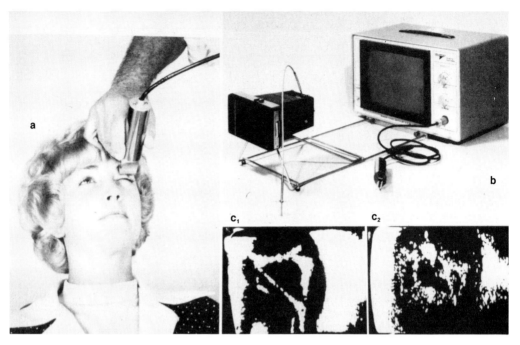

Figure 9.32   Ultrasonic exam of the eye (A), scanning system (B), retinal detachment with dense vitreous traction (C1), dense vitreous hemorrhage, and reaction (C2) (after Bronzino, J.: 1977 *Technology of Patient Care.* St. Louis: C. V. Mosby).

additional spatial resolution of the valve morphology as well as the cardiac chambers. The recent addition of Doppler flow measurements to cardiac echocardiography imaging hold great promise for the future. In this way the cardiologist not only will be able to visualize the movement of cardiac structures but also measure the blood flow velocity in the heart chambers and great vessels.

Superficial structures, located less than 5 cm from the skin surface, can be imaged in real-time. Since depth penetration is not a requirement, high frequency transducers with resultant submillimeter anatomic resolution are used. As an example, in the evaluation of the thyroid, it has been shown that very small lesions (2 to 3 mm) have been observed, which have only previously been observed by microscopic examinations *Fleischer & James, Jr. (1984). Other superficial anatomical structures which can be imaged include: carotid arteries, eye, scrotum, breast and subcutaneous tissue.

Ultrasonic examinations of the eye are important especially when an ophthamologist cannot visually examine the eye (in situations in which opaque material such as blood is present or when the patient has cataracts). It would be unfortunate to have a situation in which a cataract was removed only to find that the patient had a retinal detachment or a large melanoma. The major application of ultrasonic examinations of the eye is in the evaluation of nonmetallic foreign bodies, retinal detachment, and intraocular tumors. The availability of high-frequency transducers makes evaluating the eye for periorbital and intraorbital disorders possible

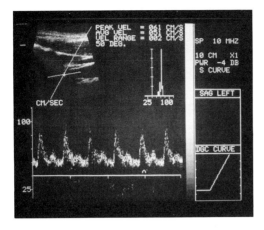

Figure 9.33 Normal duplex scan of carotid vessels.

(Fleischer and James 1984). Figure 9.32 shows an ultrasonic examination of the eye and the ultrasonic images.

In many clinical vascular laboratories a duplex scanner images and quantifies blood velocity in superficial blood vessels. These systems employ a real-time scanner to image the blood vessel and a pulsed Doppler system to measure the blood velocity in any desired location within the blood vessel. Duplex imaging is especially useful for evaluating patients with a suspected carotid lesion. These patients are normally sent to the vascular lab for a duplex evaluation if they have experienced a transient ischemic attack or if their primary physician has heard a bruit over the carotid artery.

Duplex imaging of the carotid arteries is a useful screening technique when compared with other currently available radioliographic techniques such as digital subraction angiography (DSA). Although DSA shows carotid atherosclerotic lesions with high resolution, if a patient moves or swallows during the examination, less than diagnostic images will result. Some patients are sensitive to contrast material composed of iodide, which is used for intravenous injection.

Cardullo and associates (1984) have shown that three-dimensional real-time duplex scanning of the carotid arteries is a highly accurate technique for detecting the presence of occlusive disease at the carotid bifurcation. The duplex scanner uses a combined 7.5-MHz imaging transducer and 3-MHz single-gate pulsed Doppler transducer. Real-time images are displayed at a rate of 20 frames per second; the image display rate is reduced to 4 frames per second when both the Doppler and real-time B-mode images are presented. The maximum ultrasound penetration depths for the image and Doppler fields are 8 and 5.5 cm, respectively. The axial and lateral image resolutions are 0.25 and 0.8 mm, respectively. The Doppler ultrasound sample volume is 3 by 2 mm.

Typical duplex scans are shown in Figures 9.33 and 9.34 for normal and diseased vessels, respectively. The real-time B-mode image is shown in the upper left corner. The cursor indicates the position at which the Doppler velocity measurement is taken. The lower graph is the Doppler blood velocity versus time. The upper right graph is a fast Fourier transform (FFT) of the blood velocity. In comparing the normal and abnormal duplex scans, note that the abnormal stenotic vessel has a full spread of velocities from the lowest to a high of approximately 150 cm/s.

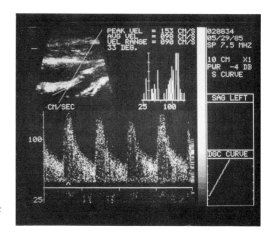

Figure 9.34 Duplex scan of stenotic internal carotid.

The normal, on the other hand, tends to have more high velocity components, with a lower maximum value of approximately 100 cm/s. The reason for this difference is that a stenotic, or narrowed, vessel causes an increase in velocity and resultant turbulence effects, whereas with undisturbed flow the velocity profile may be considered to be more laminar, with predominantly high velocities in the center of the flow stream. The FFT of the stenotic vessel also shows a broad spectrum of frequency components, whereas the normal vessel produces a narrower frequency spectrum.

Cardullo and associates (1984) point out that a relative disadvantage of the duplex scanning technique is its subjective nature. They found that the results are dependent on the experience and skill of the technologist. High-level results may be attained after 6 months of experience using the duplex scanner.

FUTURE OF ULTRASONIC IMAGING

The future of the medical applications of diagnostic ultrasound is tied to the progress of electronic and computer technology. As electronic and computer circuits become more powerful for the same hardware volume and cost, we will see more sophisticated ultrasonic imagers being developed and new medical applications being employed.

The future of diagnostic ultrasonic applications in medicine is contingent on the development of improved digital processing of the ultrasonic data. New image processing algorithms will handle and quantify the large amounts of ultrasonic data. In present-day systems, once the data are stored in relatively inexpensive digital memory devices, they can be manipulated to improve the image quality and to make simple calculations of tissue dimensions. Further work remains in terms of improving the image quality, extracting information about the nature of the tissue, and making accurate calculations of tissue dimensions, including volumes, from three-dimensional measurements.

McDicken (1981) has outlined the following areas for future ultrasound developments: computerized tomography, transmission imaging, three-dimensional imaging, holography, microscopy, and tissue characterization.

Computerized ultrasonic imaging is analogous to x-ray computerized tomography (CT). However, the ultrasound CT has the advantage that, in addition to looking at the attenuation of ultrasound by tissue, it is possible to measure the ultrasound propagation velocity through tissue and the ultrasonic scattering properties of tissue. One difficulty with ultrasound CT is that ultrasound beams cannot be transmitted equally well in all directions through the body.

Imaging transmission ultrasound is analogous to x-ray imaging of tissues: the ultrasound waves are transmitted from a source on one side of the structure and detected by a receiver on the other side. The magnitude of the received signal is proportional to the attenuation of the tissue. Problems with this, as well as any type of transmission device, are the multiple reflections, scattering, and other distortions that occur because of complex tissue structures. Ultrasonic cameras have been built using several hundred piezoelectric sensors to display the ultrasound transmission images in video format. These cameras have given a 1-mm-diameter resolution in clinical evaluations.

Ultrasonic microscopy is a technique in which biological specimens are transmission scanned by high-frequency (500 MHz) sound waves. These high-resolution images, related to the acoustic properties of the objects under study, are complementary to optical micrographs. Wells (1977) gives a historical development of this area.

Ultrasonic holography has generated much enthusiasm for its potential application. In theory the holographic technique could produce high-resolution, three-dimensional images in real time, allowing the observation of tissue movement. Wells (1977) has indicated that difficulties, due to poor signal-to-noise ratio, the difference between the ultrasound and light wavelengths, specular reflections, poor phase coherence, and physiological movements, have produced disappointing results.

The development of three-dimensional ultrasonic scanners is slow. One problem with displaying a three-dimensional image is the high density of ultrasonic echoes present. The echoes from superficial structures obscure those from deeper structures. In addition, large inexpensive computer memories are necessary to store the ultrasonic data from a three-dimensional scan. This would allow the call-up and display of any two-dimensional plane for the operator.

Perhaps one of the most exciting and challenging areas of ultrasonic imaging deals with tissue characterization. Wells (1978) reviewed the early work in this area. Basically the research relates to whether the difference between the ultrasonic signal (or signature) is different when normal or abnormal tissue is studied. A number of ultrasound parameters have been investigated, including attenuation, scattering, and velocity of propagation. Put in terms of a physiological example, is there a way to determine from an appropriate ultrasonic scan of the heart whether a myocardial infarction has taken place, and if so, how severe it was? Similar questions could be posed for benign and cancerous tissue.

Another area of future development deals with the development of specialized transducers that would be placed inside the body for better imaging of a specific organ. For instance, approximately 30 percent of all men aged 50 or over have prostate cancer. It has been proposed that a high-resolution ultrasonic transducer operating at 10 MHz when placed in the rectum could provide high-resolution ultrasound images of prostate cancer. This should give more definitive results than those available with the normal digital examination for prostate cancer.

REFERENCES

Banks, L. W. 1983. An ultrasound imaging system. *Hewlett-Packard J,* October 1983, p. 6.

Brown, P. M., et al. 1982. Detection of occlusive disease of the carotid artery spectral analysis patterns. *Surg Gynecol Obstet* 155(8):183–186.

Bronzino, J. D. 1977. *Technology for patient care: Applications for today, implications for tomorrow.* St. Louis: Mosby.

Callagan, D. A., Rowland, T. C., Goldman, D. E. 1964. Ultrasonic Doppler observation of the fetal heart. *Obstet Gynecol* 23:637.

Cardullo, P. A., Cutler, B.S., Wheeler, H. B., et al. 1984. Accuracy of duplex scanning in the detection of carotid artery disease. *Bruit* 8(6), p. 181, 1984.

Desch, C. H., Sproule, D. O., Dawson, W. J. 1946. The detection of cracks in steel by means of supersonic waves. *J Iron Steel Inst* 153:319.

De Vlieger, M. (ed.). 1978. *Handbook of clinical ultrasound.* New York: Wiley.

Donald, I. 1964. Sonar—The story of an experiment. *Ultrasound Med Biol* 1:109.

Edler, I. 1961. Ultrasoundcardiography. *Acta Med Scand [Suppl]* 170.

Farrall, W. R. 1959. Design considerations for ultrasonic flowmeters. *IRE Trans Med Electron* ME-6(4):201.

Feigenbaum, H. 1981. *Echocardiography,* (3d ed.). Philadelphia: Lea & Febiger.

Firestone, F. A. 1946. The supersonic reflectoscope, an instrument for inspecting the interior of solid parts by means of sound waves. *J Acoust Soc Am* 17:287.

Flaherty, J. J., Strauts, E. J. 1969. Ultrasonic pulse Doppler instrumentation. In Proceedings of the 8th International Conference on Medical and Biomedical Engineering. Chicago, p. 10.

Fleischer, A. C., James A. E. 1984. *Real-time sonography.* Textbook with accompanying videotape. Norwalk, Appleton-Century-Crofts.

Hagen-Ansert, S. L. 1983. *Textbook of diagnostic ultrasonography,* (2d ed.). St. Louis: Mosby.

Hajjar, W. M. 1981. *Multi-focus multi elements matrix ultrasonic transducer for real-time Doppler imaging design, construction and evaluation.* Dissertation, Worcester Polytechnic Institute.

Hill, C. R. 1978. Ultrasonic attenuation and scattering by tissues. In deVlieger, M., Holmes, J. H., Kazner, E., Kossoff, G., et al. (eds.) *Handbook of Clinical Ultrasound.* New York: Wiley. p. 91.

Histand, M. B., Miller, C. W., McLeod, F. D. 1973. Transcutaneous measurement of blood velocity profiles and flow. *Cardiovasc Res* 7:703.

Howry, D. H. 1957. Techniques used in ultrasonic visualization of soft tissues. In Kelly, E. (ed.) *Ultrasound in Biology and Medicine.* Washington: American Institute of Biological Sciences. p. 4.

Howry, D. H., Bliss, W. R. 1952. Ultrasonic visualization of soft tissue structures of the body. *J Lab Clin Med* 40:579.

Keil, O. R. 1982. Ultrasound and its various modes in use. Part II: Real-time scanners. *Med Instrum* 16(2):107.

Kremkau, F. K. 1984. *Diagnostic ultrasound: Principles, instrumentation, and exercises,* (2d ed.). New York: Grune & Stratton.

Leksell, L. 1956. Echo-encephalography: Detection of intracranial complications following head surgery. *Acta Chir Scand* 110:301.

Ludwig, G. D., Struthers, F. W. 1950. Detecting gall-stones with ultrasonics. *Electronics* 23(2):172.

McDicken, W. N. 1981. *Diagnostic ultrasonics: Principles and use of instruments.* (2d ed.). New York: Wiley.

McLeod, F. D. 1967. A directional Doppler flowmeter. *Dig Int Conf Med Biol Eng* (Stock) p. 213.

McLeod, F. D. 1964. A Doppler ultrasonic physiological flowmeter. In Proceedings of the 17th Annual Conference on Engineering in Medicine and Biology. Cleveland, p. 81.

Mozersky, D. J., Hokanson, D. E., Baker, D. W., et al. 1971. Ultrasonic arteriography. *Arch Surg* 103:663.

Mundt, G. H., Hughes, W. F. 1956. Ultrasonics in ocular diagnosis. *Am J Ophthamol* 41:488.

Peronneau, P. A., Leger, F. 1969. Doppler ultrasonic pulsed Doppler flowmeter. In Proceedings of the 8th International Conference on Medical and Biomedical Engineering, Chicago. p. 10–11.

Powis, R. L., Powis, W. J. 1984. *A thinker's guide to ultrasonic imaging.* Baltimore: Urban & Schwarzenberg.

St. Thomas, M. L. 1984. Ultrasound Doppler spectral analysis: comparison of continuous and pulsed wave techniques. M.S. thesis, Worcester Polytechnic Institute.

Satomura, S. 1957. Ultrasonic Doppler method for the inspection of cardiac functions. *J Acoust Soc Am* 29:1181.

Siedband, M. P., Holden, J. E. 1978. Medical imaging systems. In Webster, J. G. (ed.) *Medical instrumentation applications and design.* Boston: Houghton Mifflin.

Strandness, D. E., Schultz, R. D., Sumner, D. S., et al. 1966. Ultrasonic flow detection: A useful technic in the evaluation of peripheral vascular disease. *Am J Surg* 113:311.

Strutt, J. W. 1877. Third Baron Rayleigh: The Theory of Sound. London: Macmillan. vol. 1, 1877, vol. 2, 1878.

Sumner, D. S. 1982. Ultrasound. In Kempezinski, Y. (ed.) *Practical noninvasive vascular diagnosis.* Chicago. Year Book. chap. 2.

Webster, J. G. 1978. Measurement of flow and volume of blood. In Webster, J. G. (ed.) *Medical instrumentation: Application and design.,* Boston: Houghton Mifflin. chap. 8.

Wells, P. N. T. 1964. Developments in medical ultrasonics. *World Med Electron* 4:272.

Wells, P. N. T. 1969. A range-gated ultrasonic Doppler system. *Med Biol Eng* 7:641.

Wells, P. N. T. 1969. Physical principles of ultrasonic diagnosis. London: Academic Press.

Wells, P. N. T. 1977. Biomedical ultrasonics. London: Academic Press.

Wells, P. N. T. 1983. Ultrasound imaging. In Rolfe, P. (ed.) *Non-Invasive Physiological Measurements,* (2d ed.). London: Academic. chap. 9.

Wild, J. J., Reid, J. M. 1952. Further pilot echographic studies of the histologic structure of tumors of the living intact human breast. *Am J Pathol* 28:839.

Wild, J. J., Reid, J. M. 1955. Echographic tissue diagnosis. In Proceedings of the Fourth Annual Conference on Ultrasonic Therapy. p. 1.

CHAPTER 10

Radiographic and Nuclear Magnetic Resonance Imaging

Kenneth D. Taylor, Ph.D.

United Technologies Corporation

INTRODUCTION

Almost a century ago Wilhelm Roentgen described a new type of radiation, which he called *x-rays,* that ultimately led to the birth of a new medical specialty, radiology and the medical imaging industry. Initially, these systems were very rudimentary, primarily providing images of broken bones. However, in the last 20 yr widespread changes in imaging techniques and in particular, the use of the computer, have accelerated the application of imaging techniques in medical diagnosis. These changes include the ability to derive physiological as well as anatomical information from images, the ability to trade off risk, cost, and benefit via the choice of imaging modality; and the introduction of new imaging media.

For example, radiographic imaging systems rely upon the differential attenuation of x-rays to produce an image. Initial systems required sizeable amounts of radiation to produce distinct images of tissues with good contrast (that is, widely different x-ray attenuation) such as bone and muscle. However, with the advent of better film and other types of detectors, the radiation dosage decreased. Perhaps even more significant was the development of the computerized axial tomography (CAT) scanner in the 1970s. This device produces a cross-sectional view of a patient instead of the traditional shadowgraph produced by conventional x-ray systems, thus providing the ability to image a single body plane without interference by other body planes. This technique required the use of a computer to reconstruct the x-ray attenuation data but also, for the first time, provided the clinician with high-resolution, high-contrast images of virtually any body plane. Further, these data could be used to reconstruct three-dimensional images if desired.

Although the development of the CAT scanner revolutionized radiographic imaging the development of the *nuclear magnetic resonance* (NMR) imaging promises to alter the application of imaging techniques by providing a noninvasive method for biochemical assays. NMR imaging systems rely on the alteration of magnetic moments of atoms to produce an image. Presently, NMR imagers primarily use the magnetic moment of hydrogen and hence image differences in water content and relaxation parameters of water molecules, of different tissues, to produce an image. Ultimately NMR imaging systems offer the ability to image other nuclear species such as iron, sodium, and potassium. Therefore, NMR could provide information not only about tissue morphology but also about tissue biochemistry and body metabolism that heretofore no other imaging system has provided. This has obvious advantages over traditional biochemical assays in that one could visualize metabolic events as they occur.

Needless to say, both x-ray and NMR imaging systems have evolved significantly since their invention and currently provide powerful tools for the clinician. Further, future advances in these imaging modalities will enhance medical practice and provide significant engineering challenges. The purpose of this chapter is to discuss the basic operating principles of these imaging techniques, to describe the current implementations of these methods in clinical use, and to present perspectives related to future advances in these imaging techniques.

RADIOGRAPHIC (X-RAY) IMAGING SYSTEMS

Types of X-ray Imaging Systems

X-ray imaging systems use the highest energy source of any medical imaging system, having energies between 50 and 200 KeV corresponding to wavelengths of 0.5 to 10 nm. All x-ray imaging systems consist of an x-ray source, a collimator, and a x-ray detector (as shown in Figure 10.1), with the distinction between the different radiological systems being the use of different detectors. In general, an x-ray image is produced by a point source x-ray tube that generates a beam of x-rays when excited by a high-voltage power supply. This beam is truncated by a collimator and passes through the patient, creating a shadow image in the image plane. This shadow image is detected by x-ray film, an image intensifier, or a set of x-ray detectors, depending upon the type of radiographic system employed.

In projection (conventional) radiography systems, the detector is photographic film inserted into a cassette with fluorescent screens (Barrett 1981). This technique has the advantages of offering high-resolution, high-contrast images with small patient dosage and a permanent record of the image. It has the disadvantage of having significant geometric distortion, no ability to discern depth information, and no real-time imaging capability. Conventional radiography is the

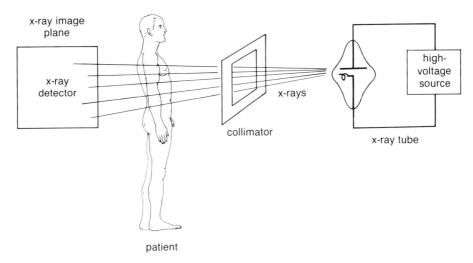

Figure 10.1   Generic x-ray imaging system.

imaging method of choice for such tasks as dental, chest, and bone imaging, since bone strongly absorbs x-ray. Therefore, fractures and caries are readily discernible by this standard radiographic technique.

In fluoroscopic radiographic systems, the detector is a fluorescent screen or an image intensifier-television camera combination (Webster 1978). This technique has the advantage of real-time imaging and is particularly useful in viewing blood vessels and in other organ examinations in which a contrast medium is injected into the body. Fluoroscopic radiographic systems are therefore extensively used in imaging of the heart and blood vessels. They have disadvantages in that geometric distortion is still evident, depth discrimination is not available, and an invasive procedure, injection of contrast medium, is necessary.

The third major radiographic system uses a set of x-ray detectors and mathematical reconstruction techniques to produce an image. These types of imaging systems, known as computerized axial tomography (CAT) scanners, have the ability to develop and display cross-sectional slices of the internal organs of the body and do not exhibit geometrical distortion (Scudder 1978). Although commercially available scanners do not yet have real-time imaging capability, experimental devices that have been developed or are under development do offer real-time or near-real-time imaging (Robb 1982). The primary disadvantage of existing CAT scanners is the relatively high cost for installation and operation of a CAT scanner facility as compared to a projection radiographic or fluoroscopic imaging system. Although CAT scanners were originally used for brain imaging they are now used for body scanning (for example, abdominal examinations) as well.

X-ray Image Formation

X-ray images are produced by the differential attenuation of x-ray transmission through the body due to differences in density and the mass attenuation coefficient of different tissues. X-ray attenuation is predicted by *Lambert-Beer's law* (Barrett 1981), in which the intensity *I(z)*, is expressed by

$$I(z) \; = \; I_0 \exp(-\mu \rho z) \tag{1}$$

where

I_0 = initial x-ray intensity

μ = linear attenuation coefficient

ρ = density

z = distance between the source plane and the measurement plane

This relation presumes a monoenergetic x-ray source producing a uniform x-ray field. The mass attenuation coefficient, μ/ρ, is often used instead of the linear attenuation coefficient in x-ray energy calculations. Either attenuation coefficient depends upon the photon energy of the source and the atomic numbers of the elements in the tissues. For x-ray photon energies in the diagnostic range (below 200 keV), three mechanisms dominate x-ray attenuation: (1) coherent scatter, (2) photoelectric absorption, and (3) Compton scatter (Macovski 1983).

Coherent or *Rayleigh scatter* results from the deflection of x-ray beams caused by atoms being excited by incident radiation and then reemitting waves at the same wavelengths. This phenomenon occurs primarily at low photon energies (below 50 keV) and hence is relatively insignificant in the image formation process. This is apparent in Figure 10.2, which shows the relative contributions of each attenuation mechanism.

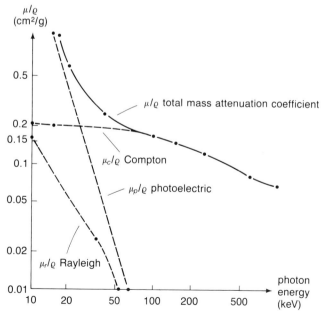

Figure 10.2   Total and components of the mass attenuation coefficient of water (after Macovski, A. 1983. *Medical imaging systems.* Englewood Cliffs, N.J.: Prentice-Hall).

Photoelectric absorption occurs when the x-ray photon is absorbed by the ejection of a tightly bound electron. The kinetic energy of the displaced electron is dissipated as heat, and the vacancy created in the electron shell is filled by an electron from an adjacent shell. This electron movement is accompanied by emission of fluorescent radiation due to the energy state change of the electron. The mass attenuation coefficient due to photoelectric absorption varies approximately as the third power of the atomic number of the matter and thus is increasingly important for higher-atomic-number materials such as radiopaque dyes. Photoelectric absorption has a major impact on the imaging process for photon energies of 20 to 50 keV.

Scattering due to the Compton effect results from a collision between an x-ray photon and either a free or loosely bound electron in an outer shell. This collision causes a change in the direction and a slight loss of energy for the x-ray photon and the scattering of the electron. Thus the energy of the scattered photons is comparable to that of the incident photons. Because of this, Compton scattering is not only a significant contributor to x-ray attenuation, but also has a significant effect on x-ray image degradation. Absorption due to Compton scattering has a major impact on the imaging process for photon energies of 50 to 200 keV.

The different attenuation mechanisms result in significant differences in mass attenuation coefficients for different tissue types. Typically the photoelectric effect predominates in low-atomic-number materials at low energies, whereas Compton scattering predominates for high energies. This is indicated in Figure

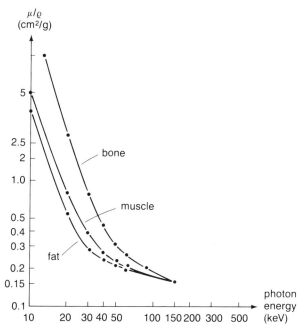

Figure 10.3 Mass attenuation coefficients for bone, fat, and muscle as a function of photon energy (after Macovski, A. 1983. *Medical Imaging Systems.* Englewood Cliffs, N.J.: Prentice-Hall).

10.3, which shows the mass attenuation coefficient of different tissues in the body as a function of x-ray photon energy.

The differences in mass attenuation coefficient govern the image formation process in radiology. An example of this would be a typical skeletal x-ray taken to find a broken bone. Generally skeletal x-rays are taken at medium photon energies (50 to 70 keV) to take advantage of the mass attenuation coefficient differences between bone and other soft tissue. Image contrast is improved further because bone is more dense than soft tissue. Using Lambert-Beer's law, the amount of x-rays absorped by the bone should be considerably higher than that of the surrounding soft tissue. Consequently, fewer x-ray photons reach the image plane, behind the bone, than in other areas.

Differences in tissue mass attenuation coefficient can be enhanced by contrast media. There are two types of contrast media, negative and positive. *Negative contrast medium* has a lower density and mass attenuation than surrounding tissue, whereas *positive contrast medium* has a higher density and mass attenuation coefficient than the surrounding tissue. Examples of negative contrast media include carbon dioxide and air, which have been used for image enhancement in ventriculography (x-rays of the ventricles in the brain). Examples of positive contrast media include high-atomic-number materials such as barium and iodine, which have been used extensively in radiopaque dyes for angiography (x-rays of the blood vessels).

X-ray Image Quality

All imaging systems are usually compared in terms of two parameters: system resolution and signal-to-noise ratio (SNR). *System resolution* determines the amount of detail the imaging system can discern, whereas the system signal-to-noise ratio determines the image dynamic range and ultimately image contrast. Both parameters limit the amount of information contained within the image and its diagnostic value. All images consist of a number of discrete picture elements called *pixels*, and generally each pixel has a finite amplitude associated with it. The maximum and minimum pixel amplitudes encompass the image signal-to-noise ratio.

System resolution can be specified by a number of techniques. An image can be considered to be a surface having a spatial resolution expressed in either line pairs per millimeter (lp/mm) or cycles per millimeter (cycles/mm). Resolution is defined in this manner so that objects and the spaces between them receive equal weight. For example, presume we have a target consisting of a matrix of holes, spaced 1 mm apart as shown in Figure 10.4. To reproduce the target faithfully, an imaging system must resolve one pixel per millimeter (1 p/mm) and have 2 pixels/millimeter to display each hole and the surrounding area.

The resolution of an imaging system can be determined by a theoretical analysis of the diffraction properties of the system or by measurement of its spatial frequency response. A theoretical analysis of the diffraction properties of an imaging system is beyond the scope of this text, although the more commonly used measures of resolution will be presented. However, the reader is cautioned to note that an exact analytical prediction of resolution of a system requires a diffraction anal-

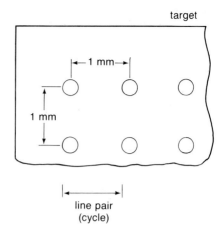

Figure 10.4 Spatial frequency example.

ysis of all system components involved with image formation and can be quite complicated.

One commonly used measurement of resolution is the Rayleigh two-point resolution criteria (Goodman 1968), which can be used to determine the minimum resolvable separation between two objects. Using Figure 10.5, presume we have two circular objects of diameter,l, which are separated by a distance,Δ, from each other. The minimum resovable separation according to the Rayleigh criterion is

$$\Delta = 1.22\lambda d/l \tag{2}$$

where

λ = the illumination source wavelength

d = distance between the object and image (observation) plane,

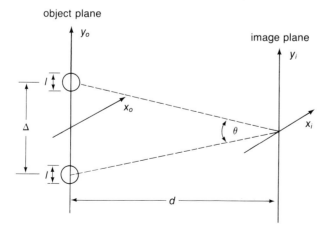

Figure 10.5 Rayleigh two-point resolution limit.

The angle, Θ, is defined by

$$\Theta = 1.22\lambda/l \qquad\qquad (3)$$

presuming that $d >> l$. The Rayleigh resolution criteria is not a particularly good indicator of system performance with respect to resolution since it does not take into account the contrast at the resolution limit. Hence a system could have high resolution, according to the Rayleigh limit, but not produce well-resolved images because of poor contrast characteristics. Better measures of system resolution use the spatial frequency response of the system to take into account contrast.

The *modulation transfer function* (MTF) is a normalized version of the spatial frequency response of an imaging system or its components (Goodman 1968). The MTF m(f) is derived analytically via diffraction theory or is measured by using a set of image phantoms (objects of known spatial frequency) with the response normalized to the value at zero spatial frequency. Generally these image phantoms are bar patterns, made with lead, that start at low spatial frequencies (large spaces between bars) and increase in spatial frequency. Using image phantoms appropriate for the imaging system produces a MTF curve such as that shown in Figure 10.6. Given a MTF, the limiting resolution point is usually considered to be the 0.05 contrast level, which corresponds to a spatial frequency of 4 cycles/mm for the imaging system in Figure 10.6.

Another property of the MTF is that if the MTFs of the individual components are known and are linear, then the system MTF can be found by multiplying the individual MTFs together, so that

$$\text{MTF(system)} = \text{MTF1} \times \text{MTF2} \times \text{MTF3} \times \ldots \times \text{MTF}n \qquad (4)$$

Figures 10.7 and 10.8 show the individual component and system MTFs for a projection radiography system and a fluoroscopic radiography system. As is

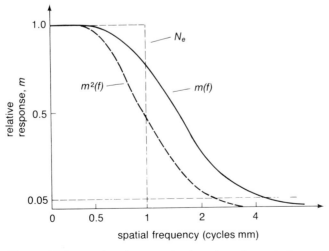

Figure 10.6 Modulation transfer function of a typical imaging system.

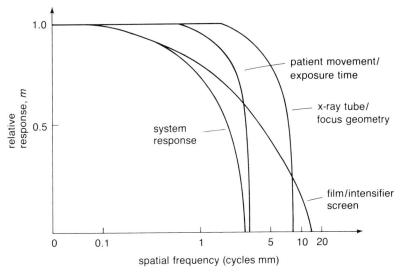

Figure 10.7 Modulation transfer function of a projection radiography system.

shown in the figures, each component places a limitation on the overall spatial frequency response of the system. For example, in the projection radiography system, although the tube has spatial frequencies extending to 8 cycles/mm, system frequency response is limited to about 3 cycles/mm by the spatial frequencies caused by patient movement/exposure time. In the fluoroscopic system, either the television camera or the image intensifier screen limits system resolution, as is shown in Figure 10.8.

A single number derived from the MTF, known as the *noise equivalent bandwidth, N_e,* is a useful method of describing component or system resolution (Web-

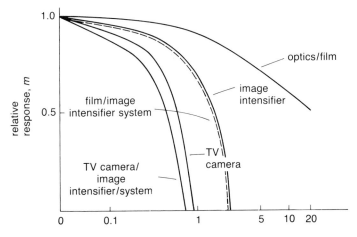

Figure 10.8 Modulation transfer function of a fluoroscopic radiography system.

ster 1978). The N_e is found by integrating the square of the MTF response, m^2, such that

$$N_e = \int_0^\infty m^2(f)df \tag{5}$$

This parameter modifies the spatial frequency response so that it has 100% amplitude response from zero frequency to N_e and zero response above N_e, as shown in Figure 10.6. Given the N_{es} of the system components, the system $N_{e,s}$ can be estimated via

$$1/N_{e,s} = [(1/N_{e,1})^2 + (1/N_{e,2})^2 + (1/N_{e,3})^2 + \ldots (1/N_{e,n})^2]^{1/2} \tag{6}$$

For example, consider a typical fluoroscopic imaging system, in which the N_e of the image intensifier and the TV camera/monitor are 1.5 and 1 cycles/mm, respectively. By equation (6), the fluoroscopic image viewed on the TV monitor has an N_e of 0.83. A similar analysis of the same fluoroscopic imaging system, using the image intensifier and film (N_e of 3) to view the image, shows that the image has an N_e of 1.34. As expected, this predicts that the image intensifier film combination will produce a more highly resolved image.

The other imaging system parameter of interest is the signal-to-noise ratio. The ability to visualize a structure in an image depends largely on the contrast, defined as

$$C = \Delta I/\bar{I}, \tag{7}$$

where $\bar{I}$ is the average background intensity and ΔI is the intensity differential in the region of interest on the image. Contrast, however, is not a fundamental limit on image visualization since it can be artificially enhanced. However, noise provides a fundamental limitation on the ability to see image information. Image signal-to-noise ratio can be related to contrast by the expression

$$\text{SNR} = C\bar{I}/\sigma \tag{8}$$

where σ is the rms noise level. Since x-ray radiation is a quantum phenomenon, it follows a Poisson statistical distribution, which has a standard deviation of σ. Hence, the generic SNR of an x-ray imaging system is defined by

$$\text{SNR} = N/(N)^{1/2} = C(N)^{1/2} \tag{9}$$

where N is the x-ray photon flux (Barrett 1981). In this expression N represents the variation in the number of photons per element defining the image structure, and $[N]^{1/2}$ is the image noise. Thus the image SNR can be made arbitrarily high except for the need to limit patient radiation dosage. Since not all x-ray photons contribute to the image, this feature reduces the value of N. Hence a generic expression for SNR is

$$\text{SNR} = C(\eta N)^{1/2} \tag{10}$$

where η is the quantum efficiency or the percentage of x-rays impinging on the detector that contribute to the image. This can be related to patient x-ray dosage, measured in roentgens (R), and the area, A, of the detector pixel to determine the number of x-ray photons per pixel by

$$N = \Phi AR \, \exp(\int_\theta -\mu dz) \qquad (11)$$

where Φ is the photon density per roentgen and the relation $\exp(-\int \mu dz)$ equals t, the x-ray transmission through the body. Then from equation (10) the SNR is

$$SNR = C(\eta \Phi ARt)^{1/2} \qquad (12)$$

For example, for a typical chest x-ray, R is 50 milliroentgens (mR) and t is 0.05 for regions devoid of bone. Presuming a detector area, A, of 1 mm^2 and a C of 0.1, the SNR is about 16 dB.

A similar expression can be derived for fluoroscopic or other types of x-ray imaging systems using ancillary electronic components in the detector by considering the noise sources contributed by these electronic components. Since typically this noise is not Poisson-distributed and is independent of the x-ray noise, it can be added to the x-ray noise so that the SNR becomes,

$$SNR = C\eta N/(N_a^2 + \eta N)^{1/2} \qquad (13)$$

where N_a is the rms value of the additive noise.

Signal-to-noise ratio in CAT scanners is analyzed slightly differently because of the method of image formation. Since CAT scanner images are reconstructions of the attenuation coefficients of the organ(s) imaged, the SNR expression of equation (8) becomes

$$SNR = C\bar{\mu}/\sigma_\mu \qquad (14)$$

where

$\bar{\mu}$ = average attenuation

σ_μ = rms attenuation noise level.

Presuming the use of the convolution back projection reconstruction method with M projections, it can be shown (Macovski 1983) that the SNR is

$$SNR = KC\bar{\mu}(N_m M)^{1/2}w \qquad (15)$$

where

K = constant dependent on the CAT scanner MTF

N = average number of x-ray photons detected per projection

w = detector width

This expression neglects electronic noise. Note that the expression is very similar to equation (9) in that the SNR increases as x-ray photon flux increases. But it also illustrates that in CAT scanner imaging, a higher-resolution system suffers a SNR penalty due to a reduced detector width.

As mentioned in the previous discussion, one method to increase the SNR is to increase the x-ray photon flux. Unfortunately, x-rays, like other forms of ionizing radiation, affect living tissue, and exposure to x-rays must be limited to minimize tissue damage. X-ray radiation can disrupt the normal molecular structure of tissue through its high-energy particles. At low doses, the biological effect is to change cell metabolism and structure. This effect appears only after some latency period, which decreases as the radiation dose increases. Higher radiation doses can result in cell death. Further, different tissues have different levels of sensitivity to radiation exposure, with the most sensitive tissues being bone and lymph nodes. Early signs of radiation damage include anemia and decreases in the number of and morphological changes to white cells. Fetal tissues, sex glands, skin, and mucosal tissues are also sensitive. The effect of radiation is cumulative, with small doses received at long intervals having an additive effect. Hence, it is very important that x-ray imaging systems use the minimum amount of x-ray energy consistent with obtaining a good image.

X-ray exposure is measured in roentgens (R), where 1 R is defined as producing ionization of 2.58×10^{-4} coulomb per kilogram (C/kg) in air (Barrett 1981). The absorbed dose unit is the radiation absorbed dose (rad), which is defined as the amount of x-ray exposure that imparts 100 ergs of energy per gram of tissue. In air, 1 R is equivalent to an absorbed dose of 0.87 rad. However, the number of rads per roentgen varies with the material and the x-ray photon energy, as is illustrated in Figure 10.9. Two other units of absorbed dose are used: the gray and the rem. A *gray* is the amount of x-ray exposure that imparts 1 joule (J) of energy per kilogram of tissue; hence, 1 gray equals 100 rads. The roentgen equivalent man (rem)

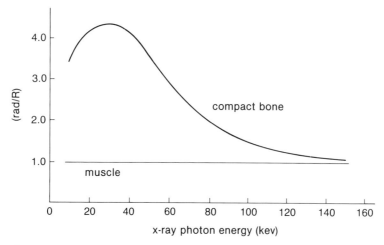

Figure 10.9 The relationship between rads and roentgen as a function of photon energy for different tissues (after Macovski, A. 1983. *Medical imaging systems.* Englewood Cliffs, N.J.: Prentice-Hall).

represents the absorbed dose of radiation that has the same biological effect as 1 rad of x-rays and is a unit used to compare the biological effects of different forms of ionizing radiation (x-rays, gamma rays, and so on). The rem is related to the rad by the expression

$$REM = RAD \times RBE \tag{16}$$

where RBE is the relative biological effect. In the case of x-rays, the RBE is 1.

General limits for radiation exposure have been established, so that the general public has an absorbed dose less than 0.5 rad per year. In the case of people who work with ionizing radiation such as nuclear power plant or radiological personnel, the limit is 0.1 rad per week with an annual limit of 5 rads. Since the effect of x-ray radiation is cumulative, the recommended upper limit for accumulated dose is defined by the relationship

$$D = 5(n - 18) \, \text{rads} \tag{17}$$

where n is the age in years. For example, for a person working in radiology at age 40, D is 110 rads, with a typical lifetime upper limit (presuming retirement at age 65) of 235 rads. This is compared to a lifetime exposure to other types of radiation (cosmic radiation, radiation from natural radioisotopes, and so on) of 5 to 15 rems.

A typical x-ray examination generally requires from 10 to 100 millirads (mrad), whereas a one-time exposure of 50 rads is required to cause the onset of noticeable radiation effects. A one-time exposure of 200 to 500 rads is required to produce radiation death. The long-term effects of large-dose radiation have been studied extensively in relation to the types of tissue damage induced and the exposure required, with some of the more significant effects being cataracts, birth defects, and cancer (Beebe 1982).

Projection Radiography Systems

The most commonly used x-ray imaging systems are projection (transmission) radiography systems, which are configured as shown in Figure 10.10. These systems consist of a high-voltage power supply, x-ray tube, aluminum filter, collimator, grid, and film cassette. An x-ray image of the body is generated by placing the patient between the collimator and the grid so that the differential x-ray attenuation of the patient's organs causes the film to be exposed and produce an image of the organs. In operation, the x-ray tube generates x-rays that are restricted to the aperture formed by the collimator. The aluminum filter removes low-energy x-rays that would not penetrate the body and hence would not contribute to the image. Scattered secondary radiation is trapped by the grid, whereas the primary radiation strikes the film cassette. The exposed film is developed to get a typical x-ray image, as shown in Figure 10.11. Because x-rays pass through the entire depth of the body, it is not possible to discern depth information in the developed radiograph.

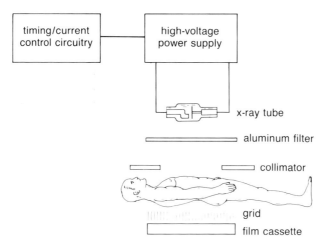

Figure 10.10 Projection radiography system.

X-rays are generated by a three-phase full-wave rectifier high-voltage dc power supply whose output current, voltage, and timing can be remotely controlled at the machine console. The x-ray tube is a temperature-limited vacuum tube diode, with a rotating anode, operated in a high vacuum as shown in Figure 10.12. In the x-ray tube, electrons are emitted by a hot filament cathode and are focused onto a restricted area of the anode that is typically made of tungsten or a tungsten alloy. X-ray photons are emitted when the electrons penetrate the anode surface. Tungsten is used as the anode material because of its high melting point and high atomic number. Since the tube is typically 1 percent efficient at 100 kV, the remainder of the energy is dissipated by thermal radiation. A rotating anode, driven electromagnetically via a stator coil, aids in the heat dissipation process and prevents the electron beam from burning one spot on the anode. The output energy of the tube Q (Webster 1978) is defined by

$$Q = kItV^2 \tag{18}$$

where

k = constant dependent upon the tube
I = anode current
t = exposure time
V = tube voltage

X-ray tube output is generally expressed, in the clinical environment, as the product of the exposure time and current. The anode current is typically controlled by adjusting the filament current.

The wavelength of the x-rays produced depends on the kinetic energy of the electrons striking the anode. However, the emitted radiation is not monoenergetic and consists of two types of x-ray emissions: bremsstrahlung and characteristic ra-

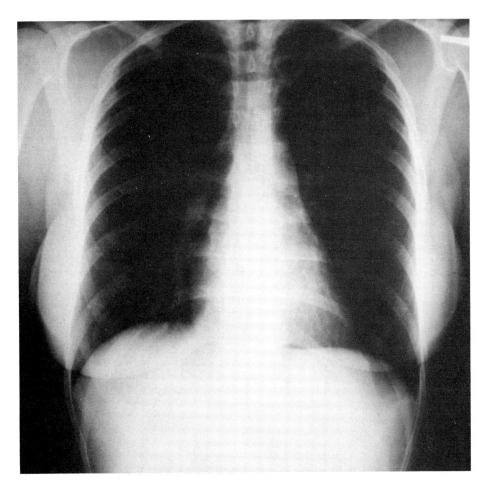

Figure 10.11   Typical chest x-ray (courtesy of General
Electric Medical System).

diation (Jacobson and Webster 1977). *Bremsstrahlung* (also known as *braking,* or
white, radiation) is produced by the deflection of the electrons by the nuclei of the
anode atoms and has a wide energy distribution. Characteristic radiation is produced when the anode atoms' innermost electrons, displaced by the arriving electrons, are replaced by outer shell electrons. The outer shell electrons emit x-rays in a
narrow band of wavelengths. Bremsstrahlung radiation spectra are dependent on the
tube voltage, whereas only the intensity of the characteristic radiation is voltage-
dependent. The effects of both types of x-ray emission are shown in Figure 10.13.

Generally, lower-energy (below 20 keV), or "soft," x-rays are filtered by the
primary filter in the tube since they will not penetrate the patient's skin and hence
will not contribute to the image and will only result in unnecessary skin dosage.
The aluminum filter between the x-ray tube and the collimator provides additional
filtration for certain diagnostic procedures.

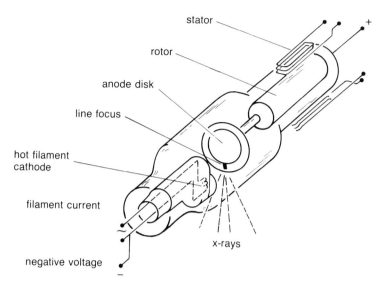

Figure 10.12   X-ray tube construction (after Jacobson, B., and Webster, J. G., 1977. *Medicine and clinical engineering.* Englewood Cliffs, N.J.: Prentice-Hall).

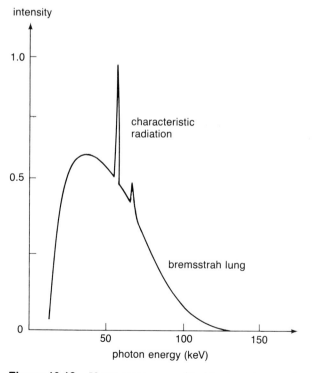

Figure 10.13   X-ray spectrum emitted by tungsten anode at 130 kV.

Two other devices, collimators and grids, increase image contrast and reduce unnecessary patient dosage. A *collimator* is a piece of lead, with a circular or rectangular aperture in it, used to truncate the x-ray beam. Most modern collimators are adjustable, so that the size of the aperture can be varied. Also, they usually incorporate an optical source that determines the size of the x-ray beam and aids in patient positioning. Choosing the smallest possible x-ray field size by appropriate collimator adjustment decreases the loss of contrast due to scattered radiation and reduces the x-ray dosage.

Grids consist of thin lead strips separated by spacers made of low mass attenuation coefficient material that are placed between the patient and the film cassette. The lead strips are angled and directed toward the x-ray tube focus so that the primary radiation from the focus that contains the image information passes through the grid, whereas the scattered radiation is attenuated. Because of the shadow of the lead strips, the resultant filmed image would be striped. To eliminate the striped appearance, a *Bucky grid* is moved back and forth during the x-ray exposure so that the time average of the grid image on the film is zero.

The film cassette consists of a double-emulsion type of photographic film sandwiched in between two fluorescent intensifier screens as shown in Figure 10.14. The film cassette is constructed in this manner since the photographic efficiency of x-rays is extremely low for two reasons: First, photographic film absorbs only a small portion of the x-rays since it contains only small amounts of substances with a high atomic number. Second, each absorbed x-ray photon represents a much higher energy level than is required to render a silver bromide grain developable. Therefore, photographic film is only used alone for special purposes such as high-resolution imaging.

Normal x-ray film cassette uses fluorescent intensifying screens placed on each side of the film to increase the film efficiency. In operation, when a x-ray pho-

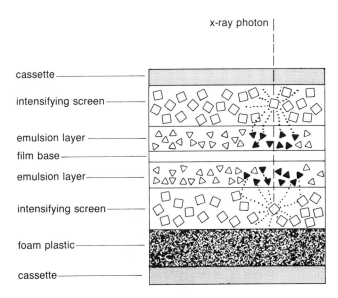

Figure 10.14 X-ray film cassette construction.

ton hits the intensifier screen, the screen fluoresces, producing many visible-light photons. Intensifier screens increase the efficiency through two mechanisms: (1) enhanced x-ray absorption (a factor of 20 to 130 times that of film), and (2) light wavelengths have 60 times more developing power than x-ray wavelengths. Therefore, an overall gain of 100 to 1,000 is possible over conventional film, although 20 to 100 is generally attainable in practice. The gain in sensitivity is obtained at the expense of resolution because the thickness of the intensifier screen causes screen scatter and loss of image detail. As a result, different types of screens are used for different clinical imaging tasks. Fine-grain screens, which have small fluorescent grains and thin layers, have a low sensitivity but high resolution (N_e = 7 lp/mm). Conversely, screens with large fluorescent grains and thick layers have a high sensitivity but low resolution (N_e = 2.5 1 p/mm).

The intensifying screens are typically made of calcium tungstate that fluoresces, producing blue light that closely corresponds to the peak wavelength of the photographic film. The photographic film is of the high-contrast type to provide good image quality.

Fluoroscopic Radiography Systems

Fluoroscopic radiography systems use the same components as projection radiography systems, except for the detector. Generally fluoroscopic systems are used for real-time x-ray imaging for surveillance or observation purposes such as observing the movement of a catheter. Since fluoroscopic units are used more for such purposes, resolution requirements are generally lower than those of projection radiography units. However, it is important to limit total patient radiation exposure.

The first fluoroscopic systems used as the detector a fluoroscopic screen that the physician viewed directly (Figure 10.15). In these systems, the x-ray photons

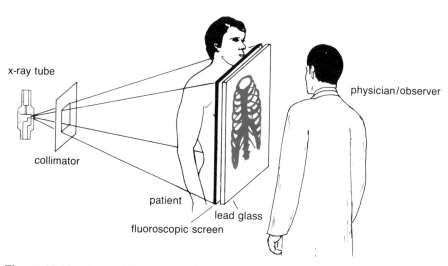

Figure 10.15   Original fluoroscopic imaging system.

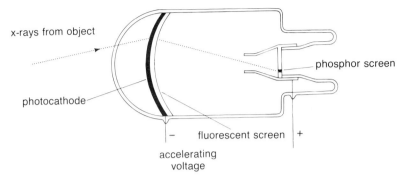

x-rays from object

phosphor screen

photocathode

fluorescent screen

accelerating
voltage

Figure 10.16   X-ray image intensifier tube construction.

reaching the screen are converted to visible light photons viewed by the observer. The screens used for this purpose were usually constructed of zinc cadmium sulfide, which emits a yellowish green light, thus closely matching the spectral response of the eye. The lead glass behind the screen protected the observer from excessive x-ray exposure and also contributed to scattering, thus reducing resolution. This technique has a number of disadvantages since the efficiency of the fluoroscopic screen (x-ray to visible light conversion) is typically 5 to 7 percent. Since the screen emits a weak light, it must be observed in a darkened room, and physicians must dark-adapt their eyes before the examination. Further, at these low brightness levels, the resolution and contrast discrimination of the eye are poor. Hence fluoroscopic screens for direct-viewing fluoroscopy are no longer used.

Modern fluoroscopic radiographic imaging systems use an image intensifier tube as the detector (Figure 10.16). The image intensifier tube contains a fluorescent screen, a photocathode, and a phosphor screen, all within an evacuated glass enclosure. X-rays hitting the fluorescent screen convert the x-ray photons into light photons. When these strike the photocathode, which is mounted behind the screen, photoelectrons are emitted. These photoelectrons are accelerated by a 25kV potential and focused, via an electrostatic lens, onto a small phosphor screen. The image can then be viewed via a television camera or simple optical enlarging system. The use of the image intensifier tube typically results in a gain of 5,000 over the use of a fluoroscopic screen alone.

Typically image intensifiers are incorporated into a fluoroscopic system, such as that shown in Figure 10.17, that uses multiple methods of viewing the image (Garrett 1980). In this system, the output of the image intensifier is optically coupled to a 16-mm movie camera and to a television camera via a beam splitter and lens optical system. This technique is used because the 16-mm camera has better resolution than the television camera and can provide a high-resolution permanent record of the fluoroscopic procedure. However, the television camera is used extensively for viewing purposes during the actual radiographic examination. Note that the x-ray source and the image intensifier are mechanically connected so that the two units move together during the patient examination. These systems often include, as an option, a videocassette recorder for recording the fluoroscopic procedure without the need to develop the film.

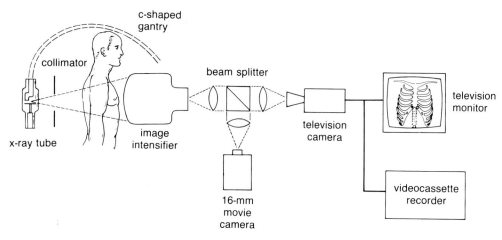

Figure 10.17 Modern fluoroscopic imaging system.

Recently, a variation of the modern fluoroscopic radiographic system that incorporates image processing hardware and software to improve the radiographic image quality (Weinstein 1981) has been developed. These systems, known as *digital radiography* or *digital subtraction radiography systems,* convert the detected x-ray image information into a digital format for image processing before display. The digital radiography system, shown in Figure 10.18, uses an image memory with integral arithmetic operation capabilities that is coupled to a computer to process image data digitally. Typically this processing is in the form of subtracting a "mask" image from subsequent images to produce a contrast-enhanced image that is viewed on the television monitor. If an artifact, such as patient motion, is introduced during the imaging process, a new mask is defined and the processing continues. Image subtraction is performed primarily to eliminate noise or undesired image information and thus increase image contrast. There are two subtraction methods used with this system: temporal and energy subtraction.

In *temporal subtraction,* an image is acquired before the introduction of a contrast agent such as radiopaque dye. A second image is acquired after the contrast agent has been administered, and the two images are subtracted from each other. Theoretically, this is the optimum way to enhance an image, but image enhancement is usually limited by misregistration of the two images due to patient motion.

In *energy subtraction,* images acquired at two different x-ray energies are subtracted from one another. Energy subtraction depends on the differences in attenuation properties between the contrast agent and the surrounding tissues for image improvement. Typically, the x-ray source is switched between two energies near the characteristic energies of the contrast material to maximize the energy-dependent differences in mass attenuation coefficient. Since this method is not time-dependent, presuming the x-ray source is rapidly switched, it is less susceptible to motion artifact.

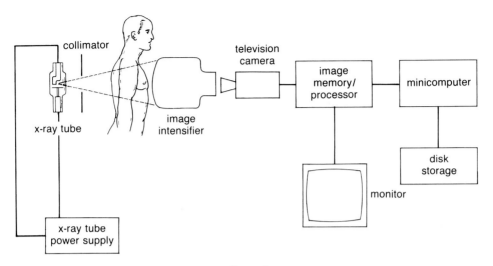

Figure 10.18 Digital subtraction radiography system.

Because of the need for x-ray source energy switching and image processing, the components used in digital radiography systems require better performance than those used in a fluoroscopic unit. Typically, the x-ray tube has more power and heat dissipation capacity, and the television camera has higher spatial resolution, improved linearity, and lower noise than those in fluoroscopic x-ray systems.

Motion Tomography Systems

Conventional (projection) radiographs and fluoroscopic images show all object planes within the same image, thus losing depth information. However, depth information is very valuable, and several techniques have been developed for producing a *tomogram*, or an image of one plane in the body. One technique, known as *motion tomography or body section radiography*, produces intentional movement-induced lack of sharpness or blurring in all planes except the one to be visualized (Macovski 1983). This is accomplished by moving the x-ray tube and film during the exposure about an axis located at the desired patient plane (Figure 10.19), via a circular, helical, or linear scanning motion. The larger the distance the tube and film cassette travel, the greater the movement nonsharpness becomes for undesired patient planes, and hence thinner tomographic sections can be observed.

However, motion tomography is limited in its ability to isolate a specific plane in the body since it is only capable of blurring the undesired planes. In general, the contrast of the desired image plane is unchanged from that of a conventional projection radiograph. Hence, the plane of interest is not visibly enhanced. A revolutionary concept in tomography, *computerized axial tomography*, provides a significant improvement over motion tomography in that it can produce an isolated image of a body section, completely eliminating all other body planes.

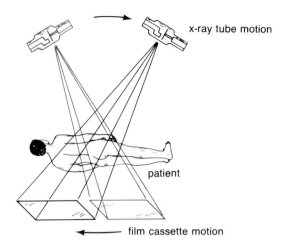

x-ray tube motion

patient

film cassette motion

Figure 10.19   Principle of motion tomography.

Computerized Axial Tomography (CAT) Scanners

Computerized axial tomography or computer-assisted tomography (CAT) scanners provide the ability to reconstruct cross-sectional images of the body from x-ray attenuation data. One of the major advantages of this technique is that since isolated cross-sectional images can be produced, intervening structures do not diminish the contrast of the desired planes as in motion tomography. Also, since only the section of interest is irradiated, patient x-ray dosage can be reduced. Additionally, tissue attenuation differences of less than 1 percent can be seen, which is much smaller than that of other radiographic imaging systems, which typically require a 10 percent or greater tissue attenuation difference to visualize a structure. The first CAT system was developed by Hounsfield (circa 1972), and a CAT scanner for brain imaging was first commercially produced by EMI Ltd of England (Hounsfield 1973). Since EMI's initial system, other scanners, by EMI Ltd and other medical imaging manufacturers, have been developed to allow imaging of the whole body. Significant improvements with respect to image reconstruction time, image resolution, and system SNR have resulted.

CAT scanner evolution

Figure 10.20 is a block diagram of the first-generation scanner, consisting of a x-ray tube mounted on an electromechanical scanning mechanism, whose output is collimated into a narrow beam. This configuration is commonly known as the *pencil beam source.* The patient is placed on a sliding table with the head resting on a rubber cup to fix it in a known position. The rim of this rubber cup is attached to the side of a plastic enclosure filled with water. The water provides a consistent medium through which x-rays pass, thereby reducing the possibility of large discrepancies in the x-ray intensity levels measured by the detector. A scintillation detector consisting of a scintillation crystal (such as sodium iodide) and a photomultiplier

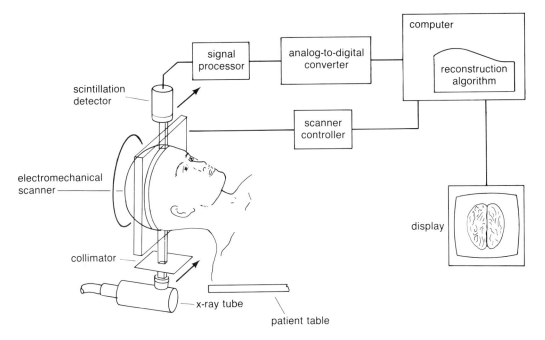

Figure 10.20   First-generation CAT scanner.

tube detects the transmitted x-ray photons. The scintillation detector is mounted on the scanning mechanism directly opposite the x-ray source. In this detector, x-ray photons that impinge on the crystal cause the emission of visible light photons that the photomultiplier tube detects. The source-detector combination is translated through 160 equally spaced positions, and a set of attenuation projection data is obtained for all positions. The scanning mechanism is then rotated about 1° and the translation/data acquisition process is repeated.

This procedure is repeated until the unit has been rotated a full 180°. Multiple sections can be examined by moving the patient table to the desired location and repeating the process. The output of the detector is processed, digitized, and stored in a computer. These projection data are operated on by a reconstruction algorithm to produce a two-dimensional image representing the linear attenuation coefficients in the section of interest. The original system used a single source-single detector combination, and since then other scanning geometries have been employed to reduce errors and scan time. Also, the original reconstruction algorithm used an iterative approach known as the *algebraic reconstruction technique* (ART) to reconstruct the image; since then other techniques have been developed with the goal of increasing reconstruction accuracy and decreasing time required for image reconstruction (Brooks and DiChiro 1975; Gilbert and Kenve 1981).

First-generation scanners used a two-motion translate-rotate scan with a single detector, as shown in Figure 10.21(a) (Scudder 1978). The major disadvantage of this technique is its relatively long scan time, typically requiring 4 to 5 min to complete a scan. Only a small portion of the total x-ray output of the tube is used, hence requiring long scan times to achieve a suitable image SNR. These long scan

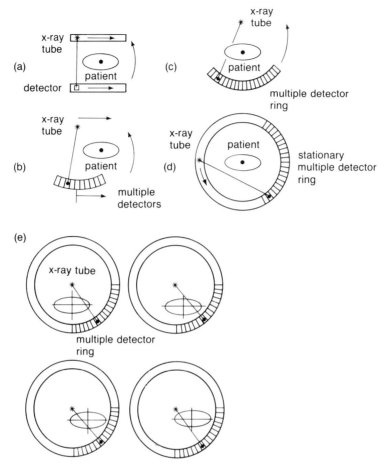

Figure 10.21   Scanner configurations (after Barrett, H., and Swindell, W., 1981. *Radiological imaging.* New York: Academic Press).

times were acceptable for stationary regions such as the head but are undesirable for abdominal imaging or imaging uncooperative patients or those having poor motor control. Further, the reconstruction computational time is 5 to 20 min. Image resolution was on the order of 0.5 cycles per millimeter.

Second-generation scanners use the same rotate-translate motions as the first-generation units except for the substitution of a multiple detector system, similar to that shown in Figure 10.21(b), which is used in place of a single detector. With this system, several projections are acquired during each linear scan. For example, if there are ten detectors, spaced 1° apart, a single translation acquires all ten projections. During the subsequent rotation, the scanning mechanism is indexed 10° instead of 1°, therefore resulting in a 10:1 time savings. Using this approach, scan times were reduced to 20 to 30 seconds. Additionally, new reconstruction techniques were used in conjunction with array processors attached to the computer to reduce reconstruction time to 1 to 3 min.

Third-generation scanners used a fan beam x-ray source and a ring of detectors to acquire attenuation data (Kak 1979). In this scanner, shown in Figure 10.21(c), both the source and the detector are rotated about an axis centered within the patient. The x-ray source produces a beam with a divergence angle between 30° and 45°, and the detector ring consists of 300 to 700 contiguous xenon gas detectors. Since the source and detector rotate together, the detectors can be relatively deep and positioned along the rays radiating from the source. The xenon gas detectors are essentially ionization chambers whereby x-ray photons entering the chamber cause ionization of the xenon gas. This increases the current flowing between two electrodes maintained at a high voltage so that detector current is directly proportional to x-ray intensity. The primary advantage this scanner approach has over first- and second-generation scanners is its mechanical simplicity in that only rotation is required. Because of its mechanical simplicity, high-speed scanning is possible with scan times of 1 to 10. Further advances in reconstruction algorithms and computer hardware reduced the reconstruction time to 30 seconds to 1 min.

One advantage that first- and second-generation scanners have over third-generation scanners is self-calibration of the system. Either before or after each linear translation, each x-ray beam impinges on the detector(s) with no intervening material, thus establishing a reference intensity level, I_0. This value is required to determine the attenuation coefficients of the image accurately. Although I_0 theoretically is constant, detector and source drift require frequent measurement in practice. Because third-generation scanners lack the self-calibration feature, these systems are susceptible to image "ring artifacts" due to calibration errors and the radial nature of the scan.

Fourth-generation scanners use a rotating fan beam x-ray source with a stationary 360° ring of detectors, as shown in Figure 10.21(d). The fan beam source is rotated around the patient, and the transmitted x-rays are detected by the stationary detector ring. Since, in this scanner scheme, rays strike the detector at different angles dependent upon the source position, the detectors must be relatively shallow to minimize cross-talk (undesirable rays entering adjacent detectors). To provide high quantum efficiency with the shallow detector requirement, scintillation detectors with high mass attenuation coefficient crystals (such as calcium fluoride or bismuth germanate) are used. Fourth-generation systems are also self-calibrating, since, at different portions of the scan, each detector is irradiated by the source without any intervening material. Fourth-generation scanners have scan times of approximately 1 second or less with reconstruction times of 30 seconds or less. Also, image resolution has improved considerably over that of first-generation units to 3 to 4 cycles per millimeter. A fourth-generation scanner and its body scan image are shown in Figure 10.22.

A variation of the fourth-generation scanner, which might be called a fifth-generation scanner, uses a complete ring of detectors translated as shown in Figure 10.21(e) (Barrett 1981). The x-ray source is located at the center of the detector array and produces a wide fan beam that is directed toward the patient. The detector ring is translated so that its center makes a complete circular path around the patient. Each detector is collimated toward the source to minimize detector cross-talk. This system is also self-calibrating.

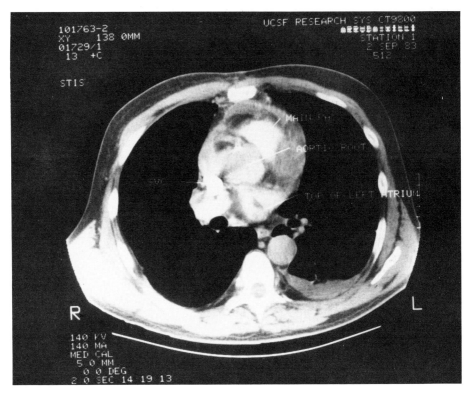

a

Figure 10.22 (a) CAT scan image of a slice through the chest, showing ribs, heart, and blood vessels (courtesy of General Electric Medical Systems). (b) Fourth-generation CAT scanner: the General Electric CT9800 computed tomography system (courtesy of General Electric Medical systems).

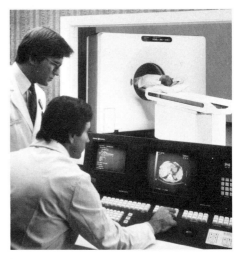

b

Reconstruction algorithms

Mathematical algorithms for taking the attenuation projection data and reconstructing an image can be classified into two categories: iterative and analytic. The *iterative* techniques (also known as the *algebraic reconstruction technique* [ART]), such as the one used by Hounsfield in the first-generation scanner, require an initial guess of the two-dimensional pattern of x-ray absorption. The attenuation projection data predicted by this guess are then calculated and the results compared with the measured data. The difference between the measured data and predicted values is used in an iterative manner so that the initial guess is modified and that difference goes to zero. The method of operation is illustrated in Figure 10.23.

The iterative process is started with all reconstruction elements r_i set to a constant such as $\bar{r}$ (the mean of r) or zero. In each iteration, the difference between the measured data for an attenuation projection p and the sum of the reconstruction elements along that ray is calculated. Here r_{ij} represents an element in the jth line forming the projection ray p_j. The difference is calculated, evenly divided among the N reconstruction elements, and then used in the next iteration so that the iterative equation is

$$r_{ij}^{q+1} = r_{ij}^{q} + \frac{p_j - \sum_{i=1}^{N} r_{ij}^{q}}{N} \qquad (19)$$

where the superscript q indicates the iteration number. This process is repeated so that the original elements are reconstructed. In general, a large number of iterations is required for convergence, with the process usually halted when the difference between the calculated and the measured data is below an error limit. A number of different versions of the ART were developed and used with first- and second-generation CAT scanners. Later-generation scanners used analytic reconstruction techniques since the iterative methods are computationally slow and have convergence problems in the presence of noise.

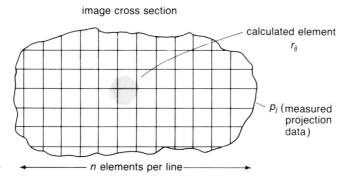

Figure 10.23 Sample reconstruction image–iterative reconstruction technique.

Analytic techniques include the Fourier transform, back projection, filtered back projection, and convolution back projection approaches (Macovski 1983). All of the analytic methods differ from the iterative methods in that the image is reconstructed directly from the attenuation projection data. Analytic techniques use the central section theorem and the two-dimensional Fourier transform, which is illustrated with the aid of Figure 10.24. Given an image $f(x, y)$, a single projection is taken along the x direction, forming a projection $g(y)$ described by

$$g(y) = \int_{-\infty}^{\infty} f(x, y)dx \tag{20}$$

This projection represents an array of line integrals as shown in Figure 10.24. The two-dimensional Fourier transform of $f(x, y)$ is given by

$$F(u, v) = \int\int_{-\infty}^{\infty} f(x, y)\exp[-j2\pi(ux + vy)]dxdy \tag{21}$$

In the Fourier domain, along the line $u = 0$, this transform becomes

$$F(0, v) = \int\int_{-\infty}^{\infty} f(x, y)\exp(-j2\pi vy)dxdy \tag{22}$$

which can be rewritten as

$$F(0, v) = \int_{-\infty}^{\infty} [\int_{-\infty}^{\infty} f(x, y)dx]\exp(-j2\pi vy)dy \quad \text{or} \tag{23}$$

$$F(0, v) = F_1[g(y)], \tag{24}$$

where $F_1[\ ]$ represents a one-dimensional Fourier transform. It can be shown that the transform of each projection forms a radial line in $F(u, v)$, and therefore $F(u, v)$ can be determined by taking projections at many angles and taking there transforms. When $F(u, v)$ is completely described, the reconstructed image can be found by taking the inverse Fourier transform to obtain $f(x, y)$.

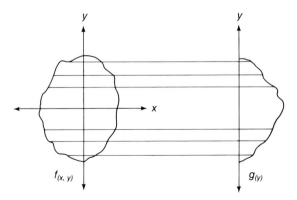

Figure 10.24 Illustration of a projection via the central section theorem.

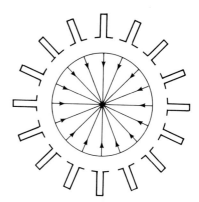

Figure 10.25   Radial back projection of a point.

The image reconstruction method used by most modern CAT scanners is the filtered back-projection reconstruction method. In this method, attenuation projection data for a given ray or scan angle are convolved with a spatial filter function either in the Fourier domain or by direct spatial convolution. The filtered data are then back-projected along the same line, using the measured value for each point along the line, as shown in Figure 10.25. The total back-projected image is made by summing the contributions from all scan angles. Depending upon the filter technique, the image is obtained directly after back-projection summation or via the inverse Fourier transform of the back-projected image.

Future perspectives in CAT scanning

As mentioned previously, CAT scanners have revolutionized radiographic imaging in much the same manner in which integrated circuits revolutionized electronic circuit design. CAT scanners are routinely and increasingly used in diagnostic imaging for many different clinical examinations. Current research and development efforts in CAT scanners are concentrated in the following areas: (1) development of fast or real-time scanners particularly for cardiac imaging, (2) use of dual-energy imaging to enhance tissue contrast in a manner similar to that in digital radiography, (3) reconstruction of a volume image, and (4) use of quantitative CAT scanning for the detection and identification of pathological tissues.

A number of research efforts are in progress toward the development of CAT scanners capable of dynamically imaging the heart, primarily because of its great diagnostic value in relation to detecting cardiovascular disease in its early stages. Further, a real-time CAT scanner could possibly supplant angiography, which is an invasive procedure requiring the injection of contrast dye, which presents a significant patient risk. However, the heart raises difficulties in imaging because of its motion, which limits data acquisition time to less than 0.1 s. One technique used to overcome this motion is *gating,* or synchronizing the scan to one point in the cardiac cycle via the use of the electrocardiogram, so that data are only collected during the same phase of the cardiac cycle (Nassi 1981). Other techniques whereby data acquisition is not limited to a specific phase in the cardiac cycle have been proposed. Two fast CAT scanner systems, which do not rely on gating, will be briefly discussed.

Another technique, in development at the Mayo Clinic, is the *dynamic spatial reconstructor* (DSR), which uses an array of x-ray tubes to scan in less than 0.1 s (Robb 1982). The DSR provides images of body sections in less than 1 s, stores them on a videodisk, and produces images of body organs in motion. The DSR has two unique capabilities: (1) high temporal resolution (very fast scanning) and (2) synchronous, true three-dimensional scanning. Therefore, it eliminates the need for successive breathholding and gated scanning required by other fast scanning techniques. The system is expected to be very useful in the early detection of lung cancer and heart disease.

The DSR is basically a multiple-channel CAT scanner designed to scan a cylindrical volume of up to 30 cm in diameter and 25 cm in height. It is designed around the use of the Mayo Mark 2 single-source imaging source-detector chain, which is shown schematically in Figure 10.26(a). The DSR consists of 28 x-ray sources mounted at 6° intervals in a semicircular arrangement with an opposing semicircular arc of 28 x-ray imaging detector systems mounted in the same gantry, as shown in Figure 10.26(b). The x-ray sources are sequentially activated and can complete a scan in 0.01 s. One scan can generate data for the reconstruction of up to 250 images of parallel, 1-mm-thick transverse sections over the full 25-cm axial range. This electronic circumferential scan can be repeated up to 60 times per second with the resultant data stored on videodisk for further processing. This device is currently undergoing clinical evaluation at the Mayo Clinic.

Another proposed fast CAT scanner, the *cardiovascular computed tomographic scanner* (CVCT) (Boyd and Gould 1979), uses a multiple-anode, scanning electron beam, x-ray source that enables the instrument to obtain two adjacent tomographic slices in 50 ms. The scanner uses a stationary scintillation detector array with 210 detectors to provide dynamic scanning at a frame rate of one per second. This particular design does not require a motor to scan the x-ray source or detector.

Another CAT scanner advance on the horizon, *dual-energy subtraction,* uses a modified version of the energy subtraction technique used in digital radiography systems. In digital radiography systems, the two x-ray energies chosen are usually just above and below the 33-keV characteristic absorption band for iodine. For CAT scanners, this is not practical since the tube voltages required are too low for efficient production of x-rays. Instead, energy subtraction is accomplished by operating the x-ray tube at widely different voltages, such as 100 and 150 kV. This technique provides increased image contrast with the use of contrast agents and also can be useful in removing bony structures without contrast agents. In most energy subtraction approaches, the tube voltage is changed between successive scans, and the two sets of attenuation data are stored in separate memory locations. In one novel approach, two detectors are positioned with different amounts of x-ray absorber between the detector and the patient. Because the detectors receive different x-ray spectra, the outputs can be subtracted from one another to obtain subtraction images (Brooks and DiChiro 1978).

Volume imaging is another area in which research is occurring. Present systems acquire an axial image representing a slice of body approximately 5 to 10 mm

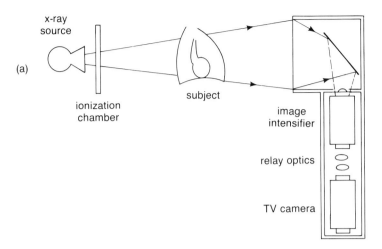

Figure 10.26a Mayo Clinic Mark 2 imaging source-detector (after Hamilton, B. (ed.). 1982. *Medical diagnostic imaging systems.* New York: F & S Press.).

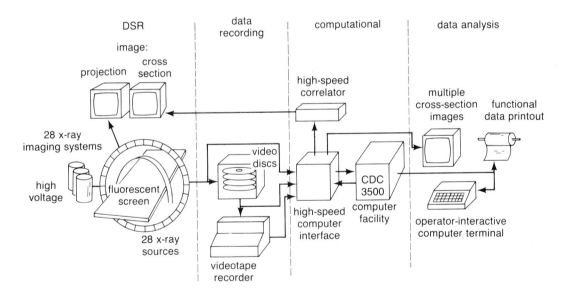

Figure 10.26b Schematic diagram of the DSR system (after Hamilton, B. (ed.). 1982. *Medical diagnostic imaging systems.* New York: F & S Press.).

thick. Generally, a number of slices of this size are acquired by moving the patient a few millimeters and repeating the process so that the region of interest is completely scanned. The set of axial images is displayed one at a time or used to create sagittal or coronal displays by the juxtaposition of data from corresponding locations in adjacent axial images. However, the derived nonaxial images are limited in spatial resolution by the slice width and slice separation. CAT scanning systems in which x-ray attenuation data would be acquired through a volume, rather than through a section, to increase the resolution in nonaxial images have been proposed. One approach for doing this is to send a cone-shaped beam of x-rays into the patient with an image intensifier/television camera serving as the detector mounted on the opposite side of the patient. The output of the television camera is digitized and stored in a computer for reconstruction processing.

Another use of the CAT scanner is in the characterization of tissues by x-ray attenuation data. X-ray attenuation data collected by the scanner are converted to hounsfields (H), which are described by the relationship

$$H = 1,000 \left[(\mu_t - \mu_w)/\mu_w \right], \tag{25}$$

where μ_t and μ_w are the linear x-ray attenuation coefficients of the tissue and water, respectively. Because of the nature of the interactions of x-rays with tissues, the number of hounsfields should be directly related to fundamental characteristics of the tissue comprising the axial slice; hence it would be useful both for identification of pathological tissues and for treatment planning in radiation planning. One application in which quantitative CAT scanning appears to be useful is in distinguishing between benign and malignant lung nodules (Siegelman and Zerhovni 1980).

Although not discussed, these advanced systems all have disadvantages or problems with respect to implementation, including high system cost, large computer memory requirements, or the need to develop new detectors or sources. It is anticipated that further developments in computer and x-ray technology will provide for additional advancements in CAT scanners, including those mentioned here.

NUCLEAR MAGNETIC RESONANCE (NMR) IMAGING SYSTEMS

NMR Operating Principles

Nuclear magnetic imaging (NMR), which is often called *magnetic resonance imaging* (MRI), is a noninvasive method of obtaining organ images without ionizing radiation. NMR imaging is based on the existence of a magnetic moment in nuclei containing an odd number of protons. The requirement of containing an odd number of protons is met by a large percentage of stable nuclei, radioisotopes,

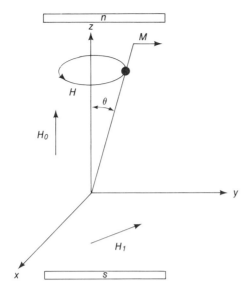

Figure 10.27   Nuclear magnetic moment precession.

and, in particular, hydrogen. Virtually every such nucleus has a natural spin, making it, in effect, a tiny magnet that can be detected. This basic effect was discovered by Bloch (circa 1946) and has been used in analytic chemistry and physics since its discovery. Lauterbur (1973) produced the first NMR images in the early 1970s, using signals received from hydrogen nuclei contained in water molecules. Since water is contained in all body tissues, it is the source of most NMR images currently produced.

The presence of a magnetic moment means that such nuclei are essentially arrays of tiny magnets. When these nuclei are placed into an external magnetic field, the nuclear magnetic moments tend to become aligned parallel with the external field. Since the nucleus is spinning, the magnetic moment, M, responds to the field like a gyroscope processing around the direction of the field, as shown in Figure 10.27 (Kaufman and Crooks 1981). The precessional or rotating angular frequency is known as the *Larmor frequency*, ω_0, and is given by the expression

$$\omega_0 = \gamma H_0 \tag{26}$$

where γ is the gyromagnetic ratio, which is constant for each nuclear species, and H_0 is the external magnetic field. Equation (26) is the fundamental NMR relationship in that it describes the magnetic field and the precessional frequency for a given nuclear species. This relationship forms the basis of both analytical and imaging NMR modalities.

To perform either imaging or material analysis, the nuclei must emit a signal at the precession frequency. This is done by exciting the precessing nuclei into resonance with a radio frequency magnetic field, H_1, in the *xy* plane, at the same frequency as the Larmor frequency, in addition to the static field, H_0, in the z direction (refer to Figure 10.27). The total magnetic field vector is given by

$$\mathbf{H} = H_0\mathbf{z} + H_1(\mathbf{x} \cos w_0 t + \mathbf{y} \sin w_0 t), \tag{27}$$

where $\mathbf{x}$, $\mathbf{y}$, and $\mathbf{z}$ are unit vectors. Note that $H_0 >> H_1$. The precessional angle, Θ, is given by the expression

$$\Theta = \gamma H_1 t_p \tag{28}$$

where t_p is the duration of the radio frequency magnetic field. When H_1 is turned off, the rotating magnetic moment undergoes what is known as "free induction decay" (FID) as the nuclei return to the ground state. In this process, a signal emitted at the resonant frequency is usually detected by the same coils used to produce H_1. Nuclei lose their energy through two distinct relaxation processes: (1) spin-lattice or longitudinal relaxation, characterized by the spin-lattice relaxation time, T_1; (2) spin-spin or transverse relaxation, characterized by the spin-spin relaxation time, T_2. *Spin-lattice relaxation* involves the transfer of the excess energy from the excited nuclei to the molecular lattice by thermal interaction, whereas *spin-spin relaxation* involves the transfer of energy between excited nuclei and adjacent nuclei in the ground state. Typically T_1 is on the order of 1 s $T_1 >> T_2$, and therefore the FID signals induced in the coils primarily decay at the T_1 time constant as shown in Figure 10.28. The voltage induced in the coils is described by

$$V = k\rho\exp(-t/T_1)\cos(w_0 t) \tag{29}$$

where k is a constant depending on coil construction, and ρ is the *spin density* (number of nuclei resonating per unit volume) of the nuclear species.

In most imaging systems, as will be discussed in the next section, repeated excitations are necessary to realize an adequate image SNR. When a region that has

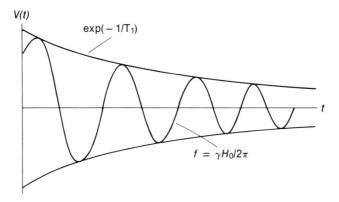

Figure 10.28   FID signal.

not fully relaxed to the ground state is excited, the resultant FID amplitude is diminished; equation (26) becomes

$$V = k\rho[1 - \exp(-t_a/T_1)]\cos(w_0 t) \tag{30}$$

where t_a is the time interval between excitations. As equation (30) indicates, the resultant signal amplitude, from repeated excitation, is dependent on the time between excitation. To provide a large portion of the maximum signal, t_a must be a reasonable fraction of a second. As a result, many imaging procedures require a few minutes for data acquisition. To resolve tissues spatially, complex magnetic field distributions are used for H_1 instead of a uniform field. In this manner, each spatial region has a unique magnetic field and hence a unique resonance and unique FID signals. In most instruments, the FID signals are analyzed via Fourier spectral analysis to generate an image. Some of the methods of generating the requisite magnetic fields are discussed in the next section.

NMR Image Formation

Figure 10.29 shows a typical NMR imaging system, which consists of a large generally circular magnet, with field strengths of 300 to 15,000 gauss (G), contained in a shielding enclosure into which the patient is placed. Also contained within this enclosure are the radio frequency (RF) excitation coils and auxiliary coils for producing image slices. These coils are excited by the RF transmitter with the emitted signals amplified by the receiver. These signals are then digitized and sent to the computer for further signal processing (usually Fourier transformation) and image reconstruction. One method of NMR image formation uses a controlled uniform field gradient so that nuclei in different parts of the patient resonate at different frequencies (Watson 1979), as illustrated in Figure 10.30, in which H has a constant component and a linear gradient G_x in the x direction, such that

$$\mathbf{H} = \mathbf{z}H_0 + \mathbf{x}G \tag{31}$$

and the associated Larmor frequency becomes

$$\omega = \omega_0 + \gamma G_x \tag{32}$$

Thus the resonant spin frequency is now a linear function of the gradient's x coordinate, and the NMR spectrum is now a one-dimensional projection of nuclei density. The spectrum can be obtained by performing a Fourier transform on the FID signals. This technique to generate one-dimensional nuclei density (or relaxation time) data can form a two-dimensional image by repeating the sequence and each time using a slightly different field gradient direction. If these directions are equally spaced around an 180° arc, then one of the standard techniques used in CAT scanners of reconstructing an image from projection data can be employed. Typically, reconstruction methods using convolution or back projection, such as

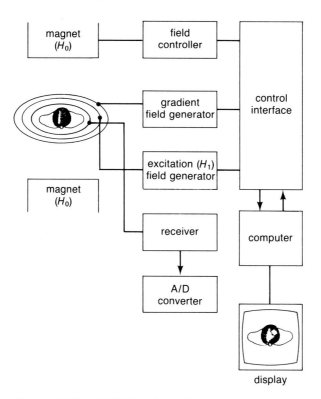

Figure 10.29   NMR imaging system.

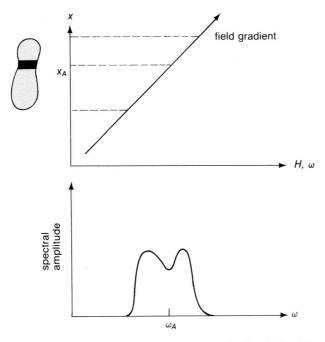

Figure 10.30   Field gradient spectral amplitude relationship.

those described previously, have been used since Fourier transforms were used and are also required as part of the data acquisition processing chain. A number of techniques have been developed to acquire image data that can be classified by the volume used to produce the image. These techniques are (1) a single point, (2) a line, and (3) a plane.

The *single point method* is the simplest way to generate an image. One method for accomplishing this, described by Damadian and associates (1971), is to use an inhomogenous main magnet field. The FONAR device, which uses this technique, has a focus or stationary point in the field pattern described by equation (27). In this fashion, a field gradient that defines the spatial region, slice, or volume element (voxel) from which FID signals are being acquired is established. The patient is then moved through the focus, via a mechanical scanner, to acquire all of the FID data. Another single point method, described by Hinshaw (1976), uses three gradient coils to generate the sensitive spatial region. This method is based on a NMR technique known as *steady-state free precession,* which uses a rapidly repeating sequence of RF pulses to produce a nearly continuous free induction signal. This technique is a radical departure from the usual examination of the FID signal in that the NMR signal is present during almost 100 percent of the data acquisition time, rather than approximately 1 percent of the time, as is normal. To produce the sensitive spatial region, the field used is described by

$$H(x, y, z, t) = \mathbf{z}H_0 + \mathbf{x}G_x(t) + \mathbf{y}G_y(t) + \mathbf{z}G_z(t) \tag{33}$$

where the three gradient fields are G_x, G_y, and G_z. It can be seen that there is only one point where H is constant, and that is at $x = y = z = 0$. Hence signals can be obtained only at this point. The sensitive point can be varied by changing the drive signal to the three coils. One of the primary disadvantages of either single point method is long data acquisition time due to the need to acquire each data point separately.

The major advantage of using a line technique to generate an image is increased data acquisition speed. One technique for accomplishing this is an extension of Hinshaw's single point technique (Holland et al. 1980). Instead of three time-dependent field gradients, only two are used; the field is described by

$$H(x, y, z, t) = \mathbf{z}H_0 + \mathbf{z}G_z + \mathbf{x}G_x(t) + \mathbf{y}G_y(t) \tag{34}$$

Since the third gradient, G_z, is fixed, now a line of points experiences a constant field from which free induction signals can be obtained. The free induction signals are Fourier analyzed to provide the response at each frequency simultaneously, indicating the nuclear density of each point along the line.

Kumar (1975) has proposed one planar imaging technique, known as *Fourier zeugmatography* or *Fourier transform zeugmatography,* to obtain an image from signals emitted from an entire plane of nuclei, via the use of pulsed orthogonal gradients. In this technique, pulses applied to the gradient coils produces a 90° precessional angle. Then a gradient G_x is applied for some time t_x; it is switched off and replaced by a gradient G_y while the FID signal is acquired. This sequence is repeated, using a range of values of the product $G_x t_x$, so that FID signals that are a function

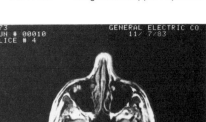

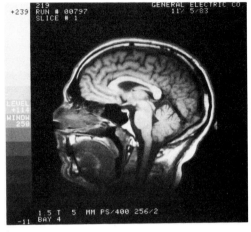

a   b

Figure 10.31   NMR brain images. (a) Top view. (b) Side view
(courtesy of General Electric Medical Systems).

of both time and $G_x t_x$ are obtained. A two-dimensional Fourier transform is performed on these data to generate the image.

Many approaches have been used to acquire NMR image data, and only a
few have been discussed here. Typical NMR images are shown in Figure 10.31(a)
and (b).

NMR Image Quality

As in other imaging systems, system resolution and signal-to-noise ratio are the
two parameters that affect and determine image quality. In NMR imaging, resolution is defined by the strength of the gradient fields used. For an imaging system to
achieve a specific spatial resolution, the separation of each volume element, in the
frequency domain, must be greater than or equal to the spectral width of the nuclei
species contributing to the image. Presuming that a voxel is a cube with sides of dimension Δ, then this condition is satisfied (Mansfield and Morris 1982) when the
field strength is

$$\gamma G \, \Delta > 1/T_2 \tag{35}$$

For biological tissue, T_2, the spin-spin relaxation time, is on the order of 50 ms, requiring that $G > 20/\gamma \, \Delta$. It is generally undesirable to increase the field strength
more than is necessary to achieve the required resolution since this spreads the signal information over a wider bandwidth, potentially degrading the image SNR.
Further, as the field strength increases, the resonant frequency also increases. This
imposes another limitation on the field strength since this frequency is limited to
about 10 MHz because of finite depth penetration in biological tissues. For these

and other reasons, spatial resolution in current NMR imaging systems is limited to about 1 mm.

Resolution and SNR are interrelated, and, in general, resolution can be traded for SNR, which can be improved by signal averaging. One expression for SNR, presuming the use of a solenoidal receiving coil of radius a and a NMR data acquisition technique such as the line technique previously described, is approximated by

$$SNR = k(T_2)^{1/2}(\gamma H)^{7/4}\Delta^3/a \tag{36}$$

where k is a system-dependent constant and Δ^3 is the voxel volume (and the resolution limit) (Mansfield and Morris 1982). From this expression, it is apparent that decreases in the voxel dimension result in a SNR decrease to the third power. This can be ameliorated to some extent by signal averaging, which increases the SNR by the $(N)^{1/2}$, N being the number of averages, such that equation (33) becomes

$$SNR = k(T_2)^{1/2}(\gamma H)^{7/4}(N)^{1/2}\Delta^3/a \tag{37}$$

Further, resolution and SNR affect the time to acquire an image, which is ultimately related to the last controllable factor in achieving higher resolution: patient motion. The time to acquire data from a given voxel of dimension, with a specific SNR is (Mansfield and Morris 1982)

$$t_{Vol} = (SNR)^2 a^2 (T_1/T_2)k/\{[\gamma H]^{7/2}\Delta^6\} \tag{38}$$

This expression shows the sixth-order dependence of the imaging time on spatial resolution and emphasizes the difficulty in improving resolution. Further it shows that increases in SNR require an increase in the data acquisition time to the second power, requiring that the patient lie still for longer periods to prevent image blur.

The preceding discussion alludes to some of the issues surrounding NMR image quality. The resolution and SNR of NMR systems are difficult to analyze because of the large variety of NMR configurations and different operating conditions. The reader is referred to Crooks and Coworkers (1984) and Mansfield and Morris (1982) for a more complete discussion of NMR image resolution and SNR.

Comparison of CAT Scanners and NMR Imaging Systems

NMR imaging systems have a number of advantages over x-ray-based CAT scanners, with one major advantage being the use of nonionizing radiation. Because NMR uses only magnetic fields, multiple NMR scans can be performed without the fear of radiation overexposure or any of the other biological effects of long-term ionizing radiation exposure. Another important advantage of NMR is that since hydrogen nuclei are imaged, dense substances such as bone that normally block x-rays become transparent since bone contains little water. Soft tissues like the gray and white matter of the brain are imaged very well as a result of their high water content, and NMR imagers can distinguish between gray and white matter, whereas CAT scanners cannot.

Further, since NMR provides some indication of tissue biochemistry, it also can differentiate some tumors that CAT scanners cannot. Additionally, it does offer the promise of being able to image other nuclear species besides hydrogen, such as fluorine, iron, phosphorus, and sodium, to provide considerable information about body metabolism. Other advantages are that blood flow can be measured without contrast agents, and that patient motion in NMR only degrades image resolution, whereas in CAT scanners it can degrade resolution and cause image artifacts.

However, NMR imaging systems also have a number of disadvantages. Although NMR does not use ionizing radiation, the large magnetic fields used can cause other problems. For example, pacemaker wearers cannot be examined because of interference with pacemaker operation or programming, and patients whose bodies contain metal surgical clips are also ruled out because the field may cause hazardous clip movement. Further, although extensive testing on the biological effects of large magnetic fields has indicated no danger, conceivably there are long-term effects.

Another disadvantage of NMR is high acquisition and operating costs. NMR imaging systems use large magnets that are either permanent, resistive, or superconducting. Permanent magnets are very heavy (greater than 100 tons) and thus require special attention to the structural bracing for the imaging facility. Resistive magnets require large amounts of electrical power and water cooling systems, whereas superconducting magnets require power only to start current flow but need cryogenic cooling with expensive liquid helium for proper operation. All magnet types require shielding, with the superconducting type needing extraordinary care in shielding to minimize the extent of the fringe field so that relatively innocuous objects are not turned into deadly projectiles. Because of the facility requirements, NMR installations tend to be more costly than CAT scanner installations because of shielding and auxiliary equipment and usually require more space. Also power and cooling requirements make NMR imaging systems' operating cost higher than that of CAT scanners.

Additionally, although one of NMR's advantages in brain imaging is the characteristic that bone is transparent, as a result, NMR cannot be used for bone imaging, which CAT scanners can readily perform. Further, NMR imagers need long scan times (10 to 30 min is typical for a hydrogen scan) for an adequate SNR, requiring that the patient be immobile for long periods. Present-day CAT scanners are almost instantaneous with respect to scan time, and patient motion is less of a problem. Since immobility is difficult for some NMR patients, image blurring due to patient motion often occurs. Additionally some patients become claustrophobic from being confined to the inside of the magnet for long periods.

One other disadvantage is that CAT scanners presently have an edge on NMR imaging systems with respect to resolution (Crooks et al. 1984). Modern CAT scanners have a limiting resolution of approximately 3 to 4 cycles per millimeter, whereas NMR systems have a limiting resolution of approximately 1 cycle per millimeter.

In view of the evolution of other medical imaging systems, it appears that improvements in NMR imaging systems will be made at least to mitigate some of these disadvantages. However, in the near future, it seems that the two imaging systems will be complementary clinical tools for those institutions that can afford their installation and operation.

Future Perspectives in NMR Imaging

Although NMR imagers have been in existence for more than 10 yrs, NMR imaging as a diagnostic tool is still in its infancy and has yet to find its niche in the medical diagnostic imaging arena. Current research and development efforts are concentrated in the following areas: (1) the use of NMR to image other nuclear species besides hydrogen, (2) cardiac and blood flow NMR imaging studies, and (3) determination of the optimal field strength for NMR imaging (Portugal 1984).

One of the most promising aspects of NMR is the potential to obtain information about body metabolism and biochemical reactions directly from NMR data. With respect to NMR imaging, the human body is an aqueous mixture of elements, with some of the more important ones being carbon, iron, nitrogen, phosphorus, sodium, and sulfur. By manipulating these nuclei with the appropriate RF field, NMR imaging promises to enable the physician to identify which elements are present along with their chemical forms, concentrations, and locations. For example, iron deficiency causes anemia, which conceivably could be detected and measured noninvasively with NMR instead of using the conventional technique of drawing a blood sample and performing a test for iron content. However, iron is beyond the sensitivity of today's instrumentation since only about 2 percent of the body's iron is present as the isotope iron 57, the odd-numbered form detectable by NMR methods. Also iron's gyromagnetic ratio is very low compared to that of hydrogen and requires a much higher field to generate a reasonable NMR signal. Sodium is another element of interest, which may be useful in localizing the site of infarction in strokes and heart attacks. Sodium concentrations increase dramatically at the site of infarcted tissues; therefore, NMR using sodium as the nuclear species measured could readily locate the damaged area in the brain or the heart. Phosphorus is also of interest because it is a key element to a number of biochemical reactions. For example, it is contained within adenosine triphosphate (ATP), a major energy source for body cells. Phosphorus also plays a role in muscle contraction and may also be useful in NMR tumor detection.

Another nuclear species of interest, which occurs in the body in trace amounts only, is fluorine. NMR imaging using fluorine is of interest in studying the effects of surgical anesthetics, many of which contain fluorine. NMR is helpful in studying the ways anesthetics are absorbed and distributed, the portions of the brain that are affected, and the length of time they take to produce anesthesia. Also fluorine has been used as a NMR contrast agent in blood flow studies. Biologically inert fluorinated hydrocarbons have been used as blood substitutes and theoretically could determine flow rates within small blood vessels deep within the body. One advantage of fluorine imaging is that fluorine 19 gives almost as large a

NMR signal as hydrogen, as compared to the relatively weak signals of iron and sodium.

Cardiac imaging is another new area for NMR imaging (Hamilton 1982). Presently this is accomplished by the gating technique described for CAT scanners, whereby snapshots of the heart are taken at different points of the cardiac cycle. The image is reconstructed by using data from the snapshots and produces cardiac images with minimal blurring. Cardiac imaging offers the promise, in conjunction with sodium and phosporus NMR, of providing new information about the heart's structure, tissue characteristics, and metabolism. This is potentially important for studying the alterations in cardiac metabolism in heart attack patients.

Additionally, the use of fluorine in blood flow measurements has already been discussed. Blood flow can also be measured without fluorine by taking NMR snapshots, 50 to 500 milliseconds apart, of the blood vessel of interest (Portugal 1984). The average cross-sectional area of the blood vessel can be calculated from the image, whereas flow velocity can be determined from the NMR data. This technique offers some advantages over other noninvasive flowmeters such as ultrasonic flowmeters in that it does not require laminar flow conditions to measure blood flow accurately.

Another area of interest is determining the optimal field strength for NMR imaging. On the basis of equation (36), most researchers concede that NMR image signal-to-noise improves with field strength and that image resolution and SNR tradeoffs can be made. Moreover, higher fields allow imaging of more nuclear species. However, there is no consensus as to how strong a field is really needed for imaging. For example, whole body images have been produced with permanent magnets producing a magnetic field of 3,000 G (0.3 T) and images have been produced by using superconducting magnets with field strengths of 24,000 G (2.4 T) and higher. Although higher field strengths do offer the promise of imaging of nuclear species other than hydrogen, it is questionable whether the added capital and operating cost are justifiable for most clinical applications.

As stated previously, NMR imaging is in its infancy, and undoubtedly the aforementioned advances and research activities will be expanded upon in the coming years. Since NMR images can be produced without ionizing radiation but with resolution that approaches that of radiographic imaging, it can be said that a new era has arrived in diagnostic imaging that shows great promise in redefining the clinician's expectations regarding the type of information available in the imaging process.

REFERENCES

Barrett, H., and Swindell, W. 1981. *Radiological imaging.* New York: Academic.

Bates, R. H. T., Garden, K. L., and Peters, T. M. 1983. Overview of computerized tomography with emphasis on future developments. *Proc. IEEE* 71:356–372.

Beebe, G. W. 1982. Ionizing radiation and health. *Am Sci* 70:35–44.

Boyd, D. P., Gould, R. G., et al. 1979. A proposed dynamic cardiac 3-d densitometer for early detection and evaluation of heart disease. *IEEE Trans Nucl Sci* 26:2845–2847.

Brooks, R. A., and DiChiro, G. 1975. Theory of image reconstruction in computed tomography. *Radiology* 117:561–572.

Brooks, R. A., and DiChiro, G. 1978. Split detector computed tomography. *Radiology* 126:255.

Crooks, L. E., Kaufman, L., Hoenninger, J. et al. 1984. Spatial resolution in NMR imaging. *IEEE Trans Med Imaging* MI–3:51–53.

Damadian, R., Goldsmith, M., and Minkoff, L. 1978. NMR in cancer. XX: FONAR scans of patients with cancer. *Physiol Chem Phys* 10:285–286.

Garrett, D. A., and Bracher, D. A. 1980. *Real-time radiologic imaging: Medical and industrial applications.* Philadelphia: American Society for Testing and Materials.

Gilbert, B. K., Kenue, S. K. et al. 1981. Rapid execution of fan beam image reconstruction algorithms using efficient computational techniques and special-purpose processors *IEEE Trans Biomed Eng* 28:98–115.

Goodman, J. W. 1968. *Introduction to Fourier optics.* New York: McGraw Hill.

Hamilton, B. (ed.). 1982. *Medical diagnostic imaging systems.* New York: F&S Press.

Hinshaw, W. S. 1976. Image formation by nuclear magnetic resonance. *J Appl Phys* 47:3709–3721.

Holland, G. N., Moore, W. S., and Hawks, R. L. 1980. Nuclear magnetic resonance tomography of the brain. *J Comput Assist Tomo* 4:1–3.

Hounsfield, G. N. 1973. Computerized transverse axial scanning, (part I). *Br J Radiol* 46:1016–1022.

Jacobson, B., and Webster, J. G. 1977. *Medicine and clinical engineering.* Englewood Cliffs N.J.: Prentice-Hall.

Kak, A. C. 1979. Computerized tomography with X-ray, emission, and ultrasound sources. *Proc IEEE* 67:1245–1272.

Kaufman, L., Crooks, L. E., and Margulis, A. R. (eds.). 1981. *NMR imaging in medicine.* New York: Igaku-Shoin.

Kaufman, L., and Crooks, L. E. 1983. Realistic expectations for the near term development of clinical NMR imaging. *IEEE Trans Med Imaging* MI–2:57–65.

Kumar, A., Welti, D., and Ernst, R. 1975. NMR Fourier zeugmatography. J *Magnet Reson* vol. 18; 69-85.

Lauterbur, P. 1973. Image formation by induced local interactions: Examples employing nuclear magnetic resonance. *Nature* 242:190–191.

Macovski, A. 1983. *Medical imaging systems.* Englewood Cliffs, N.J.: Prentice-Hall.

Mansfield, P., and Morris, P. G. 1982. *NMR imaging in biomedicine.* New York: Academic.

Nassi, M., Brody, W. R., Cipriano, P. R., and Macovski, A. 1981. A method for stop-action imaging of the heart using gated computer tomography *IEEE Trans Biomed Eng* BME-28:116–122.

Portugal, F. R. 1984. NMR promises to keep. *High Technology* 4(8):66–78.

Robb, R. A. 1982. The dynamic spatial reconstructor: An x-ray video fluoroscopic CT scanner for dynamic volume imaging of moving organs. *IEEE Trans Med Imaging* MI-1:22–33.

Scudder, H. J. 1978. Introduction to computer-aided tomography *Proc. IEEE* 66:628–637.

Siegelman, S. S., Zerhouni, E. A., et al. 1980. CT of the solitary pulmonary nodule. Am J Radiol 135:1.

Watson, B. W. (ed.). 1979. *IEE medical electronics, Monographs 28–33, Medical Imaging Techniques-Imaging by Nuclear Magnetic Resonance.* London: Peter Peregrinus pp. 79–93.

Webster, J. G. (ed.). 1978. *Medical instrumentation—application and design.* Boston: Houghton Mifflin.

Weinstein, M., M.T., Modic, E. Buonocore, T.F. Meaney, Digital Subtraction Angiography: Clinical Experience at the *Cleveland Clinic Foundation Applied Radiology,* vol. 10, Nov/Dec 1981, 53-69.

Part Six

Medical Technology and Ethical Issues

The Moral and Ethical Aspects of Technology in Medicine

Joseph D. Bronzino

Trinity College
Hartford, CT

INTRODUCTION

The intense infusion of technology into the practice of medicine during the past 25 years has enabled us to enter a new medical era. The leading causes of death in the early 1900s—pneumonia, tuberculosis, and influenza—are largely restrained. In the United States, vaccines have nearly eradicated four other diseases: smallpox, whooping cough, diphtheria, and poliomyelitis. Advances in material science have produced artificial limbs, heart valves, and blood vessels, thereby permitting "spare-parts" surgery. Numerous patient disorders are now routinely diagnosed with highly sophisticated machinery, and the lives of critically ill patients are being "maintained" through significant improvements in resuscitative and supportive devices, such as respirators, pacemakers, and artificial kidneys. Significant improvements in modern health care have resulted from these medical and technological innovations.

However, in spite of all these benefits, these biomedical and technical advances have also touched the moral fiber of the medical world. As a result of their newly acquired power over life and death, health professionals are confronting essentially new and monumental decisions. Provided with the ability to perform organ transplants, medical experts have been forced to consider moral questions such as the definition of death, the psychological impact of this procedure on the donor's family, and the emotional trauma recipients experience as they wait patiently for someone to die so they may live. Provided with the technology to maintain the breath and heartbeat of a patient with irreversible brain damage, health professionals have had to re-examine the meaning of such terms as the *quality of life, heroic efforts,* and *acts of mercy.* Typical of the questions those responsible for the care of critically ill patients are raising are the following: What are my primary responsibilities? Should any patient without hope of regaining a meaningful existence be permitted to die peacefully? Does this responsibility lie solely with the patient? These questions remain essentially unanswered.

Science and technology have precipitated most of the moral issues confronting our modern society. As Alvin Toffler in *Future Shock* (1970) and *The Third Wave* (1980) indicates, it is not only "the change" brought about by this technology that is so confounding, it is the rate at which this change is taking place. Consequently, the acceleration of scientific and technologic discoveries and their impact on our lives is awesome. Medicine, science, and technology have expanded human control over life and death and have added new dimensions to the power and capability of the medical profession. However, in the process they have also posed new issues about what is right and wrong, good and evil, and desirable and undesirable in the practice of medicine. The purpose of this chapter is to examine some of these vital moral issues relating to the use of the new technologies in caring for patients. It is not the objective of this presentation, however, to provide solutions or recommendations for these issues. Rather, the intent is to demonstrate that each technological miracle has consequences that affect the very core of human values. Ideally, individuals engaged in the development of new medical devices and in the care of patients will be stimulated to examine and evaluate critically "accepted views" and to reach their own conclusions.

To begin such a process, the following section presents definitions of morality and ethics, followed by a more detailed discussion highlighting the impact of technology in the following areas:

1 The definition of death
2 Care of the critically ill and the concept of euthanasia
3 Human experimentation
4 Organ transplantation

MORALITY AND ETHICS: A DEFINITION OF TERMS

From the very beginning, individuals have raised concerns about the nature of life, its significance, and the manner in which one's life energies should be expended. Many of these humanitarian issues have been incorporated into the four fundamental questions of Immanuel Kant: What can I know? What ought I to do? What can I hope? What is man? Evidence that early societies have raised these questions can be found in the generation of rather complex codes of conduct embedded in the customs of the earliest human social organization, the tribe. By 600 B.C., the

Greeks were successful in reducing many of these primitive speculations, attitudes, and views on many of these questions to some type of order or system and integrating them into the general body of wisdom called *philosophy* (Fagothey 1976). Being seafarers and colonizers, the Greeks had close contact with many different peoples and cultures. In the process, struck by the variety of customs, laws, and institutions that prevailed in the societies that surrounded them, they began to examine and compare all human conduct in these societies. This part of philosophy they called *ethics.*

The term *ethics,* therefore, comes from the Greek *ethos,* meaning "custom." On the other hand, the Latin word for custom is *mos,* and its plural, *mores,* is the equivalent of the Greek *ethos* and the root of the words *moral* and *morality.* Although both terms (*ethics* and *morality*) are often used interchangeably, there is a distinction between them that should be made.

Customs that result from some abiding principle in people's being and not from some arbitrary whim are called *morals.* Some examples of morals in our present society (although some readers may actually question their existence) are telling the truth, paying one's debts, honoring one's parents, and respecting the rights and property of others. Most members of society usually consider such conduct not only customary but right; to deviate from it is wrong. Thus morality encompasses what people *believe to be right and good and the reasons they give for it* (Fletcher 1974). These judgments, which constitute the morality of our culture, are the cornerstone of our existence as a human society. Their impact on our lives is all-encompassing. Most of us follow these rules of conduct and adjust our lifestyles in accordance with the principles they represent; many even sacrifice life itself rather than diverge from them, applying them not only to their own conduct but also to the behavior of others. Individuals who disregard these "accepted customs" are considered deviants, and in many cases are punished for engaging in an activity the society as a whole considers unacceptable. For example, individuals committing criminal acts with no regard for society are often "outlawed" and in many cases severely punished. These judgments, however, are not viewed as inflexible; they must continually be modified to fit changing conditions and thereby avoid the trauma of revolution as the vehicle for change. Because men and women make judgments of right or wrong, ethics has its place.

Thus ethics is the study of right and wrong, of good and evil in human conduct. It is critical reflection about morality and rational analysis of it. Ethics is not concerned with providing any judgments or specific rules for human behavior, but rather with providing an objective analysis about what individuals "ought to do." Defined in this way, it represents the philosophical view of morals and therefore is often referred to as *moral philosophy.* To emphasize further the distinction between morals and ethics, let us consider the following three questions that have been raised in the practice of medicine in the recent years: (1) Should badly deformed infants be kept alive? (2) When should a particular pregnancy be terminated? (3) Should treatment cease to allow an incurably ill patient to die? If someone were to ask whether these are questions of morality or ethics, what would be your response? In terms of the definitions just provided, all three of these inquiries are considered moral questions. The ethical problem, on the other hand, involves determining how these moral decisions are to be made.

In medicine, moral dilemmas arise in those situations that raise fundamental questions about right and wrong in the treatment of sickness and the promotion of health. In many of these situations, the health professional usually faces two alternative choices, neither of which seems to be a satisfactory solution to the problem. For example, Is it more important to preserve life or prevent pain? Is artificial insemination more meaningful to the prospective mother than adoption? Is sterilization of the mentally retarded warranted? All these situations seem to have no clearcut imperative based on our present set of convictions about right and wrong. That is the dilemma: What ought I to do?

In the practice of medicine moral dilemmas are certainly not new; they have been present throughout medical history. Is it right to withhold treatment when withholding it may lead to a shortening of life? Does an individual have the right to refuse treatment when refusing it may lead to death? Consider the situation in which doctors certain of the benefit of penicillin did not use it for a severely mentally retarded person. Their decision could be construed as running counter to the basic rule of the physician, that the primary concern is the well being of the patient (Spicker and Englehardt 1977). As a result, over the years individuals have attempted to provide a set of guidelines for those responsible for patient care. These efforts have resulted in the development of specific codes of professional conduct for health professionals. Let us examine some of these guidelines to ascertain whether they are appropriate today in an era of modern technologically based medical care.

For the medical profession, the World Medical Association adopted a version of the Hippocratic Oath entitled the *Geneva Convention Code of Medical Ethics* in 1949. This declaration contains the following statements:

I solemnly pledge myself to consecrate my life to the services of humanity;
I will give to my teachers the respect and gratitude which is their due;
I will practice my profession with conscience and dignity;
The health of my patient will be my first consideration;
I will respect the secrets which are confided in me;
I will maintain by all the means in my power, the honour and the noble traditions of the medical profession;
My colleagues will be my brothers;
I will not permit considerations of religion, nationality, race, party politics or social standing to intervene between my duty and my patient.
I will maintain the utmost respect for human life from the time of conception; even under threat. I will not use my medical knowledge contrary to the laws of humanity.
I make these promises solemnly, freely and upon my honour.

More recently, in 1980 the House of Delegates of the American Medical Association (AMA) adopted the following Principles of Medical Ethics:

Principles of Medical Ethics

PREAMBLE: The medical profession has long subscribed to a body of ethical statements developed primarily for the benefit of the patient. As a member of this profession, a physician must recognize responsibility not only to patients, but also to society, to other health professionals, and to self.

I A physician shall be dedicated to providing competent medical service with compassion and respect for human dignity.

II A physician shall deal honestly with patients and colleagues, and strive to expose those physicians deficient in character or competence, or who engage in fraud or deception.

III A physician shall respect the law and also recognize a responsibility to seek changes in those requirements which are contrary to the best interests of the patient.

IV A physician shall respect the rights of patients, of colleagues, and of other health professionals, and shall safeguard patient confidences within the constraints of the law.

V A physician shall continue to study, apply and advance scientific knowledge, make relevant information available to patients, colleagues and the public, obtain consultation, and use the talents of other health professionals when indicated.

VI A physician shall, in the provision of appropriate patient care, except in emergencies, be free to choose whom to serve, with whom to associate, and the environment in which to provide medical services.

VII A physician shall recognize a responsibility to participate in activities contributing to an improved community.

For the nursing profession, the American Nurses Association formally adopted in 1976 the *Code For Nurses* whose statements and interpretations provide guidance for conduct and relationships in carrying out nursing responsibilities consistently with the ethical obligations of the profession and the quality in nursing care (Abrams and Buckner 1983).

Code for Nurses

PREAMBLE: The *Code for Nurses* is based on belief about the nature of individuals, nursing, health, and society. Recipients and providers of nursing services are viewed as individuals and groups who possess basic rights and responsibilities, and whose values and circumstances command respect at all times. Nursing encompasses the promotion and restoration of health, the prevention of illness, and the alleviation of suffering. The statements of the *Code* and their interpretation provide guidance for conduct and relationships in carrying out nursing responsibilities consistent with the ethical obligations of the profession and quality in nursing care.

1 The nurse provides services with respect for human dignity and the uniqueness of the client unrestricted by considerations of social or economic status, personal attributes, or the nature of health problems.

2 The nurse safeguards the client's right to privacy by judiciously protecting information of a confidential nature.

3 The nurse acts to safeguard the client and the public when health care and safety are affected by the incompetent, unethical, or illegal practice of any person.

4 The nurse assumes responsibility and accountability for individual nursing judgments and actions.

5 The nurse maintains competence in nursing.

6 The nurse exercises informed judgment and uses individual competence and qualifications as criteria in seeking consultation, accepting responsibilities, and delegating nursing activities to others.

7 The nurse participates in activities that contribute to the ongoing development of the profession's body of knowledge.

8 The nurse participates in the profession's efforts to implement and improve standards of nursing.

9 The nurse participates in the profession's efforts to establish and maintain conditions of employment conducive to high-quality nursing care.

10 The nurse participates in the profession's effort to protect the public from misinformation and misrepresentation and to maintain the integrity of nursing.

11 The nurse collaborates with members of the health professions and other citizens in promoting community and national efforts to meet the health needs of the public.

Both the Hippocratic Oath and the Code for Nurses take as their guiding principle the concepts of service to humankind and respect for human life. When reading these codes of conduct it is difficult to imagine that anyone could improve on them as summary statements of the primary goals of individuals responsible for the care of patients. However, some believe that such codes fail to provide answers to many of the difficult moral dilemmas confronting health professionals today. For example, in many situations all the fundamental responsibilities of the nurse cannot be met at the same time. When a patient suffering from a massive insult to the brain is kept alive by artificial means and this equipment is needed elsewhere, it is not clear from these guidelines how "nursing competence is to be maintained to conserve life and promote health." Although it may be argued that the decision to treat or not to treat is a medical and not a nursing decision, both professions are so intimately involved in the care of patients that they are both concerned with the ultimate implications of any such decision.

Faced with the kind of medical dilemma just illustrated, health professionals are reviewing their role in a continually changing medical arena. The codes themselves do not provide all the answers, rather a starting point to analyze the important concepts on which they are based. In employing the new technologies, health professionals are being forced to reexamine their code of conduct and the so-called commonsense ideas that are presently widely accepted. The thrust of the scientific explosion in medicine has resulted in the reawakening of the philosopher within all of those engaged in health care delivery. It is a necessary process, one that is to be encouraged. For only with critical review and evaluation can health professionals use the new miracles of science to improve the quality of human life in our society.

DEFINITION OF DEATH

Until recently, only philosophers and theologians cared to discuss the topic of death. Although medicine has long been involved in the observation and certification of death, many of its practitioners have not always expressed philosophical concerns regarding the beginning of life and the onset of death. Since medicine is a clinical and empirical science, it was thought that health professionals had no medical need to consider the concept of death: the fact of death was sufficient. The distinction between life and death was viewed as the comparison of two extreme conditions separated by an infinite chasm. With the advent of technological advances in medicine to assist health professionals prolong life, this view has changed (Gaylin 1974; Weir 1977).

There is no doubt that the use of technology in medical care has in many instances warded off the coming of the grim reaper. One need only look at the trends in "average life expectancy" for confirmation. For example, in the United States today, the average life expectancy for white males is 74.3 yr and for white females 76 yrs, whereas at the turn of the century the average life expectancy for both sexes was only 47 yr. Infant mortality has been significantly reduced in developed nations, where technology is an integral part of the culture. Premature births no longer constitute a threat to life because of the artificial environment that medical technology can provide. Many infants who have been safely brought to the point of celebrating their first birthday would not have survived 25 years ago. Today, technology has not only helped individuals to avoid early death but has also been effective in delaying the inevitable. Pacemakers, artificial kidneys, and a variety of other medical devices enabled individuals to add many more productive years to their life. Technology has been so successful that health professionals responsible for the care of critically ill patients have been able to maintain their "vital signs of life" for extensive periods of time. In the process, however, serious philosophical questions concerning the quality of the life provided these patients have arisen.

Consider the case of the patient who sustains multiple cuts, bruises, and a serious injury to the head in an automobile accident. To the attendants in the ambulance who reached the scene of the accident, the patient was unconscious but still alive: his heart was beating. After the victim was rushed to the hospital and into the emergency room, the resident in charge verified the stability of the vital signs of heartbeat and respiration during examination and ordered x-ray films to indicate the extent of the head injury. The results of this procedure clearly showed extensive brain damage. When the EEG was obtained from the scalp electrodes placed about the head, it was noted to be significantly abnormal. In this situation, then, the obvious questions arise: What is the status of the patient? Is he alive?

Or consider the events encountered during a recent open heart surgery procedure. During this procedure, the patient was placed on the heart bypass machine, while the surgeon attempted to correct a malfunctioning valve. As the complex and long operation continued, the EEG monitors that had indicated a normal pattern of electrical activity at the onset of the operation suddenly displayed a relatively straight line indicative of feeble electrical activity. However, since the patient's so-called vital signs were being maintained by the heart-lung bypass, what should the surgeon do? Should the medical staff continue on the basis that the patient is alive or is the patient dead?

The increasing occurrence of these situations has stimulated health professionals to reexamine the definition of death. In essence, technology by delaying death has precipitated its redefinition by the medical world.

This should not be so surprising because the definition of death has always been closely related to the extent of medical knowledge and available technology. For many centuries, death was defined solely as the absence of breathing. Moviegoers are sure to recall at least one scene in which a mirror is held to the mouth or nostrils of a dying person to determine the cessation of breathing. Since is was felt that the spirit of the human being resided in the spiritus (breath), its absence became indicative of death. With the continuing proliferation of scientific information regarding human physiology and the development of techniques to revive a nonbreathing person, attention turned to the pulsating heart as the focal point in determination of death. In essence, most of us have been raised in this tradition. However, once again this view was to change through additional medical and technological advances in supportive therapy, resuscitation, and organ transplantation.

As understanding of the human organism increased, it became obvious that one of the primary constituents of the blood is oxygen and that any organ deprived of oxygen for a specified period of time will cease to function and die. The higher functions of the brain are particularly vulnerable to this type of insult, since the removal of oxygen from the blood supply even for a short period of time (3 min) produces irreversible damage to the brain tissues. Consequently, the evidence of "death" began to shift from the pulsating heart to the vital, functioning brain. Once medicine was provided with the means to monitor the brain's activity (EEG), another factor was introduced in the definition of death. Advocates of the concept of brain death argued that the human brain is truly essential to life as we prefer to define it. When the brain is irreversibly damaged, so are the functions that are identified with self and our own "humanness": memory, feeling, thinking, knowledge, and so on.

In the past all of these concepts were included in the meaning of clinical death. As a result, it was widely accepted that the meaning of clinical death implies that the spontaneous activity of the lungs, heart, and brain is no longer present. The irreversible cessation of functioning of all three major organs—heart, lungs, and brain—was required before anyone was pronounced dead. Although damage to any other organ system such as the liver or kidney may ultimately cause the death of the individual through a fatal effect on the essential functions of the heart, lungs, or brain, this aspect was not included in the definition of clinical death (Ramsey 1968; Veatch 1976).

With the development of modern respirators, however, the medical profession has encountered an increasing number of situations in which a patient with irreversible brain damage can be maintained almost indefinitely. This situation, coupled with those experienced during the "intense heart transplantation era" of the 1960s, clearly demonstrated the need to reexamine the definition of death once more: to decide whether persons die when their brains cease to function or whether death occurs only with the permanent cessation of function of major organ systems.

The movement toward redefining death received considerable impetus with the publication of a report sponsored by the Ad Hoc Committee of the Harvard

Medical School in 1968, in which the committee offered an alternative definition of death based on the functioning of the brain. The report of this committee was considered such a landmark attempt to deal with death in light of technology that it is highlighted here:

A Definition of Irreversible Coma

Irreversible coma is defined as a new criterion for death. There are two reasons why there is need for a definition: (1) Improvements in resuscitative and supportive measures have led to increased efforts to save those who are desperately injured. Sometimes these efforts have only partial success so that the result is an individual whose heart continues to beat but whose brain is irreversibly damaged. The burden is great on patients who suffer permanent loss of intellect, on their families, on the hospitals, and on those in need of hospital beds already occupied by these comatose patients. (2) Obsolete criteria for the definition of death can lead to controversy in obtaining organs for transplantation.

Irreversible coma has many causes, but we are concerned here only with those comatose individuals who have no discernable central nervous system activity. If the characteristics can be defined in satisfactory terms, translatable into action—and we believe this is possible—then several problems will either disappear or will become more readily soluble.

More than medical problems are present. There are moral, ethical, religious, and legal issues. Adequate definition here will prepare the way for better insight into all of these matters as well as for better law than is currently applicable.

Characteristics of irreversible coma

An organ, brain or other, that no longer functions and has no possibility of functioning again is for all practical purposes dead. Our first problem is to determine the characteristics of a permanently nonfunctioning brain.

A patient in this state appears to be in deep coma. The condition can be satisfactorily diagnosed by points 1, 2, and 3 to follow. The electroencephalogram (point 4) provides confirmatory data, and when available it should be utilized. In situations where for one reason or another electroencephalographic monitoring is not available, the absence of cerebral function has to be determined by purely clinical signs, to be described, or by absence of circulation as judged by standstill of blood in the retinal vessels, or by absence of cardiac activity.

1 Unreceptivity and unresponsively—There is a total unawareness to externally applied stimuli and inner need and complete unresponsiveness— our definition of irreversible coma. Even the most intensely painful stimuli evoke no vocal or other response, not even a groan, withdrawal of a limb, or quickening of respiration.

2 No movements of breathing—Observations covering a period of at least one hour by physicians is adequate to satisfy the criteria of no spontane-

ous respiration or response to stimuli such as pain, touch, sound, or light. After the patient is on a mechanical respirator, the total absence of spontaneous breathing may be established by turning off the respirator for 3 minutes and observing whether there is any effort on the part of the subject to breathe spontaneously. (The respirator may be turned off of this time provided that at the start of the trial period the patient's carbon dioxide tension is within the normal range, and provided also that the patient has been breathing room air for at least 10 minutes prior to the trial.)

3 No reflexes—Irreversible coma with abolition of central nervous system activity is evidenced in part by the absence of elicitable reflexes. The pupil will be fixed and dilated and will not respond to a direct source of bright light. Since the establishment of a fixed, dilated pupil is clear-cut in clinical practice, there should be no uncertainty as to its presence. Ocular movement (to head turning and to irrigation of the ears with ice water) and blinking are absent. There is no evidence of postural activity (decerebrate or other). Swallowing, yawning, vocalization are in abeyance. Corneal and pharyngeal reflexes are absent.

As a rule the stretch of tendon reflexes cannot be elicited; i.e., tapping the tendons of the biceps, triceps, and pronaor muscles, quadriceps and gastrocnemius muscles with the reflex hammer elicits no contraction of the respective muscles. Plantar or noxious stimulation gives no response.

4 Flat electroencephalogram—Of great confirmatory value is the flat or isoelectric EEG. We must assume that the electrodes have been properly applied, that the apparatus is functioning normally, and that the personnel in charge is competent. We consider it prudent to have one channel of the apparatus used for an electrocardiogram. This channel will monitor the ECG so that, if it appears in the electroencephalographic leads because of high resistance, it can be readily identified. It also establishes the presence of the active heart in the absence of the EEG. It is recommended that another channel be used for a noncephalic lead. This will pick up space-borne or vibration-borne artifacts and identify them. The simplest form of such a monitoring noncephalic electrode has two leads over the dorsum of the hand, preferably the right hand, so the ECG will be minimal or absent. Since one of the requirements of this state is that there be no muscle activity, these two dorsal hand electrodes will not be bothered by muscle artifact. The apparatus should be run at standard gains 10 v/mm, 50 v/5 mm. Also it should be isoelectric at double this standard gain which is 5 v/mm or 25 v/5 mm. At least 10 full minutes of recording are desirable, but twice that would be better.

It is also suggested that the gains at some point be opened to their full amplitude for a brief period (5 to 100 seconds) to see what is going on. Usually in an intensive care unit artifacts will dominate the picture, but these are readily identifiable. There shall be no electroencephalographic response to noise or pinch.

All of the above tests shall be repeated at least 24 hours later with no change.

The validity of such data as indications of irreversible cerebral damage depends on the exclusion of two conditions: hypothermia (temperature below 90 °F [32.2 °C]) or central nervous system depressants, such as barbiturates.

Other procedures

The patient's condition can be determined only by a physician. When the patient is hopelessly damaged as defined above, the family and all colleagues who have participated in major decisions concerning the patient, and all nurses involved, should be so informed. Death is to be declared and then the respirator turned off. The decision to do this and the responsibility for it are to be taken by the physician-in-charge, in consultation with one or more physicians who have been directly involved in the case. It is unsound and undesirable to force the family to make the decision.*

In summary, the criteria established by this committee were (1) that if an individual is unreceptive and unresponsive, that is, in a state of irreversible coma; (2) if the patient has no movements of breathing when the mechanical respirator is turned off; (3) if the patient demonstrates no reflexes; and (4) if the individual has a flat EEG for at least 24 h indicating no electrical brain activity, then death may be declared.

The committee also strongly recommended that the decision to declare the person dead and then to turn off the respirator not be made by physicians involved in any later efforts to transplant organs or tissues from the deceased individual. This last point seems to be opinion of a great number of professionals who have written or spoken on this subject. In this way, a prospective donor's death will not be hastened merely for the purpose of transplantation. Thus the complete separation of authority and responsibility for the care of the recipient and the physician or group of physicians who are responsible for the care of the patient who is the prospective donor is absolutely essential. It is necessary, therefore, that this procedure be included among the "checks and balances" already established in medical institutions to monitor professional conduct. In addition to the medical interpretation of death, one must be concerned also about its legal definition.

The contrast between the new medical concept and the legal definition of death came to the fore when courts upheld definitions of death in terms of cessation of all vital functions (Halley and Harvey 1968). For example, the Supreme Court of Kansas held in 1967 that "Death is the complete cessation of all vital functions without the possibility of resuscitation." This stress on cessation of all vital functions, however, implies that removing the heart from or turning off the ventilator sustaining a brain-dead body would involve taking the life of a person. As a result, there developed an open conflict between definitions of the death of a person based on brain death and legal definitions based on biological death, or cessation of all vital functions.

The traditional legal criteria for death as presented in Black's *Law Dictionary* are "The cessation of life; the ceasing to exist; defined by physicians as the total stoppage of the circulation of the blood, and the cessation of the animal and vi-

---

*Report of the Ad Hoc Committee of the Harvard Medical School: 1968. A definition of irreversible coma, *JAMA 205*:85–88.

tal functions consequent therein such as respiration, pulsation, etc."*(Black's Law Dictionary* 1968). According to this legal definition, a person might be held to be "alive," even though the brain is completely destroyed and all possibility of personal human life has ceased.

The shift to a brain-oriented concept, however, involved deciding that much more than just biological life is necessary to be a human person. Thus, when the reports of the Ad Hoc Committee of the Harvard Medical School and the Ad Hoc Committee of the American Electroencephalographic Society on EEG Criteria for Determination of Cerebral Death recommended support of the brain death concept they were essentially saying that mere vegetative human life is not personal human life. In other words, an otherwise intact and alive but brain-dead person is not a human person. Many of us have taken for granted the assertion that being truly alive in this world requires an "intact functioning brain." Yet precisely this issue was at stake in the gradual movement from using heart beat and respiration as indices of life to using brain-oriented indices instead. However, this movement took time.

Experience with the Harvard criteria has indicated that they are clearly not overinclusive, since there has not been one patient who has met all of the criteria and survived. In fact, they may indeed be underinclusive, raising the issue of whether it is necessary to retain one or more of the following requirements of the Harvard criteria: the absence of spinal cord reflexes, the requirement that the pupils be dilated, and the requirement of a flat EEG.

A set of criteria developed in Minnesota and applied retrospectively to a group of 503 patients in what is known as *The Collaborative Study* also met the standard that no patient who satisfied all of the criteria should survive (Taub 1981). The Minnesota criteria included l) cerebral unresponsivity and absence of spontaneous movement, 2) absence of spontaneous respiration when the patient was removed from the mechanical respirator for up to 4 min, and 3) absence of brain stem reflexes. These criteria had to be met at two different times, at least 12 h apart. It is interesting to note that of the 141 patients who fulfilled the Minnesota criteria and eventually died, 11 had shown some EEG activity.

Not all clinicians agreed that the flat EEG should be eliminated, however. Some believed that it provided useful objective documentation of the finding of brain death, provided that other possible causes of a flat EEG, such as drug overdosage, were ruled out. Angiography was suggested as a substitute, but its relative complexity, compared to that of the EEG, was recognized. There was also disagreement as to whether the official time of death should be the time of the first or the second set of observations.

Most clinicians took the position that brain death should be defined as death of the entire brain, including the brain stem, rather than death of the cortex alone. Dr. William Sweet, Professor Emeritus at the Harvard Medical School and one of the original members of the Harvard Committee on Brain Death, appeared to be alone in espousing the more radical view that cortical death should suffice. He stated, "It certainly seems to a number of us that an individual whose cerebral hemispheres are dead is no more worthy of another erg of effort or a farthing of money than a person whose brain stem is dead." He admitted that the practical problems of diagnosing death of the cerebral hemispheres might be greater but suggested that this might be done by measuring the uptake of labeled glucose molecules in the cells of the cortex (Taub 1981).

Those who favored the whole-brain definition of brain death stated that this would provide a built-in safety factor, since the brain stem is generally more resistant to destruction of function than the cortex. They also believed that such a definition of brain death would be more readily accepted by both the public and the medical profession. Consequently, this concept of brain death has been endorsed by the President's Commission on Biomedical Ethics (Taub 1981).

Many of the brain-death statutes now in force in 27 states refer to "irreversible cessation of spontaneous brain function," without specifying whether total brain function is meant. The statutes generally leave to physicians the question of the criteria to be used to determine whether brain function has been lost. In an effort to standardize these efforts within the United States a Uniform Brain Death Act, proposed by the National Conference of Commissioners on Uniform State Laws with the approval of representatives of the American Medical Association and the American Bar Association, reads as follows: "An individual who has sustained either 1) irreversible cessation of circulatory and respiratory function or 2) irreversible cessation of all functions of the entire brain including the brain stem is dead. The determination of death must be made in accordance with accepted medical standards." It was clear that definition of the criteria should be left to the medical profession, because of the time lag involved in enacting legislation that recognizes advances in medicine and technology. Adoption of a uniform statute by all states would eliminate the admittedly remote possibility that a person declared dead in Kansas, for example, could not legally be declared dead in California. Agreement on a uniform statute would encourage those states which have not yet enacted brain-death legislation (of which Connecticut is one) to do so. Ever since the President's Commission on Biomedical Ethics recommended that all 50 states adopt the uniform act, in a letter prepared for President Reagan and the leaders of the United States Senate and House of Representatives (Taub 1981), it has been viewed that it is only a matter of time before all states will agree to this policy.

THE CRITICALLY ILL PATIENT AND EUTHANASIA

The concept of death is, in general, one that most people consider evil and frightening. To others, however, it can prove to be a blessing in disguise, putting an end to intolerable suffering. Critically ill patients today often find themselves in a strange world of institutions and surrounded by technology that may be of assistance in their fight against death. However, at the same time, this modern technologically oriented medical system may cause the patient and family considerable economic, psychological, and physical pain. In enabling medical science to prolong life, modern technology has in many cases made dying slower, more painful, and more undignified than it has ever been before. As a result of this situation, there is a moral dilemma in medicine for all health professionals when the pain of these critically ill patients is unbearable, but *death* is not spontaneous. Is it then right or wrong under these circumstances to deliver or wish the death blow on oneself or on another?

The increasing significance of this problem becomes apparent once it is realized that the majority of Americans today will die of chronic illness in a rather slow, lingering fashion. Although death is all about us in the form of accidents, drug overdose, alcoholism, murder, and suicide, for most of us the end lies in growing older and succumbing to some form of chronic illness. As the aged approach the end of life's journey, they may eventually wish for the day when all troubles can be brought to an end. Such a desire, frequently shared by a compassionate family, is often shattered by therapies provided with only one concern: to prolong life no matter what else is involved. As a result, many claim that a dignified death is often not compatible with today's medical view.

Dying patients frequently find themselves institutionalized, possessing little control over their own lives. Consider the situation of a woman in her forties dying of leukemia in a public hospital. Her last hours were spent in an intensive care ward surrounded by bright lights and attached to tubes and machines. Her family were restricted to a room down the hall, where they were forced to wait for the 5 min they were allowed with her each hour. There was another example of an expert horsewoman who for 18 yr was a patient, decerebrate at midlevel, with quadraplegia as the result of a riding accident. Her treatment in a general community hospital lasted 18 yr. In reviewing this particular case, one raises questions concerning the moral issues of maintaining life where there is little hope for enhancing the quality of the life of the patient (Field and Romanus 1977). Such a situation reflects little concern of the medical system for a human, philosophical approach to death (Paris 1981).

There is no doubt that in many respects the fight for life is a correct professional view. The forces of medicine should always be committed to utilizing innovative ways of prolonging life for the individual. However, this cannot be the only approach to caring for the *critically ill*. Certain moral questions regarding the extent to which heroic efforts may prolong life must be addressed if the individual is to have any right to question or control these decisions.

Consider the plight the thousands of Americans who die each year from primary kidney disease experience. For these individuals, death can be averted only through a kidney transplant or treatment on an artificial kidney machine that removes poisons from the blood. The main function of the kidney is to adjust the electrolyte and water content of the body to maintain it within constant limits and to make certain that wastes derived from protein metabolism are eliminated. If the kidneys cannot perform this function, death results. However, life can be maintained even in the absence of kidney function by circulating the blood through an artificial kidney. Unfortunately, since there are not enough artificial kidney machines, more than half these patients are unable to receive any dialysis care. Deciding who will receive such care and treatment is a difficult problem in itself. In addition, individuals considered fortunate to be undergoing dialysis treatment may experience demoralizing side effects such as infections, severe headaches, disease of the bones, impotence, neurological disease, and a host of other complications. These factors, combined with the additional financial hardship resulting from such care, have led many patients to decide that they have had enough. Consequently, some dialysis patients have voluntarily removed themselves from treatment. The number of individuals making this decision has been increasing.

Over the years, many individuals have considered these questions and have expressed the point of view that the goal of those responsible for patient care should not solely be the prolongation of life as long as possible by the extensive use of drugs, operations, respirators, hemodialyzers, pacemakers, and the like, but rather the provision of a "quality of life" necessary for each patient. It is out of this new concern that the concept of euthanasia has once again become a controversial issue in the practice of medicine.

The term *euthanasia* is derived from two Greek words meaning "good" and "death." Euthanasia was practiced in many primitive societies in varying degrees. For example, on the island of Cos, the ancient Greeks assembled elderly and sick people at an annual banquet to consume a poisonous potion. Even Aristotle advocated euthanasia for gravely deformed children. Other cultures acted in a similar manner toward their aged by abandoning them when they felt these individuals no longer served any useful purpose. However, with the spread of Christianity in the Western world, a new attitude developed toward euthanasia. Because of the Judeo-Christian belief in the biblical statements "Thou shalt not kill" (Exodus 20:13) and "He who kills a man should be put to death" (Leviticus 24:17), the practice of euthanasia decreased. As a result of these moral judgments, killing was considered a sin, and the decision whether someone should live or die was viewed solely as God's responsibility—not humans'.

At present, the availability of numerous methods to prolong life has resulted in a rekindling of an interest in euthanasia in certain situations. In today's society, euthanasia implies to many "death with dignity," a practice to be followed when life is merely being prolonged by machines and no longer seems to have value. In many instances, it has come to mean a contract for the termination of life in order to avoid unnecessary suffering at the end of a fatal illness and therefore has the connotation of relief from pain (Krant 1974; Horan and Mall 1977; Abrams and Buckner 1983).

Opinions expressed by individuals, as well as specific groups, regarding the issue of euthanasia vary, depending on the type of euthanasia under discussion, that is, whether active or passive euthanasia is being advocated. The distinction between them is extremely important. *Passive euthanasia* is the planned omission of therapies that probably would prolong life. An example of passive euthanasia is the withdrawal of life-sustaining treatments to allow a hopelessly ill patient to die. *Active euthanasia,* on the other hand, is much more controversial, since it involves the institution of therapy that promotes the onset of death; in this situation, the health professional knowingly administers a drug or other modality to hasten death.

Both active and passive euthanasia can be administered either voluntarily or involuntarily, depending on whether the patient (or the family of an incapacitated person) has consented to the action. The Euthanasia Society has advocated that any individual has the right to a dignified death by requesting that no extraordinary means be used to extend biological life when death from a fatal illness is close. The following is the living will of the Euthanasia Society.

The Living Will
To my family, my physician, my clergyman,
my lawyer

If the time comes when I can no longer take part in decisions for my own future, let this statement stand as the testament of my wishes.

If there is no reasonable expectation of my recovery from physical or mental disability, I, _____, request that I be allowed to die and not be kept alive by artificial means or heroic gestures. Death is as much a reality as birth, growth, maturity and old age—it is the one certainty. I do not fear death as much as I fear the indignity of deterioration, dependence, and hopeless pain. I ask that drugs be mercifully administered to me for terminal suffering even if they hasten the moment of death.

This request is made after careful consideration. Although this document is not legally binding, you who care for me will, I hope, feel morally bound to follow its mandate. I recognize that it places a heavy burden of responsibility upon you, and it is with the intention of sharing that responsibility and of mitigating any feelings of guilt that this statement is made.

Date _____   Signature_____

Witnessed by

_____

_____

As the living will itself states, it is not a legally binding document. It is essentially a passive request and depends on moral persuasion. Proponents of the will, however, believe that it is valuable in relieving the burden of guilt carried by health professionals and the family (Horan and Mall 1977). Even a person who also disagrees with the aims of the Euthanasia Educational Council must admit that the publication of the Council's Living Will arouses the interest of many people.

A survey designed to ascertain the attitudes of health professionals, as well as members of the lay community, regarding active and passive euthanasia had some startling results. With the establishment of certain prerequisites, that is, (1) appropriate changes in law, (2) consent of the patient or appropriate relative, and (3) sufficient consultation regarding the status of the patient, about 80 percent of the physicians and the lay group favored passive euthanasia. About 80 percent of the physicians claimed that they had practiced passive euthanasia, and about 18 percent of the physicians and 35 percent of the lay group favored active euthanasia (Williams 1973).

Those who favor euthanasia look on it as a kindness ending the misery endured by the patient. The thought of a dignified death is much more attractive than the process of continuous suffering and gradual decay into nothingness. Viewing each person as a rational being possessing a unique mind and personality, proponents argue that critically ill patients should have the right to control the ending of their own life. In addition to this concept of individual rights and freedom of choice, arguments concerning the financial burden of keeping a person in a state of suspended life are used. Since hospital bills are so outrageously expensive, it is argued that keeping a patient alive with irreversible brain damage is not worth the cost and effort. Conscious of what awaits them, elderly citizens are becoming more concerned about squandering their life's savings to squeeze out a "nothing existence."

Maintaining a critically ill patient is expensive in terms other than money. Hospital facilities are often overcrowded and understaffed; many cannot be used to care for the hopelessly sick. Advocates of passive euthanasia argue further that since it is being practiced anyway, it should become accepted practice. They are quick to point out that decisions regarding which patients should receive the required treatments and care are made every day without the fanfare or attention usually aroused by the word *euthanasia.*

On the other hand, those opposed to euthanasia demand to know who has the right to end the life of another (Maguire 1974). Using religious arguments, they emphasize that euthanasia is in direct conflict with the belief that God, and God alone, has the power to decide when a human life ends. Their view is that if anyone who practices euthanasia is essentially acting in the place of God, and that no human should ever be considered so omnipotent.

These individuals also turn to the established codes, reminding those responsible for the care of patients that they must do whatever is in their power to save a life. Their argument is that health professionals cannot honor their pledge and still believe that euthanasia is justified. Why end all chance of recovery by killing those considered hopeless today who may be curable tomorrow? If such patients are kept alive, there is at least a chance of finding a cure that might be useful to them (Maguire 1974). Opponents of euthanasia feel that legalizing it would destroy the bonds of trust between doctor and patient. After all, how would sick individuals feel if they couldn't be sure that their physician and nurse would try everything possible to cure them, knowing that if their condition worsened, they would just lose faith and decide that death would be better. It is thought that most people must continually be reassured that they are being well taken care of. If euthanasia were condoned, it is argued that this reassurance would be lost. Opponents of euthanasia also question whether it will be truly beneficial to the suffering person or will only be a means to relieve the agony of the family. They believe that destroying life (no matter how minimal) merely to ease the emotional suffering of others is indeed unjust.

Many fear that if euthanasia is legalized, it will be difficult to control. That is, can definite and clear-cut guidelines to make these decisions be established? The answer here is obviously no. Once any form of euthanasia is accepted by society, its detractors fear that many other problems will arise (St. John-Stevas 1964). Even the acceptance of passive euthanasia could, if carried to its logical conclusion, be applied in state hospitals and institutions for the mentally retarded and the elderly. Such places currently house thousands of people who have neither hope nor any prospect of a life that even approaches normality. Legalization of passive euthanasia could prompt an increased number of suits by parents seeking to end the agony of incurably afflicted children or by children seeking to shorten the suffering of aged and terminally ill parents. In Nazi Germany, for example, mercy killing was initially practiced to end the suffering of the terminally ill. Eventually, however, the practice spread, so that even persons with the slightest deviation from the norm (the mentally ill, minority groups, and others) were destroyed. If euthanasia should be permitted, answers to the following questions must be given: How will it be controlled? What should the criteria be? Who will have the "divine right" to make such judgments? Since these questions are by no means quickly answered, the situation is delicate and thought-provoking.

Many of these arguments have been dramatized by the media in the last decade because of the much publicized Karen Quinlan case. Because this New Jersey case deals with some of the most fundamental aspects of human existence, as well as the moral and legal issues already present in this chapter, it has become the focus of increasing attention from health professionals, lawyers, and moral thinkers. The major issue in question is the "quality of life" of Karen Quinlan. As a result of the accidental mixing of tranquilizers and alcohol one night in April 1975, Karen fell into a coma from which she did not recover, and her life had to be supported by artificial means. Mechanical devices assisted her to breathe and provided her with adequate nourishment to survive. However, her brain was irreversibly injured, and her body steadily deteriorated: she initially lost 60 of her 120 lb. (Bereck 1975a).

Her adoptive parents, Mr. and Mrs. Joseph Quinlan, felt that she should be allowed to die with dignity, rather than suffer through life in a coma and undergo a slow and undignified death. For a while, the family kept hoping she would recover. Although the doctors told them that if she survived she would probably never be normal, they kept their faith. However, as the months passed and Karen did not show satisfactory signs of improvement, her family decided it was best to let her die peacefully. Oddly enough, the Catholic Church, which normally took the stand against euthanasia, sided with the parents in this case. The pastor of the parish to which the Quinlans belong told them that ending a life being sustained by extraordinary means is not wrong: Life does not end with death but rather just begins (Bereck 1975b).

The Quinlans signed a statement authorizing the physicians involved to shut off the respirator. Unsure of the legal and moral implications of such an act and unwilling to risk a charge of malpractice, the physicians refused. The Quinlans then turned to the law and requested that Karen's father be named her guardian so that he could authorize her removal from the machine. In response, the Superior Court judge in charge of the case took action. He requested that the county prosecutor show cause why he should not be prevented from prosecuting if the machine were stopped and also appointed a public defender to protect the legal rights of unconscious Karen Quinlan. Establishing a hearing so that all voices could be heard in the fall of 1975, the judge set out on his difficult task to rule whether it is legally permissible to remove the artificial devices that are keeping another human being in the twilight zone between life and death (*Time* Nov. 3, 1975).

During these hearings, despite the testimony of medical experts attesting to the seriousness of Karen's condition, which was likened to a child without a brain, these same experts agreed that she did not meet the accepted criteria for determining death. She had not suffered brain death, the legal measure of death at that time in eight states, although not New Jersey. In addition, EEG records showed that there was still some brain activity, and Karen had, on occasion, breathed spontaneously for up to 30 min.

The lawyers in turn expressed their widely divergent arguments. Although retreating slightly from his initial claim that Karen could recover, her court-appointed legal guardian insisted that the court protect her constitutional "right to life." In essence, this position maintained that Karen had individual rights that no one should be able to take away simply because the sight of her sick body was troubling. It also reflected the belief that at least if she were kept alive, there might be some possibility that in her lifetime something would be discovered that could help her.

The attorney representing the Quinlans insisted that although Karen was still alive in a biological sense, she was indeed personally dead. Under these circumstances, it was felt that her parents as guardians not only had the responsibility to look after her best interests, but also a constitutional right to end her medical treatment on the basis of guarantees of religious freedom, protection against cruel and unusual punishment, and the right to privacy spelled out in the First, Eighth, and Fourteenth Amendments.

In the midst of this uncertainty, a decision was reached in April 1976, 1 yr from the date of the unfortunate accident. The New Jersey Supreme Court ruled that Karen Quinlan be permitted to die and that her constitutional right to privacy permitted the "plug to be pulled." The court declared Karen's father her guardian, providing him the legal authority to make decisions for her, subject to the agreement of physicians and hospital authorities that there is "no reasonable possibility" she might recover. This decision reflects the view that the state's interest in protecting life must under these circumstances give way to Karen's right, as exercised by her father, to decide in private.

Ironically, when the respirator was removed, Karen started to breathe for herself. With physicians unwilling to discontinue administration of life-sustaining nutrients, Karen's plight continued until June 1985, when she died.

In the early 1970s, there was little if any legal precedent for the presiding judge to follow. For instance, the New Jersey Supreme Court held that a member of Jehovah's Witnesses did not have the right to refuse a blood transfusion on religious grounds. The courts had also in several cases named doctors as guardians to assure that children received treatments that parents for whatever personal or religious reasons were unwilling to provide. Even today, the courts have yet to establish that there is any constitutional "right to die." However, there has been a growing feeling that people do have the right to refuse treatment. Quite recently fear that brain-death legislation, for example, would quickly lead to euthanasia and more permissive abortion laws initially led many religious groups to lobby against it. Also, a New York court ruled that the director of a Roman Catholic religious order could act on behalf of a member of that order who was diagnosed as being in a "permanent vegetative state," and he was authorized to direct termination of life-support systems under certain conditions. The Florida Supreme Court ruled that a 73-yr-old patient with amyotrophic lateral sclerosis had a right to disconnect the respirator keeping him alive. Since the President's Committee for the Study of Ethical Problems in Medicine and Biomedical Research determined in 1981 that the matter of "defining" death should continue to be the province of state legislatures, with the federal government reserving responsibility only for those areas of exclusive federal jurisdiction, it appears that such recent court decisions will have profound influence in the near future (Taub 1981). Still, in anticipation of the important decisions yet to be made, it is considered essential that health professionals engage in an open dialogue regarding these vital issues, which, because of technological advances, may grow more complex in the years to come.

HUMAN EXPERIMENTATION

During the past 30 years, medical research has held an exalted position in our society. It has been acclaimed for its significant achievements, which range from development of the Salk and Sabin vaccines for polio, to development of artificial and transplanted organs. This trend toward scientific medicine has had major side effects on the quality and nature of medical care. It has stimulated changes in the material content and emphasis in both nursing and medical education and has attracted a new breed of individuals interested in the further advancement of medical science on the health care scene. There is an ever-increasing interest in medical research, thereby creating an environment in which many patients (and nonpatients) may become subjects in some form of clinical experiment.

It is generally accepted that advances in medical research depend to a considerable degree on the refinement of technological developments such as pacemakers and diagnostic equipment using human subjects, which may include those suffering from illness or disability. Consequently, this is an issue of vital importance to everyone. For example, "If we say 'Yes' to Pig Valves, but 'No' to limb grafts, where do we draw the line?" (Gorovitz 1982) There is no doubt that at some point new procedures must eventually be tested on humans. This is absolutely necessary if one is to determine their effectiveness and value. After all, all the techniques and devices presently being employed were at one time new and untried. The issue is therefore not whether humans should be involved in clinical studies designed to benefit themselves or their fellow humans, clarifying or defining more precisely the conditions under which such studies are to be permitted (Pellegrino 1971; Baker 1980; Mellon et al. 1983).

For example, consider the case of a 50-yr-old female patient suffering from severe coronary artery disease. What guidelines should be followed in the process of experimenting with new drugs or devices that may or may not help her? Should only those procedures viewed as potentially beneficial to the patient be tried? Can experimental diagnostic procedures or equipment be tested to evaluate their performance against accepted techniques, even though they will not be directly beneficial to the patient?

Or consider the situation of conducting research on the human fetus. This type of research has significantly increased in recent years partly as a result of the legalization of abortion in the United States and the technological advances that have made fetal studies more practicable than in the past. Under what conditions should medical research be conducted on these subjects? For example, should potentially hazardous drugs be given to women planning to have abortions to determine the effect of these drugs on the fetus? Should the fetus, once aborted, be used in the experimental studies? Should dead fetuses be involved in research studies designed to evaluate certain types of transplantation procedures?

In such situations, the questions are difficult to answer without some reservation. However, these cases are not simply fantasy; they are the reality confronting health professionals today. As a result, clinical research teams of nurses and physicians responsible for the well-being of their patients must face the moral issues involved in testing new equipment and procedures on humans and at the same time safeguard the inviolable rights of their patients.

Definition and Purpose of Experimentation

One may ask, What exactly constitutes a human experiment? Although the experimental protocol may vary, it is generally accepted that human experimentation occurs whenever the clinical situation of the individual is consciously manipulated to gather information regarding the capability of new instruments, treatments, diagnostic procedures, and so on. Medical research projects involving human subjects are usually classified as either therapeutic or nontherapeutic. In a *therapeutic study,* such experimentation (trying out a new device, drug, operative technique, or therapeutic procedure) may have direct benefit for the patient. The basic goal of *nontherapeutic research,* on the other hand, is purely scientific, without direct benefit to the person subjected to the research (Pellegrino 1969; Campbell 1972; Baker 1980).

Throughout medical history there have been numerous examples of therapeutic research projects. The use of nonconventional radiotherapy to inhibit the progress of a malignant condition, of pacemakers to provide the necessary electrical stimulation for proper heart function, of artificial kidneys to mimic nature's function and remove poisons from the blood, and of computerized axial tomography to assist in detection of brain tumors prior to surgery were all at one time considered novel approaches that might have some value for the patient. Yet they were tried and found to have extreme value for humankind.

Nontherapeutic research on normal volunteers for the potential good of others with no immediate benefit to the subjects themselves has also been an important vehicle for medical progress. Such experiments designed to study the impact of infection from the hepatitis virus or the malarial parasite or the procedures involved in cardiac catheterization have all had significant importance in the advancement of medical science and the ultimate development of appropriate therapies for the benefit of humankind.

Unfortunately, in spite of all the advantages of human experimentation, numerous instances have caused great alarm and concern, especially when children have been involved. The involvement of human beings in nontherapeutic studies has raised fundamental questions regarding the risk and the nature of the consent obtained from the "volunteer." One such incident involved a Canadian engineering student. The student was paid $50 to permit the placement of a catheter in his arm to run some tests. At a later date the student claimed he did not know that the catheter was intended to travel through his bloodstream to his heart. During the study, the catheter caused his heart to stop. It took 90 s to restart, and the student was rendered unconscious for 4 days. On recovery, he complained of memory loss and impaired concentration. The student sued and eventually was awarded $22,500 because actual informed consent was not obtained (Pappworth 1968).

In another case, children in a school for the mentally retarded in Staten Island, New York, were involved in a research project designed to study viral hepatitis (Goldman 1970). The ultimate goal of this study was to develop an effective vaccine against the disease. Selected groups of new admissions to the school were admitted to a special experimental unit in which they were deliberately infected with the disease. One might wonder how this was possible and the method by which permission was secured. In this case, consent was gained from parents, who were convinced that since this disease was rampant at the school, their children were likely to get it anyway and that by being involved in this study, they would be cared for under the best circumstances possible. The objectionable aspect of this experiment was that it deliberately caused distress to children who could not understand what was happening to them (Campbell 1972). Unfortunately, in many cases such as these, difficulties encountered in estimating the degree of risk to the patient involved in each project or in communicating the problems involved were essentially ignored before the 1970s (Beecher 1970). Some experts have expressed concern that even when patients are totally aware of their situation and the experiment is designed to benefit them, serious moral difficulties often arise. In this situation the method by which a patient is informed and the degree of the parent's understanding are areas of major concern. Thus the primary moral issues concerning human experimentation today focus generally on whether the subject has given free and informed consent, whether the risks involved are warranted by the probable good to be achieved, and whether the individual's right to privacy is respected in conducting the study (Pellegrino 1971; Loftus and Fries 1983).

Informed consent has long been considered by many to be the most important of the issues in human experimentation (Beecher 1970; Cassileth et al. 1983). A major reason for this opinion is that it is the principal condition that must be satisfied if such research activities are to both lawful and ethical.

For experimentation to be lawful, the individual must be legally capable of giving medical consent. Since all adults have the legal capacity to give medical consent (unless it has been specifically denied through some legal process), issues concerning legal capability are usually limited to minors. Many states, if not all, have some exceptions to the rule that minors cannot give medical consent. This is not the province of the investigator. On this basis, informed consent is an attempt to increase the rights of individuals by giving them the opportunity for self-determination, that is, to determine for themselves whether they wish to participate in any experimental effort.

In an attempt to provide some guidelines in this area the World Medical Association in Finland in 1964 endorsed a code of ethics for human experimentation, which was revised by the 29th World Medical Assembly in Tokyo, Japan, in 1975:

Declaration of Helsinki
(World Medical Association)

Introduction
It is the mission of the medical doctor to safeguard the health of the people. His or her knowledge and conscience are dedicated to the fulfillment of this mission.

The Declaration of Geneva of the World Medical Association binds the doctor with the words, "The health of my patient will be my first consideration," and the International Code of Medical Ethics declares that, "Any act or advice which could weaken physical or mental resistance of a human being may be used only in his interest."

The purpose of biomedical research involving human subjects must be to improve diagnostic, therapeutic and prophylactic procedures and the understanding of the aetiology and pathogenesis of disease.

In current medical practice most diagnostic, therapeutic or prophylactic procedures involve hazards. This applies *a fortiori* to biomedical research.

Medical progress is based on research which ultimately must rest in part on experimentation involving human subjects.

In the field of biomedical research a fundamental distinction must be recognized between medical research in which the aim is essentially diagnostic or therapeutic for a patient, and medical research, the essential object of which is purely scientific and without direct diagnostic or therapeutic value to the person subjected to the research.

Special caution must be exercised in the conduct of research which may affect the environment, and the welfare of animals used for research must be respected.

Because it is essential that the results of laboratory experiments be applied to human beings to further scientific knowledge and to help suffering humanity, The World Medical Association has prepared the following recommendations as a guide to every doctor in biomedical research involving human subjects. They should be kept under review in the future. It must be stressed that the standards as drafted are only a guide to physicians all over the world. Doctors are not relieved from criminal, civil and ethical responsibilities under the laws of their own countries.

I. Basic Principles

1 Biomedical research involving human subjects must conform to generally accepted scientific principles and should be based on adequately performed laboratory and animal experimentation and on a thorough knowledge of the scientific literature.

2 The design and performance of each experimental procedure involving human subjects should be clearly formulated in an experimental protocol which should be transmitted to a specially appointed independent committee for consideration, comment and guidance.

3 Biomedical research involving human subjects should be conducted only by scientifically qualified persons and under the supervisions of a clinically competent medical person. The responsibility for the human subject must always rest with a medically qualified person and never rest on the subject of the research, even though the subject has given his or her consent.

4 Biomedical research involving human subjects cannot legitimately be carried out unless the importance of the objective is in proportion to the inherent risk to the subject.

5 Every biomedical research project involving human subjects should be preceded by careful assessment of predictable risks in comparison with foreseeable benefits to the subject or to others. Concern for the interests of the subject must always prevail over the interests of science and society.

6 The right of the research subject to safeguard his or her integrity must always be respected. Every precaution should be taken to respect the privacy of the subject and to minimize the impact of the study on the subject's physical and mental integrity and on the personality of the subject.

7 Doctors should abstain from engaging in research projects involving human subjects unless they are satisfied that the hazards involved are believed to be predictable. Doctors should cease any investigation if the hazards are found to outweigh the potential benefits.

8 In publication of the results of his or her research, the doctor is obliged to preserve the accuracy of the results. Reports of experimentation not in accordance with the principles laid down in this Declaration should not be accepted for publication.

9 In any research on human beings, each potential subject must be adequately informed of the aims, methods, anticipated benefits and potential hazards of the study and the discomfort it may entail. He or she should be informed that he or she is at liberty to abstain from participation in the study and that he or she is free to withdraw his or her consent to participation at any time. The doctor should then obtain the subject's free-given informed consent, preferably in writing.

10 When obtaining informed consent for the research project the doctor should be particularly cautious if the subject is in a dependent relationship to him or her or may consent under duress. In that case the informed consent should be obtained by a doctor who is not engaged in the investigation and who is completely independent of this official relationship.

11 In the case of legal incompetence, informed consent should be obtained from the legal guardian in accordance with national legislation. Where physical or mental incapacity makes it impossible to obtain informed consent, or when the subject is a minor, permission from the responsible relative replaces that of the subject in accordance with national legislation.

12 The research protocol should always contain a statement of the ethical considerations involved and should indicate that the principles enunciated in the present Declaration are complied with.

II. Medical Research Combined with Professional Care *(Clinical Research)*

1 In the treatment of the sick person, the doctor must be free to use a new diagnostic and therapeutic measure, if in his or her judgment it offers hope of saving life, reestablishing health or alleviating suffering.

2 The potential benefits, hazards and discomfort of a new method should be weighed against the advantages of the best current diagnostic and therapeutic methods.

3 In any medical study, every patient—including those of a control group, if any—should be assured of the best proven diagnostic and therapeutic method.

4 The refusal of the patient to participate in a study must never interfere with the doctor-patient relationship.

5 If the doctor considers it essential not to obtain informed consent, the specific reasons for this proposal should be stated in the experimental protocol for transmission to the independent committee.

6 The doctor can combine medical research with professional care, the objective being the acquisition of new medical knowledge, only to the extent that medical research is justified by its potential diagnostic or therapeutic value for the patient.

III. Non-Therapeutic Biomedical Research Involving Human Subjects (Non-Clinical Biomedical Research)

1 In the purely scientific application of medical research carried out on a human being, it is the duty of the doctor to remain the protector of the life and health of that person on whom biomedical research is being carried out.

2 The subjects should be volunteers—either healthy persons or patients from whom the experimental design is not related to the patient's illness.

3 The investigator or the investigating team should discontinue the research if in his/her or their judgment it may, if continued, be harmful to the individual.

4 In research on man, the interest of science and society should never take precedence over considerations related to the wellbeing of the subject.

Adopted by the 18th World Medical Assembly, Helsinki, Finland, 1964, and as revised by the 29th World Medical Assembly, Tokyo, Japan, 1975 (Abrams and Buckner 1983).

A strict interpretation of these criteria would automatically rule out whole classes of potential subjects from participating in nontherapeutic research. Children, the mentally retarded, and any patient whose capacity to think is affected by illness would be excluded on the grounds of their inability to comprehend exactly what is involved in the experiment, whereas those individuals having a dependent relationship to the clinical investigator, such as the investigator's patients and students, would be eliminated on the basis of constraint. Since mental capacity also includes the ability of subjects to appreciate the seriousness of the consequences of the proposed procedure, this means that even though some minors have the right to give consent for certain types of treatments, they must understand all the risks involved.

Any research study must clearly define the risks involved. Regardless of whether the effect is therapeutic or nontherapeutic, if the proposed procedure is experimental, the patient must receive a total disclosure of all known information. If the proposed procedure is new or novel, the patient must be informed of this fact along with whatever information may be necessary to make the patient aware that not everything is known about what might occur.

In the past, the evaluation of risk and benefit in many therapeutic situations belonged to the medical professional alone. Once made, it was assumed that this decision would be accepted at face value by the patient. Today, this assumption is only half valid. The medical staff still must weigh the risks and benefits involved in any procedure they suggest, but now the patient has the right to make the final determination. The patient cannot, of course, decide whether the procedure is medically correct, since that requires more medical expertise than the individual possesses. But once the procedure is recommended, the patient then must have enough information to decide whether the hoped-for-benefits are sufficient to risk the hazards (Mills 1974). Only when this is accomplished can a valid consent be given.

According to the developing concept of informed consent, it is thought that nurses must be involved not only as witnesses but as participants in the process (Meisel 1975). This is especially true when it is the nurse who is to perform a given procedure. The same applies for physician assistants and other health personnel. Thus, it is necessary to consider the guidelines for informed consent.

Once true understanding and informed consent has been obtained and recorded, then it affords the following protection:

1 It represents legal authorization to proceed; the subject cannot later claim assault and battery.
2 It usually gives legal authorization to use the data obtained for professional or research purposes; invasion of privacy cannot later be claimed.
3 It eliminates any claims in the event that the subject fails to benefit from the procedure understood and consented to.
4 It is defense against any claim of an injury when the risk of the procedure is understood and consented to.
5 It protects the investigator against any claim of an injury resulting from the subject's failure to follow safety instructions if the orders were well explained and reasonable (Ladimer 1967; Annas 1983).

Ethical issues must be carefully examined before participation of any subjects in an experiment. Even when human experimentation is viewed as possibly beneficial, it is absolutely essential to examine the nature of the experiment and the rights of the individual. This doctrine and those included in the "Declaration of Helsinki" were also reiterated by the President's Commission in 1981.

The Commission's findings and conclusions on this subject can be summarized as follows:

1 Although the informed consent doctrine has substantial foundations in law, it is essentially an ethical imperative.
2 Ethically valid consent is a process of shared decision-making based upon mutual respect and participation, not a ritual to be equated with reciting the contents of a form that details the risks of particular treatments.

3 The literature about informed consent often portrays it as a highly rational process, suitable primarily for intelligent, highly articulate, self-aware individuals. The Commission found, however, a universal desire for information, choice, and respectful communication about decisions—for all patients, in all health care settings.

4 Informed consent is based upon the principle that competent individuals are entitled to make health care decisions based upon their own personal values and in furtherance of their own personal goals. However, patient choice is not absolute:

> Patients are not entitled to insist that health care practitioners furnish them services when to do so would breach the bounds of acceptable practice or violate a professional's own deeply held moral beliefs or would draw on a limited resource to which the patient has no binding claim.
>
> In order to promote self-determination and patient well-being, individuals should be presumed to have decisionmaking capacity; only in a small minority of cases should incapacity disqualify a patient from making a decision regarding health care.
>
> Alternative arrangements should be made for decisionmaking on behalf of individuals who lack substantial capacity to make their own decisions; incapacity should be viewed, however, as specific to each particular decision.
>
> Persons lacking decisional capacity should be consulted about their own preferences, to the extent feasible, out of respect for them as individuals.

5 Health care providers should not ordinarily withhold unpleasant information simply because it is unpleasant.

6 Achieving the goal of shared decisionmaking based upon mutual respect is ultimately the responsibility of individual health care professionals. However, health care institutions such as hospitals also have important roles to play in fostering the process.

7 Patients should have access to the information they need to help them understand their conditions and make treatment decisions.

8 Improvements in the relationship between health care professionals and patients must come not primarily from the law but from changes in the teaching, examination, and training of health care professionals.

9 Family members are often of great assistance to patients in helping them to understand information about their condition and in making decisions about treatment. Their involvement should be encouraged to the extent compatible with respect for the privacy and autonomy of individual patients.

10 In order to promote a greater commitment of time to the process of shared decisionmaking, reimbursement schedules for all medical and surgical interventions should take account of the time necessarily spent in discussion with patients.

11 To protect the interests of patients who lack decisionmaking capacity:

Decisions made by others should, when possible, replicate those the patients would make if they were capable; when that is not feasible, the decisions of surrogates should protect the patients' best interests.

Health care institutions should consider using mechanisms such as"ethics committees" for review and consultation regarding decisionmaking for those who lack the capacity to decide.

State courts and legislatures should consider making provision for advance directives through which people may designate others to make health care decisions on their behalf and/or give instructions about their care should they become incapacitated.

Controversy regarding human experimentation in recent years has focused on two major areas: fetal research and organ transplantation. Each of these areas offers a number of specific issues that merit separate discussion.

Fetal Research

Fetal studies have in the past proved invaluable for medical research. For example, diagnostic ultrasound was shown to be an effective imaging tool providing valuable information regarding the size and position of the developing fetus. Experiments with fetuses in the womb led to the development of a technique to give blood transfusions to newborn babies with Rh complications. These studies made possible transfusions of the right blood type to newborns with blood diseases. In spite of these benefits, however, fetal studies have become very controversial. In fact, ethical issues surrounding fetal studies have reached a crescendo in recent years.

With the legalization of abortion, many more fetuses have become available to researchers. This increased involvement of "new life" in medical research projects has caught the attention of numerous prolife groups,who are generally opposed to fetal studies. The main argument of these groups centers about the onset of life and the belief that the fetus is a human being and as such should not be exposed to any harmful agents, regardless of the experiment. For the most part, although these groups are definitely opposed to any nontherapeutic studies involving the fetus, they do not completely oppose beneficial (therapeutic) studies or research on dead fetuses. This group believes that if one analyzes proxy consent where it is accepted as legitimate that life and health are "goods" for the child, the child would choose life. In other words, proxy consent is morally valid insofar as it is a reasonable presumption of children's wishes (McCormick 1983).

Others have expressed concern in respect to the ethical issues involved in obtaining a valid consent to conduct fetal studies. They are opposed to *any* nontherapeutic research on the fetus because such research is being imposed on one incapable of consent. Using arguments similar to those used in opposing nontherapeutic research involving children, they state that such procedures, regardless of their potentially beneficial character, are invasions of the privacy of individuals incompetent to give informed consent. Therefore attempts by parents to provide proxy consent should be judged to be violent presumptions, the extortion of charitable works from one incapable, as yet, of making such a decision (McCormick 1976).

Still others fear the extension of the philosophy endorsed by fetal research. That is, these individuals believe that the use of human fetuses as "guinea pigs" simply because they are to be aborted may be used in the future to justify research on the aged, the terminally ill, or children with terminal birth defects.

Because of these fears and the pressure exerted from antiabortion groups, various legislation has been passed on fetal research. The earliest such legislation on fetal studies concerned fetal viability, that is, the question determining at what point the fetus is considered to be a live human being. In 1971, the federal government suggested guidelines limiting research to fetuses weighing less than 500 g. However, these guidelines were not always accurate, since it has been demonstrated that a fetus weighing only 395 g can live outside the womb.

Then in 1973, the Supreme Court decided that the legal definition of life was the 24th wk of fetal life. Many medical experts believe that it is not possible for a fetus at this stage of its development to live on its own for very long. As a result, this activity has raised fundamental moral questions regarding the status of life in the womb. Is a fetus viable even if it has a very low chance of survival? Should a fetus be considered to have a low chance of survival, and therefore nonviability, if it is going to be aborted? Such questions cannot be answered easily.

During 1973 and 1974, 12 states established their own criteria for fetal viability and passed laws prohibiting or restricting live-fetus research. In this same time period, however, no laws limiting fetal research had been passed in Massachusetts. This fact was to lead to an incident concerning fetal research that awakened the entire country to the issues involved.

In 1974, researchers at Boston City Hospital reported the results of their fetal research project, which was conducted to investigate the effectiveness of two specific antibiotics against congenital syphilis. The study involved 33 women scheduled for legal abortions after 10 to 22 wk of pregnancy. With their consent, the women received doses of one or the other antibiotic before their abortions. After the abortions, the concentration of the antibiotics in the fetal tissue was measured. The results of this study determined that clindamycin, one of the antibiotics, had enough effectiveness in reaching the fetus to control congenital syphilis (*Newsweek* 1974).

On reading the results of this study, however, several groups expressed their alarm and concern about the nature of these experiments. One of these groups, the Boston Value of Life Committee, protested vigorously to Boston City Council. The Boston City Hospital reacted to the protests by starting an 8-mo study of abortions at its facilities. The Boston City Council took more drastic steps. It set up public hearings to listen to both sides of the controversy. At the conclusion of the testimony, however, the district attorney began a grand jury investigation into the matter. During this investigation, four of the researchers were indicted on the basis of a 160-yr-old law prohibiting the illegal use of human bodies for dissection (*Time* 1974).

Lawyers for the defendants argued that they had done nothing inconsistent with accepted standards of medical practice and the Supreme Court guidelines on abortion. In addition, they claimed that the district attorney had to prove that the fetuses were living as defined by law at the time the research was conducted. Because the Supreme Court guidelines established in 1973 specified that a fetus is not viable if it is less than 24 wk, the district attorney had a difficult case to prove.

Partially as a result of this fetal research trial, the federal government decided to put some controls on fetal studies. In June 1974, a Senate-House Committee temporarily banned the Department of Health, Education, and Welfare from funding fetal research on living fetuses before or after abortion. Congress also requested that an organization, the National Commission for the Protection of Human Subjects, be set up to define rules for medical research, with fetal research receiving top priority. The ban on fetal research would last until the commission presented its recommendations on whether the ban was to be extended or lifted.

The commission was set up in the late fall of 1974. Eleven members were chosen by the Secretary of Health, Education, and Welfare. The committee was chaired by J. Kenneth Ryan of Boston, Massachusetts, and included three physicians, three lawyers, two biomedical researchers, two ethicists (one Catholic and one Protestant), and one representative of the public. The commission met for the first time in December 1974 and began its work. After deciding its objective, it initiated a series of public hearings. Speakers presenting testimony on fetal research included ethicists, lawyers, physicians, antiabortion activists, medical researchers, and citizens. In addition, the commission asked several laboratories for statistics on fetal research.

With this wealth of information from various sources, the commission formulated their conclusion on fetal research. On April 28, 1975, in an eight to one vote, it recommended an immediate lift of the ban on fetal research. They also suggested that certain guidelines be established that would go into effect after the Secretary of Health, Education, and Welfare approved them. These regulations would affect all research facilities funded by the department and those facilities that generally follow the department's policies.

The commission guidelines classified fetal studies as either therapeutic or nontherapeutic research. Therapeutic measures may be directed toward the mother or toward the fetus. If an untested procedure is to be used on a fetus in a mother's uterus, the procedure must be approved by a review board. The mother's consent must also be obtained. If the therapeutic procedure is going to benefit the mother, there must be assurance that the fetus will be exposed to minimal risk.

The commission guidelines divided nontherapeutic research into five different situations. The first situation dealt with the fetus in the mother's uterus. The recommendation allowed nontherapeutic research, provided that (1) the purpose of such research is the development of important biomedical knowledge that cannot be obtained by alternative means, (2) investigation on pertinent animal models and nonpregnant humans has preceded such research, and (3) minimal or no risk to the well-being of the fetus will be imposed by the research (McCormick and Walters 1975). The consent of the mother is required for this procedure. The same conditions applicable to the fetus in utero apply to the fetus in anticipation of abortion. Any research project deviating from the guidelines would have to be approved by the national review board.

The guidelines proposed for the second and third situations, the fetus during abortion and the nonviable fetus outside the uterus, were most controversial. The commission allowed research on fetuses less than 20 wk. However, it was stressed that no significant procedural changes be introduced into the abortion procedure in the interest of pure research alone and that no intrusion into the fetus be made that alters duration of life. In essence, this means that fetal life cannot be lengthened or shortened for research purposes alone.

The last two situations deal with the viable fetus out of the uterus and with the dead fetus. The viable fetus ex utero may be the subject of nontherapeutic research only when there is minimal or no risk to the fetus. There are no limitations on dead fetus research except those normally imposed on the use of dead bodies for research.

These guidelines also included a recommendation to set up a national ethical review board to decide whether certain research procedures were risky to the fetus. The commission charged Health, Education, and Welfare with the task of appointing such a review board and added that the public should be encouraged to participate in the review process. On July 29, 1975, the Health, Education, and Welfare Secretary, then Caspar N. Weinberger, endorsed these recommendations on fetal research of the National Commission for the Protection of Human Subjects. In effect this removed the ban on fetal experiments that had existed since July 1974 (*Science News* 1975). The key restriction in the commission's recommendations on nontherapeutic research was that it pose minimal or no risk to the fetus. This process and its results clearly indicated the impact of evaluating and examining the nature of medical research on the basis of ethical concerns.

This process continues today and clearly indicates the controversy surrounding the fetal research issue. In 1980, the ethics advisory board, designed to oversee all the research on human embryos, was disbanded, with the result that no research in this area could be initiated. Recently the National Institute of Health (NIH) sent a request for the board's reestablishment to the Department of Health and Human Services (HHS), and a set of options was forwarded to HHS secretary Margaret Heckler. However, as a result of the political situation in that department recently and the "new morality" that has affected the United States lately, all perinatal research is in limbo. For instance, Senator Jeremiah Denton of Alabama has proposed a measure that could prohibit the use of federal funds for perinatal research. The proposal states, "The director of the National Institute of Health and the director of any national research institute may not conduct or support research . . . on living human fetus or infant, unless the experiment is intended to benefit the fetus or infant, or unless the risk to the fetus or infant is no greater than those encountered in daily life or during the performance or routine physical or psychological examinations or tests." It is believed that a strict interpretation of the language could limit a broad area of research (*Science* 1984). Although such attitudes may dampen researchers' hopes, they do reflect society's ethical concerns and their effects on medical research. It is important for biomedical research, and society, that such interplay, and maybe compromise, continue in the future.

Organ Transplantation

One of the most dramatic achievements of our technologically oriented medical system, especially in the last 5 yr, has been the development and use of artificial and transplanted organs. As the demand for replacement body parts grows, high-risk techniques since considered to be on the scientific fringe are beginning to enter the medical mainstream. Since 1980, transplantation of hearts, livers, kidneys, and other organs has increased dramatically. For example, the number of liver grafts rose from 15 per year in 1980 to 145 in 1983, while heart transplants jumped from 36 to 172 (*U.S. News and World Report* 1984).

With heart disease a major killer in the U.S., the potential demand for heart transplantations could run into the tens of thousands. With this in mind it is interesting to note the following:

1 Estimates by the National Institutes of Health indicate that up to 50,000 Americans could benefit from such operations.

2 At Stanford University, one of the leading heart-transplant centers, more than 90 percent of patients leave the hospital in stable condition. The patient to survive the longest is doing well 14 years after surgery.

3 At this time roughly 800 hearts have been transplanted worldwide, according to estimates by the National Center for Health Services Research. The 1-yr survival rate has risen from less than 65 percent in 1980 to more than 80 percent today.

The outlook for kidney patients is a little better:

1 Around the world, close to 1,000 livers have been transplanted.

2 At the University Health Center of Pittsburgh, the 1-yr survival rate today approaches 90 percent for children, 75 to 80 percent for adults.

3 For children born with biliary atresia, a liver defect that affects about 500 Americans a year, transplantation is becoming the recommended treatment.

4 Potential candidates for liver transplants also include persons suffering from such disease as chronic hepatitis, liver cancer, and cirrhosis.

5 Estimates by Battelle Human Affairs Research Centers suggest that up to 10,000 Americans could benefit from a liver transplant, including some 4,000 alcoholics.

6 More than 60,000 kidney transplants have been done around the world in the past 20 yr. The operations are now being performed in the United States at the rate of 5,000 a year, and there are 6,000 to 8,000 candidates waiting for a suitable donor organ.

7 Today, nearly 99 percent of the patients survive with the transplanted organs for at least 1 yr. Should a transplant fail, the patient usually can stay alive by resuming kidney dialysis.

In addition to the transplantation of these two major body organs doctors have also performed an estimated 5,300 bone-marrow transplants for anemia and leukemia patients, 4,000 pancreas transplants for diabetics, and some 15,000 cornea transplants each year.

Transplant surgery began to accelerate in 1980, after the introduction of the immunosuppressant drug cyclosporin, which prevents the body from rejecting a grafted organ. Since then, the number of hospitals in the United States performing heart and liver transplants has jumped from 6 to 35. Kidney and cornea transplants are presently performed at most medical centers.

Success in this activity has required the surmounting of many difficult problems in the fields of medicine and biomedical engineering. New surgical techniques and drugs have made the human body more hospitable to borrowed tissue, transforming organ transplantation from a kind of surgical adventure into an increasingly routine procedure. In fact recently a 58-yr-old Louisville man was the third patient to acquire an artificial heart. Because this operation lasted only 3 1/2 h, one of the nurses involved in the process quipped "God, this is a dull operation!" (*Boston Globe* 1985).

However, as transplantation procedures have moved into the clinical arena, it has become apparent that the problems associated with these techniques are not purely medical or technical in nature. They pose grave moral and ethical problems when one attempts to answer the following questions. When should transplantation be initiated? Should individuals be encouraged to be recipients, even though the chances for success are exceptionally low? How does one select the donor? Should living donors be involved in this procedure? Is it right to subject a healthy person to the risks involved in order to extend another's life, even a close relative, for a relatively short period of time? If the prospective donor is dying, when should the organ be removed? And should, as in the case of Baby Fae, a transplant include organs from another being other than a human, like a baboon? Some of the issues raised by these questions are interrelated with the previous discussion, providing further illustration of the ethical concerns in caring for the dying patient, as well as the moral dilemmas of clinical research. Therefore, when discussing problems relating to potential cadaveric (dying) donors, it is clear that moral concerns regarding the acceptable definition of death must be considered, whereas concern for the recipients of these organs requires one to examine the risk-benefit decision associated with all experimental procedures.

Since organ transplantation today refers primarily to the technique of removing a diseased organ such as a kidney, a liver, or a heart and replacing it with an organ from another human, it is clear that not one but two human beings or animals are involved in each transplantation process. It is therefore essential that the individual rights of both persons, the recipient and the donor, be respected. Some of the fundamental moral dilemmas confronting health professionals in this situation become evident. Let us proceed and examine some of the ethical and moral problems inherent in this controversy, which not too long ago was unimaginable.

The Patient Recipient

For the patient recipient, one must be concerned about the relative chances of success compared to the physical, mental, and financial risks involved in the procedure. Even though the recipient often faces the likelihood of death because of the failure of a major organ, this in itself does not justify any procedure. The ultimate decision must reside only with the patient.

Similar to the fetal experimentation, infants, who can decide nothing, represent an extremely difficult case. Since infants are incapable of giving consent, the parents legally are permitted to do so on their behalf. In Baby Fae's case what kind of consent did they give (*Time* 1984)?

The Donor

The most controversial aspect of organ transplantation is the source of the donor organ. Consequently, different moral issues arise, depending on whether live or dying donors are used. In dealing with kidney transplants, live donors have a pair of these organs and usually survive any transplantation operation. This fact, in addition to the desire to ensure tissue compatibility, has made this approach an acceptable medical technique.

However, it must be clearly understood that any individual who agrees to donate a kidney to another person submits to certain surgical and medical risks. The thought of a willing donor's dying on the operating table or having the remaining kidney eventually fail is enough to cause concern to most medical professionals. Therefore, it is absolutely essential that the prospective donor also understand the risks involved and be under no external or abnormal psychological pressures to make the donation, even though the donor may be a parent or sibling of the recipient. In addition to the obvious medical risks, other hazards should be considered. Emotional and psychological difficulties in the relationship between the donor and the recipient may also arise. For example, if the transplantation process fails, it is quite possible that the donor may feel guilty or angry at what may eventually be viewed as an unnecessary sacrifice or risk. If it is successful, on the other hand, the donor may feel unworthy of proprietary rights on the life of the other. To minimize these effects, both donor and recipient must be alerted to this possibility in advance.

On the question of how to make more organs available for transplant, two provocative remedies define the range of the debate. At one extreme is a proposal called *presumed consent,* which means that the organs of a person who enters the condition known as brain death can be donated to recipients unless the individual or the next of kin has registered specific objections. Supporters of this view argue that since organs may be seized without permission in autopsy cases, "why not pass a law allowing them to be seized for humanitarian purposes?" At the opposite extreme is the idea of letting a commercial market in human organs solve the supply-and-demand imbalance. Presumed consent is a respectable topic in medical circles; not so the market solution. One reason there is not now a market in kidneys is that leading medical societies have announced they will expel any physician who participates.

Opponents argue that organ selling cheapens life. They say that it would induce sellers to lie about their medical histories, as do sellers of blood plasma, causing a higher incidence of contamination in commercial blood. They contend, too, that a bidding war over body parts would be unjust, since it would deny the poor equal access to health care.

Besides the moral arguments against an "organ free market," there is an economic one: that it might well raise the cost of organs without doing much to increase the supply. People who now donate organs for altruistic reasons might demand payment instead or, convinced that the market was taking care of things, they might decline to part with their organs at all. The elasticity of supply and demand may not apply in the emotionally charged atmosphere of a hospital waiting room, where the next of kin are considering how to dispose of a parent.

The political bickering over what the government should do about the organ shortfall takes place well inside the extreme boundaries of commercial sales and presumed consent, but the nature of the argument is much the same: private enterprise versus government intervention.

As the momentum builds to transplant more human organs, as well as animal and synthetic parts, these advances threaten to drain the country's health resources.

Heart transplants can cost more than $110,000, a liver transplant may exceed $20,000, and postoperative drugs can run as high as $18,000 a year. Therefore, pressure is mounting on private insurance companies and government health programs to develop policies to cover these operations. The federal government pays for kidney transplants and for some liver transplants in children. California's medicaid program covers liver and heart transplants.

So far, commercial insurers and the federal government have balked at writing a blank check for all transplant procedures, forcing some patients to raise money through such devices as bake sales and media appeals. Consequently, health officials caution that although transplantation shows great promise, long-term questions over the financial costs and type of patients most likely to gain from this new technology remain. Once we develop a procedure that is very expensive and can be made available to many more people, we raise the policy issue of whether the benefits justify the costs. Unless sanity decides that cost is no object, these advances will open up an enormous moral and economic dilemma (*U.S. News and World Report* 1984).

REFERENCES

Abrams, N., and Buckner, M. D. (eds.). 1983. Appendix: Professional Codes and Statutes. In *Medical Ethics,* Cambridge, Mass: MIT Press, pp. 641–686.

A life in the balance, Time, Nov. 3, 1975, pp. 52–61.

Annas, C. J. 1983. Informed consent. Abrams, N., and Buckner, M. D. (eds.). In *Medical ethics.* Cambridge, Mass: MIT Press, pp. 254-256.

Baker, S. P. 1980. On lobbies, liberties and the public good. *American J. Public Health* 1980 June: 70(6).

Beecher, H. K. 1970. Research and the individual. In *Human studies,* Boston: Little, Brown.

Bereck, M. G. 1975a. Quinlan witnesses: Still hope. *Newsday,* Oct. 21, 1975. p. 6.

Bereck, M. G. 1975b. Prayer, then a clear decision. *Newsday,* October 22, 1975. p. 3.

Black's law dictionary, (4th ed). 1968. St. Paul, Minn.: West Publishing.

Brody, J. E. 1975. Fetal research averts abortion. *New York Times,* May 23, 1975. p. 38.

Campbell, A. V. 1972. *Moral dilemmas in medicine.* Edinburgh: Churchill Livingston.

Cassileth, B. R., Zupkis, R. V., Sutton-Smith, K. and March, V. 1983. Informed consent: Why are its goals imperfectly realized In Abrams, N. and Buckner, M. D. (eds.). *Medical Ethics,* Cambridge, Mass.: MIT Press, pp. 281–285.

Cons as guinea pigs. *Time,* March 19, 1973. p. 101.

Curren, W. J. 1969. Government regulations of the use of human subjects in medical research: the approach of two federal agencies, conference on ethical aspects of experimentation on human subjects. *Daedalus* 89:542–594.

Downing, A. B. (ed.). 1969. *Euthanasia and the right to death.* Los Angeles: Nash.

Elkinton, J. R. 1969. Moral problems in the use of borrowed organs, artificial and transplanted. *Ann Intern Med* 60:463–479.

Engelhardt, H. T., Jr. 1975. Defining death: A philosophical problem for medicine and law, *Am Rev Respi Dis* 112:587–590.

Fagothey, A. 1976. Rights and reason, (6th ed.). St.Louis: Mosby.

Field, R. E. and Romanus, R. J. 1977. A decerebrate patient: eighteen years of care. *Ill Med J* 151(2):121–123.

Fletcher, J. 1974. *The ethics of genetic control.* Garden City, N.Y.: Anchor.

Gaylin, W. 1974. Harvesting the dead. *Harpers,* September 1974. pp. 23-30.

Goldman, L. 1970. The willowbrook debate. *World Med* 6:17–25.

Gorovitz, S. 1982. *Doctors' Dilemmas: Moral Conflict and Patient Care.* New York: Macmillan

Halley, M. M., and Harvey, W. F. 1968. Medicine vs legal definitions of death. JAMA 210:103–105.

Health research aims for visibility. 1974. *Science News* 106:35–39.

Horan, D. J. 1978. Right to die laws: Creating, not clarifying problems *Hosp Prog* 59(6):62–65.

Horan, D. J. and Mall, D. 1977. *Death, Dying and Euthanasia.* Washington: University Publications of America.

Kohl, M. 1974. *The morality of killing.* Atlantic Highlands, N.J.: Humanities.

Krant, M. J. 1974. *Dying and dignity: The meaning and control of a personal death.* Springfield, Ill.: Thomas.

Ladimer, I. 1967. Human studies for safety evaluation: Medicolegal aspects. In Proceedings of a Conference on Use of Human Subjects in Safety Evaluation of Food Chemicals, Washington, D.C., 1967. National Academy of Sciences, National Research Council.

Loftus, E. F. and Fries, J. F., 1983. Informed consent may be hazardous to your health. In Abrams, N., and Buckner, M. D. (eds). *Medical Ethics,* Cambridge, Mass.: MIT Press. pp. 295–296.

Lyons, C. 1970. *Organ transplants: The moral issues.* Philadelphia: Westminster Press.

Maguire, D. C. 1974. *Death by choice.* Garden City,N.Y.: Doubleday & Co.

Mannes, M. 1973. *Last rights.* New York: Morrow.

McCormick, R. A. 1976. Experimental subjects: Who should they be? *JAMA* 235:2197.

McCormick, R. A. 1983. Bioethics in the public forum. *Millbank Mem Fund Q* 61(1):113–126.

McCormick, R. A. and Walters, L. 1975. Fetal research and public policy, *America* 132:473–476.

Meisel, A. 1975. Informed consent—the rebuttal. *JAMA* 234:615.

Mendelsohn, E., Swazey, J. P., and Traviss, I. (eds.). 1971. *Human aspects of biomedical innovation.* Cambridge, Mass.: Harvard University Press.

Mills, D. H. 1974. Whither informed consent? *JAMA* 229:305–310.

New attack on abortion, *Time,* May 27, 1974. p. 84.

O'Rourke, K. 1977. Christian affirmation of life. In Horan, D., Mall, D. (eds.) *Death, dying, and euthanasia.* Washington: University Publications of America.

Pappworth, M. H. 1967. Human guinea pigs: Experimentation on man. Boston: Beacon.

Pappworth, M. H. 1968. Ethical issues in experimental medicine. In Cutler, D. R. (ed.). *Updating life and death.* Boston: Beacon.

Paris, J. J. 1981. Sounding Board. The New York Court of Appeals rules on the rights of incompetent dying patients. The conclusion of the Brother Fox case. *N.Engl. J. Med.* June 4:304(23) 1424-5, 1981.

Pellegrino, E. D. 1969. The Necessity, promise, and dangers of human experimentation. In Weber, H., (Ed.) *Experiments with man.* Geneva: World Council of Churches.

Pellegrino, E. D. 1976. Physician, patients and society. In Mendelsohn, E., Swazey, J. P., and Traviss, I. (eds.) *Human aspects of biomedical innovation,* Cambridge, Mass.: Harvard University Press.

Ramsey, P. 1968. On updating death. In Cutler, D. R. (ed.) *Updating life and death.* Boston: Beacon.

Ramsey, P. 1970. *The patient as a person.* New Haven, Conn.: Yale University Press.

Research on fetuses: Monstorium ends. 1975. *Science News* 107:285.

Row over fetal research, *Newsweek,* June 24, 1974. p. 74.

St. John-Stevas, N. 1964. *The right to life.* New York: Holt, Rinehart & Winston. 1975.

St. John-Stevas 1975. Euthanasia—a pleasant sounding word. *America* 132:421–422.

Sidel, V. N. 1971. New technologies and the practice of medicine. In Mendelsohn, E., Swazey, J. P., and Traviss,I. (eds.) *Human aspects of biomedical innovation.* Cambridge, Mass.: Harvard University Press.

Smith, H. L. 1970. Ethics and the new medicine. Nashville, Tenn.: Abingdon.

Spicker, S. F. and Engelhardt, H. T. Jr. 1977. *Philosophical Medical Ethics: Its Nature and Significance.* Boston: Reidel.

Spicker, S. F. and Engelhardt, J. M. 1981. *The Law Medicine Relations: A Philosophical Exploration.* London: Reidel.

Taub, S. 1981. Brain Death: A reevaluation of the Harvard criteria. *Conn Med* 45(9): 597–599.

The right to live—or die. *Time,* October 27, 1975. p. 45.

Toffler, A. 1970. *Future shock.* New York: Random House

Toffler, A. 1980. *The Third Wave.* New York: Morrow.

Trubo, R. 1973. An act of mercy: Euthanasia today. Los Angeles: Nash.

United Trust Company v. Pyke 199 KAN 1, 427 P, 2d67, 71, 1967.

Veatch, R. 1976. *Death, Dying and Biological Revolution.* New Haven, Conn.: Yale University Press.

Weir, R. F. 1977. *Ethical Issues in Death and Dying.* New York: Columbia University Press.

Wertz, R. W. 1973. Readings on ethical and social issues in biomedicine. Englewood Cliffs, N.J.: Prentice-Hall.

White, L. P. (ed.). 1969. *Care of patients with fatal illness.* New York: Academy of Sciences.

Williams, R. H. 1973. Propagation, modification and termination of life; conception, abortion, suicide, euthanasia. In Williams, R. H., (ed.) *To live and to die: When, why and how.* New York: Springer-Verlag.

Woodruff, M. F. A. 1970. *The one and the many.* London: The Royal Society of Medicine.

Index